Lung Cancer: Part I

Editors

M. PATRICIA RIVERA
RICHARD A. MATTHAY

CLINICS IN
CHEST MEDICINE

www.chestmed.theclinics.com

March 2020 • Volume 41 • Number 1

ELSEVIER

1600 John F. Kennedy Boulevard • Suite 1800 • Philadelphia, Pennsylvania, 19103-2899

http://www.theclinics.com

CLINICS IN CHEST MEDICINE Volume 41, Number 1
March 2020 ISSN 0272-5231, ISBN-13: 978-0-323-79140-3

Editor: Colleen Dietzler
Developmental Editor: Casey Potter

Clinics in Chest Medicine (ISSN 0272-5231) is published quarterly by Elsevier Inc., 360 Park Avenue South, New York, NY 10010-1710. Months of issue are March, June, September, and December. Periodicals postage paid at New York, NY and additional mailing offices. Subscription prices are $388.00 per year (domestic individuals), $766.00 per year (domestic institutions), $100.00 per year (domestic students/residents), $423.00 per year (Canadian individuals), $952.00 per year (Canadian institutions), $484.00 per year (international individuals), $952.00 per year (international institutions), $100.00 per year (Canadian Students), and $230.00 per year (International Students). International air speed delivery is included in all Clinics subscription prices. All prices are subject to change without notice. **POSTMASTER:** Send address changes to Clinics in Chest Medicine, Elsevier Health Sciences Division, Subscription Customer Service, 3251 Riverport Lane, Maryland Heights, MO 63043. **Customer Service: Telephone: 1-800-654-2452** (U.S. and Canada); **1-314-447-8871** (outside U.S. and Canada). **Fax: 1-314-447-8029. E-mail: journalscustomerservice-usa@elsevier.com (for print support); journalsonlinesupport-usa@elsevier.com (for online support).**

Reprints. For copies of 100 or more of articles in this publication, please contact the Commercial Reprints Department, Elsevier Inc., 360 Park Avenue South, New York, NY 10010-1710. Tel.: 212-633-3874; Fax: 212-633-3820; E-mail: reprints@elsevier.com.

Clinics in Chest Medicine is covered in *MEDLINE/PubMed (Index Medicus), Current Contents/Clinical Medicine, EMBASE/ Excerpta Medica, Science Citation Index,* and *ISI/BIOMED.*

Contributors

EDITORS

M. PATRICIA RIVERA, MD
Professor of Medicine, Division of Pulmonary
and Critical Care Medicine, Co-Director,
Multidisciplinary Thoracic Oncology Program,
Director, Multidisciplinary Lung Cancer
Screening Program, Medical Director
Bronchoscopy and PFT Laboratory,
The University of North Carolina at Chapel Hill,
Chapel Hill, North Carolina

RICHARD A. MATTHAY, MD
Senior Research Scientist, Professor Emeritus,
Pulmonary, Critical Care and Sleep Medicine
Section, Department of Medicine, Yale School
of Medicine, New Haven, Connecticut

AUTHORS

MATT ABOUDARA, MD, FCCP
Assistant Professor of Medicine, University of
Missouri - Kansas City, Division of Pulmonary
and Critical Care, St. Luke's Health System,
Kansas City, Missouri

JASON AKULIAN, MD, MPH
Assistant Professor of Medicine, Director of
Interventional Pulmonology, Division of
Pulmonary and Critical Care Medicine,
The University of North Carolina at Chapel Hill,
Chapel Hill, North Carolina

BRETT C. BADE, MD
Assistant Professor, Department of Medicine,
Section of Pulmonary, Critical Care, and Sleep
Medicine, Yale School of Medicine,
New Haven, Connecticut

A. COLE BURKS, MD
Assistant Professor of Medicine, Interventional
Pulmonology, Division of Pulmonary and
Critical Care Medicine, The University of
North Carolina at Chapel Hill, Chapel Hill,
North Carolina

CHARLES S. DELA CRUZ, MD, PhD
Associate Professor, Department of Medicine,
Section of Pulmonary, Critical Care, and Sleep
Medicine, Yale School of Medicine,
New Haven, Connecticut

FRANK C. DETTERBECK, MD
Department of Surgery, Division of Thoracic
Surgery, Yale School of Medicine, New Haven,
Connecticut

STEVEN M. DUBINETT, MD
Chief, Division of Pulmonary, Critical Care,
Sleep Medicine, Clinical Immunology and
Allergy, Departments of Medicine,
Pathology and Laboratory Medicine, and
Molecular and Medical Pharmacology, David
Geffen School of Medicine at UCLA,
Los Angeles, California

HASMEENA KATHURIA, MD
Associate Professor, The Pulmonary Center,
Boston University Medical Center, Boston
University, Boston, Massachusetts

RUI LI, MD, PhD
Post-Doctoral Fellow, Department of Medicine,
David Geffen School of Medicine at UCLA,
Los Angeles, California

BIN LIU, PhD
Adjunct Professor, Department of Medicine,
David Geffen School of Medicine at UCLA,
Los Angeles, California

CHRISTINA R. MacROSTY, DO
Instructor, Department of Medicine, Division of Pulmonary and Critical Care Medicine, Fellow, Interventional Pulmonary Program,
The University of North Carolina at Chapel Hill, Chapel Hill, North Carolina

FABIEN MALDONADO, MD, FCCP
Associate Professor of Medicine and Thoracic Surgery, Division of Allergy, Pulmonary, and Critical Care, Vanderbilt University Medical Center, Nashville, Tennessee

VINCENT J. MASE Jr, MD
Department of Surgery, Division of Thoracic Surgery, Yale School of Medicine, New Haven, Connecticut

PETER J. MAZZONE, MD, MPH, FCCP
Director, Lung Cancer Program,
Respiratory Institute, Cleveland Clinic, Cleveland, Ohio

ENID NEPTUNE, MD
Associate Professor, Department of Internal Medicine, Division of Pulmonary and Critical Care Medicine, Johns Hopkins School of Medicine, Baltimore, Maryland

MANASH K. PAUL, PhD
Project Scientist, Department of Medicine, David Geffen School of Medicine at UCLA, Los Angeles, California

OTIS RICKMAN, DO, FCCP
Associate Professor of Medicine and Thoracic Surgery, Division of Allergy, Pulmonary, and Critical Care, Vanderbilt University Medical Center, Nashville, Tennessee

M. PATRICIA RIVERA, MD
Professor of Medicine, Division of Pulmonary and Critical Care Medicine, Co-Director, Multidisciplinary Thoracic Oncology Program, Director, Multidisciplinary Lung Cancer Screening Program, Medical Director Bronchoscopy and PFT Laboratory,
The University of North Carolina at Chapel Hill, Chapel Hill, North Carolina

RAMIN SALEHI-RAD, MD, PhD
Assistant Clinical Professor, Department of Medicine, David Geffen School of Medicine at UCLA, VA Greater Los Angeles Healthcare System, Los Angeles, California

CATHERINE R. SEARS, MD
Assistant Professor, Department of Medicine, Division of Pulmonary, Critical Care, Sleep and Occupational Medicine, Indiana University School of Medicine, Indianapolis, Indiana

NICHOLE T. TANNER, MD, MSCR, FCCP
Associate Professor of Medicine, Division of Pulmonary, Critical Care, Allergy and Sleep Medicine, Medical University of South Carolina, Health Equity and Rural Outreach Innovation Center (HEROIC), Ralph H. Johnson VA Hospital, Charleston, South Carolina

NINA A. THOMAS, MD
Pulmonary and Critical Care Fellow, Division of Pulmonary, Critical Care, Allergy and Sleep Medicine, Medical University of South Carolina, Charleston, South Carolina

WILLIAM D. TRAVIS, MD
Director, Thoracic Pathology, Department of Pathology, Memorial Sloan Kettering Cancer Center, New York, New York

Contents

> Despite advances in our understanding of risk, development, immunologic control, and treatment options for lung cancer, it remains the leading cause of cancer death. Tobacco smoking remains the predominant risk factor for lung cancer development. Nontobacco risk factors include environmental and occupational exposures, chronic lung disease, lung infections, and lifestyle factors. Because tobacco remains the leading risk factor for lung cancer, disease prevention is focused on smoking avoidance and cessation. Other prevention measures include healthy diet choices and maintaining a physically active lifestyle. Future work should focus on smoking cessation campaigns and better understanding disease development and treatment strategies in nonsmokers.

> Lung cancer is a heterogeneous disease with abundant genomic alterations. Chronic dysregulated airway inflammation facilitates lung tumorigenesis. In contrast, antitumor host immune responses apply continuous selective pressure on the tumor cells during the evolutionary course of the disease. Unprecedented advances in integrative genomic, epigenomic, and cellular profiling of lung cancer and the tumor microenvironment are enhancing the understanding of pulmonary tumorigenesis. This understanding in turn has led to advancements in lung cancer prevention and early detection strategies, and the development of effective targeted therapies and immunotherapies with survival benefit in selected patients.

> Tobacco dependence is the most consequential target to reduce the burden of lung cancer worldwide. Quitting after a cancer diagnosis can improve cancer prognosis, overall health, and quality of life. Several oncology professional organizations have issued guidelines stressing the importance of tobacco treatment for patients with cancer. Providing tobacco treatment in the context of lung cancer screening is another opportunity to further reduce death from lung cancer. In this review, the authors describe the current state of tobacco dependence treatment focusing on new paradigms and approaches and their particular relevance for persons at risk or on treatment for lung cancer.

Lung cancer in women is a modern epidemic and a major health crisis. Cigarette smoking remains the most important risk factor for lung cancer, and unfortunately smoking rates are either stabilized or continue to increase among women. Women may not be more susceptible to the carcinogenic effects of tobacco, but the biology of lung cancer differs between the sexes. This paper summarizes the biological sex differences in lung cancer, including molecular abnormalities, growth factor receptors, hormonal influences, DNA repair capacity, as well as differences in the histology and treatment outcomes of lung cancer in women.

Lung cancer can be diagnosed based on histologic biopsy or cytologic specimens. The 2015 World Health Organization Classification of Lung Tumors addressed the diagnosis of lung cancer in resection specimens and in small biopsies and cytology specimens. For these small specimens, diagnostic terms and criteria are recommended. Targetable mutations such as *EGFR* and *ALK* rearrangements emphasize the importance of managing these small specimens for molecular testing.

Robust evidence exists in support of lung cancer (LC) screening with low-dose computed tomography in patients at high risk of developing LC; however, judicious patient selection is necessary to obtain optimal benefit while minimizing harm. Several professional societies have published recommendations regarding patient selection criteria for screening. Multiple risk prediction models that include additional patient-specific risk factors have since been developed to more accurately predict risk of developing LC. Implementation of a new screening program requires thorough multidisciplinary planning and maintenance. Multisociety guidelines highlight 9 principal components to implement and maintain a successful program.

Most focal persistent ground glass nodules (GGNs) do not progress over 10 years. Research suggests that GGNs that do not progress, those that do, and solid lung cancers are fundamentally different diseases, although histologically they seem similar. Surveillance of GGNs to identify those that gradually progress is safe and does not risk losing a window. GGNs with 5 mm solid component or 10 mm consolidation (mediastinal and lung windows, respectively, on thin slice CT) are highly curable with resection. The optimal type of resection is unclear; sublobar resection is reasonable but an adequate margin is critically important.

> Biomarkers that focus on lung cancer risk assessment, detection, prognosis, diagnosis, and personalized treatment are in various stages of development. This article provides an overview of lung cancer biomarker development, focusing on clinical utility and highlighting 2 unmet clinical needs: selection of high-risk patients for lung cancer screening and differentiation of early lung cancer from benign pulmonary nodules. The authors highlight biomarkers under development and those lung cancer screening and nodule management biomarkers post-clinical validation. Finally, trends in lung cancer biomarker development that may improve accuracy and accelerate implementation in practice are discussed.

> In the diagnosis of lung cancer, pulmonologists have several tools at their disposal. From the tried and true convex probe endobronchial ultrasound (EBUS)-guided transbronchial needle aspiration to robotic bronchoscopy for peripheral lesions and new technology to unblind the biopsy tools, this article elucidates and expounds on the tools currently available and being developed for lung cancer diagnosis.

> Therapeutic bronchoscopy for both endobronchial tumors and peripheral lung cancer is rapidly evolving. The expected increase in early stage lung cancer detection and significant improvement in near real-time imaging for diagnostic bronchoscopy has led to the development of bronchoscopy-delivered ablative technologies. Therapies targeting obstructing central airway tumors for palliation and as a method of local disease control, patient selection and patient-centered outcomes have been areas of ongoing research. This review focuses on patient selection when considering therapeutic bronchoscopy and new and developing technologies for endobronchial tumors and reviews the status of bronchoscopy-delivered ablative tools for peripheral lung cancers.

CLINICS IN CHEST MEDICINE

FORTHCOMING ISSUES

June 2020
Lung Cancer: Part II
M. Patricia Rivera and Richard A. Matthay,
Editors

September 2020
**Chronic Obstructive Pulmonary Disease
(COPD)**
Gerard J. Criner and Bartolome R. Celli, *Editors*

December 2020
**Advances in Occupational and Environmental
Lung Diseases**
Carrie A. Redlich, Kristin J. Cummings, and
Peggy Lai, *Editors*

RECENT ISSUES

December 2019
Tuberculosis
Charles L. Daley and David M. Lewinsohn,
Editors

September 2019
Thoracic Manifestations of Rheumatic Disease
Danielle Antin-Ozerkis and Kristin B. Highland,
Editors

June 2019
Clinical Respiratory Physiology
Denis E. O'Donnell, *Editor*

SERIES OF RELATED INTEREST

Hematology/Oncology Clinics
https://www.hemonc.theclinics.com/

THE CLINICS ARE AVAILABLE ONLINE!
Access your subscription at:
www.theclinics.com

Preface
Passion, Perseverance, and Quantum Leaps: Lung Cancer in the Twenty-First Century

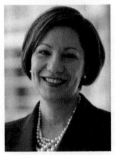   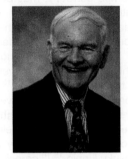

M. Patricia Rivera, MD   Richard A. Matthay, MD
Editors

At the turn of the twentieth century, lung cancer was a rare disease accounting for only 1% of all cancers and found primarily at autopsy. By the 1940s, lung cancer rates had significantly increased. It was the second most common cause of cancer death after gastric cancer, and surgery was the only available treatment. Although a connection between smoking and lung cancer had been recognized by the German physician Fritz Lickint in 1929,[1] it was not until the early 1950s, following the publication of 2 landmark studies from the United Kingdom and the United States, that cigarette smoking was identified as an important factor in the development of lung cancer.[2,3] The 1964 US Surgeon General report titled, "A Focus on Cigarette Smoking," stated that "cigarette smoking is an important health hazard in the United States and action is required to reduce its harmful effects." The first cancer prevention study initiated in 1959 demonstrated a relative risk of death from lung cancer among smokers compared with never smokers of 2.69 and 11.3 for women and men, respectively.[4] This study has been described as a "key guide to national policy and changing public attitudes" with regards to the link between cigarette smoking and lung cancer.

Unfortunately, in the decades following the Surgeon General report and the cancer prevention study results, not only have lung cancer incidence rates significantly increased, especially in women, but also the disease has become the leading cause of cancer death worldwide. It will remain a significant health problem well through the twenty-first century, particularly in women and in developing countries, which continue to observe rising incidence rates.[5,6]

Pessimistic attitudes regarding lung cancer treatment prevailed from the 1960s through the 1980s fueled by a dearth of research and federal funding and the continued negative attitudes of bias and blame surrounding the diagnosis of lung cancer. A pivotal turning point however occurred between 1990 and 1995 with the publication of 2 key studies. The first was a randomized trial comparing sequential chemotherapy and radiation therapy to radiation therapy alone in patients with unresectable stage III non–small cell lung cancer (NSCLC), which demonstrated a 5-year survival of 17% in patients treated with combination therapy.[7] The second, a metaanalysis by the NSCLC Cooperative Group (CG) evaluating 9 randomized trials that compared doublet, platinum-based chemotherapy and best supportive care in advanced NSCLC, demonstrated a 10% improvement in 1-year survival in patients treated with chemotherapy.[8]

The results of these 2 studies marked a paradigm shift in the treatment of lung cancer; they paved the way for the passion and perseverance of basic and clinical scientists to advance lung cancer research, and of dedicated pulmonologists, thoracic surgeons, and medical and radiation oncologists who embraced the inherent

Clin Chest Med 41 (2020) ix–xi
https://doi.org/10.1016/j.ccm.2019.12.001
0272-5231/20/© 2019 Published by Elsevier Inc.

complexity and heterogeneity of lung cancer to successfully develop multidisciplinary programs committed to expeditious coordination of care for lung cancer patients. For the next 15 years, multiple advances were made in the development of (1) third-generation chemotherapeutic drugs (gemcitabine, paclitaxel, pemetrexed), which led to multiple clinical trials exploring these agents in advanced NSCLC, combined multimodality therapy (surgery and adjuvant chemotherapy) in early-stage disease, and concurrent chemoradiotherapy in locally advanced disease; (2) imaging modalities, including PET with fludeoxyglucose and subsequent combined PET-computed tomographic imaging, which improved radiologic staging; (3) minimally invasive diagnostic and staging tools, such as endobronchial ultrasound (EBUS), which revolutionized the approach to mediastinal staging, and electromagnetic navigation bronchoscopy, which improved the diagnosis of peripheral lung cancers; (4) international efforts to inform future revisions in the TNM staging system, which enhanced our ability to prognosticate NSCLC; (5) minimally invasive surgical techniques, such as video-assisted thoracoscopic surgery, which resulted in decreased surgical morbidity and better options for older patients and those with advanced lung disease; (6) newer radiotherapy techniques, such as stereotactic radiotherapy (SBRT), which provided options for treatment of early-stage NSCLC in medically inoperable patients; and (7) revisions to the pathologic classification of lung tumors, giving us an early window to the heterogeneity of lung cancers, which led to eventual guidelines for how best to optimize biopsies and needle aspirations to yield histologic accuracy. Collectively, these advances led to significant improvement in the management of lung cancer such that, by the year 2005, a decade after the NSCLC-CG metaanalysis, adjuvant chemotherapy had resulted in statistically significant improvement in 5-year survival and was established as standard of care in stage II and III NSCLC.[9] Concurrent chemoradiotherapy had improved 5-year survival in unresectable stage III disease,[10] and platinum-based third-generation chemotherapy regimens provided 1- and 2-year survival rates of 33% and 11%, respectively, in advanced NSCLC.[11] Moreover, clinical trials demonstrated the importance of accurate histologic differentiation in order to select chemotherapy regimens that provided superior survival results and decreased toxicity in adenocarcinoma and squamous cell NSCLCs.

This last decade has been highlighted by quantum leaps in research that have revolutionized the care of patients across the continuum of lung cancer. These include the results of the National Lung Screening Trial,[12] which demonstrated low-dose computed tomography resulted in a 20% relative lung cancer mortality reduction in high-risk smokers; 4 decades after the first lung cancer screening (LCS), studies were conducted in the United States, and we had a formal recommendation for screening in lung cancer, one, that if implemented correctly, may be the single intervention with the largest effect on decreasing cancer deaths in our lifetime. There has been a tremendous increase in the understanding of the biology of lung cancer, including (1) genomic profiling, which led to the discovery of driver oncogenes activated by mutations,[13] fusion, and translocations,[14] leading to the development of highly effective oral tyrosine kinase inhibitors and shepherding the era of precision medicine in lung cancer; (2) the groundbreaking work by Drs James Allison and Tasuku Honjo,[15,16] corecipients of the 2018 Noble prize in Medicine, which led to the discovery of central and peripheral negative regulatory pathways known as immune checkpoints used by tumors to suppress immune surveillance and the subsequent development of checkpoint inhibitors; and (3) the development of genomic biomarkers and classifiers in plasma circulating cell-free DNA and bronchial specimens that allow prognostication, detection of relevant driver and resistance mutations, disease monitoring, and early detection,[17,18] further propelling the personalized medicine paradigm in lung cancer care.

Lung cancer is now at the forefront of diagnostic and therapeutic innovations; future research will focus on prevention, early detection, and optimizing precision therapy to improve cure and overall survival in all patients with the disease. The significant progress made in the continuum of lung cancer care could not be covered in a single issue of the *Clinics in Chest Medicine*. For the first time, a comprehensive review in lung cancer is presented in 2 separate issues, Lung Cancer Part I and Lung Cancer Part II.

Lung Cancer Part I reviews the epidemiology, biology, and pathology of lung cancer; the modern epidemic of lung cancer in women; primary and secondary prevention of lung cancer via tobacco treatment; an update of patient selection and implementation of LCS; a review of subsolid pulmonary nodules; advances in diagnostic and therapeutic bronchoscopic interventions; and a comprehensive review of biomarkers in lung cancer.

Lung Cancer Part II covers reviews on the new TNM staging system; advances in surgical techniques; alternate therapies for early-stage NSCLC, including SBRT and radioablative therapy; treatment of stage III NSCLC; advances in targeted and immunotherapies in advanced NSCLC; management of malignant pleural effusions; and small cell lung cancer. This issue also includes a review of oligometastatic disease, an important subset of patients with stage IV NSCLC who may benefit from more aggressive therapy to improve overall survival; an update on palliative care; and reviews in complications of chemotherapy, radiation, and immunotherapy.

We hope this comprehensive 2-part review of the phenomenal advances made in the last 25 years in lung cancer care will encourage readers to enhance their knowledge and skills to promote implementation of LCS in high-risk individuals, tobacco treatment and counseling for all smokers, and multidisciplinary state-of-the-art care for every patient with lung cancer.

M. Patricia Rivera, MD
Division of Pulmonary and
Critical Care Medicine
Medical Director Bronchoscopy and
PFT Laboratory
University of North Carolina
at Chapel Hill
Chapel Hill, NC 27599, USA

Richard A. Matthay, MD
Pulmonary
Critical Care and Sleep Medicine Section
Department of Medicine
Yale Medical School
333 Cedar Street
New Haven, CT 06510, USA

E-mail addresses:
Mprivera@med.unc.edu (M.P. Rivera)
richard.matthay@yale.edu (R.A. Matthay)

REFERENCES

1. Lickint F. Tabak and Tabakrauch als aetiologischer Faktor des Carcinoms. [[Tobacco and tobacco smoke as etiological factors for cancer]]. Z Krebsforsch 1929;30:349–65.
2. Doll R, Hill AB. Smoking and carcinoma of the lung; preliminary report. Br Med J 1950;2:739–48.
3. Wynder EL, Graham EA. Tobacco smoking as a possible etiologic factor in bronchogenic carcinoma; a study of 684 proved cases. J Am Med Assoc 1950; 143:329–36.
4. Garfinkel L. Selection, follow-up and analysis in the American Cancer Society prospective studies. Natl Cancer Inst Monogr 1985;67:49–52.
5. Bray F, Ferlay J, Soerjomataram I, et al. Global cancer statistics 2018: GLOBOCAN estimates of incidence and mortality worldwide for 36 cancers in 185 countries. CA Cancer J Clin 2018;68:394–424.
6. Siegel RL, Miller KD, Jemal A. Cancer statistics 2019. CA Cancer J Clin 2019;69:7–34.
7. Dilman RO, Seagren SL, Propert KJ, et al. Chemotherapy plus high-dose radiation versus radiation alone in stage III non-small cell lung cancer. N Engl J Med 1990;323:940–5.
8. Chemotherapy in non-small cell lung cancer: a metanalysis using updated data on individual patients from 52 randomized clinical trials. Br Med J 1995;311:899–909.
9. Pignon JP, Tribodet H, Scagliotti GV, et al. Lung adjuvant cisplatin evaluation: a pooled analysis by the LACE Collaborative Group. J Clin Oncol 2008; 26:3552–9.
10. Curran WJ Jr, Paulus R, Langer CJ, et al. Sequential vs. concurrent chemoradiation for stage III non-small cell lung cancer: randomized phase III trial RTOG 9410. J Natl Cancer Inst 2011;103:1452–60.
11. Schiller J, Harrington D, Belani C, et al. Comparison of four chemotherapy regimens for advanced non-small cell lung cancer. N Engl J Med 2002;346:92–8.
12. Aberle DR, Adams AM, Berg CE, et al. Reduced lung cancer mortality with low-dose computed tomographic screening. N Engl J Med 2011;365:395–409.
13. Lynch TJ, Bell DW, Sordella R, et al. Activating mutations in the epidermal growth factor receptor underlying responsiveness of non-small-cell lung cancer to gefitinib. N Engl J Med 2004;350: 2129–39.
14. Shaw AT, Kim DW, Nakagawa K, et al. Crizotinib versus chemotherapy in advanced ALK-positive lung cancer. N Engl J Med 2013;368:2385–94.
15. Korman AJ, Peggs KS, Allison JP. Checkpoint blockade in cancer immunotherapy. Adv Immunol 2006;90:297–339.
16. Okazaki T, Chikuma S, Iwai Y, et al. A rheostat for immune responses: the unique properties of PD-1 and their advantages for clinical application. Nat Immunol 2013;14:12121218.
17. Hyman DM, Taylor BS, Baselga J. Implementing genome-driven oncology. Cell 2016;168:584–99.
18. Silvestri GA, Vachani N, Whitney D, et al. A bronchial genomic classifier for the diagnostic evaluation of lung cancer. N Engl J Med 2015;373:243–51.

Lung Cancer 2020
Epidemiology, Etiology, and Prevention

Brett C. Bade, MD, Charles S. Dela Cruz, MD, PhD*

KEYWORDS

- Lung cancer • Tobacco smoking • Epidemiology • Etiology • Prevention

KEY POINTS

- Lung cancer is on the rise globally and is the most common cause of cancer death.
- Tobacco smoking remains the biggest risk factor for lung cancer.
- In the United States, lung cancer incidence, mortality, and survival are improving, although risk of disease development and outcomes vary by age, gender, race, and socioeconomic status.
- Nontobacco risk factors including environmental and occupational exposures, chronic lung disease, and lifestyle factors contribute to lung cancer risk.

Notable changes in lung cancer epidemiology and prevention have occurred over the past decade owing to changes in smoking patterns, groundbreaking advances in our understanding of the genetics of lung cancer, the immune system's role in lung cancer control, and lung cancer treatment options. Despite these advances, lung cancer remains the leading cause of cancer death.[1] Worldwide, there are more lung cancer cases and deaths since 2011, the number of smokers increased between 1980 and 2012,[2,3] and lung cancer rates are climbing in developing countries in conjunction with tobacco smoking. In the United States, lower tobacco smoking rates have led to reductions in lung cancer incidence and mortality, altered the demographics of patients developing lung cancer, and heightened the importance of nontobacco risk factors. Although disease understanding, treatment options, and outcomes for lung cancer in the United States are improving, survival continues to be low. Clinicians caring for patients with lung cancer should be familiar with current contemporary trends. This article reviews the epidemiology and etiology of lung cancer as well as preventive interventions.

EPIDEMIOLOGY OF LUNG CANCER
Global Lung Cancer Trends

Globally, lung cancer cases and deaths are rising. In 2018, GLOBOCAN estimated 2.09 million new cases (11.6% of total cancer cases) and 1.76 million deaths (18.4% of total cancer deaths),[4,5] higher than 2012 reported rates (1.8 million new cases and 1.6 million deaths),[6] making it the most frequent cancer and cause of cancer death in men and women combined (**Fig. 1**A, B),[5,7] and in women, the third most common cancer type and the second most common cause of cancer death (**Fig. 1**C).[5,7]

Between countries, significant variation in lung cancer incidence and demographic distribution are noted, and tobacco smoking rates and stage of economic development influence these patterns. Although cancer statistics in developing countries are less reliable, lung cancer incidence is expected to increase in developing regions

Funding Sources for this work: None.
Department of Medicine, Section of Pulmonary, Critical Care, and Sleep Medicine, Yale University School of Medicine, PO Box 208057, 300 Cedar Street TAC-441 South, New Haven, CT 06520-8057, USA
* Corresponding author.
E-mail address: charles.delacruz@yale.edu

Clin Chest Med 41 (2020) 1–24
https://doi.org/10.1016/j.ccm.2019.10.001
0272-5231/20/

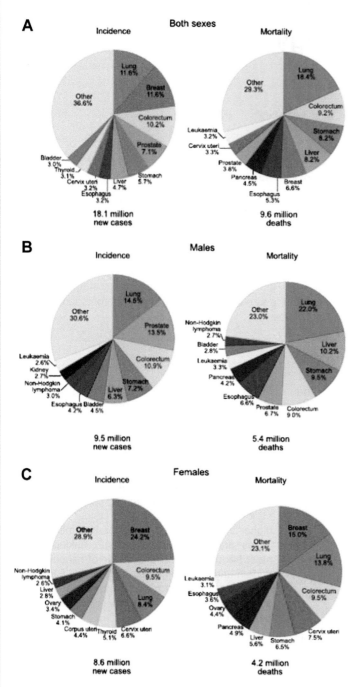

Fig. 1. Distribution of cases and deaths for the 10 most common cancers in 2018 for (A) both sexes, (B) males, and (C) females. For each sex, the area of the pie chart reflects the proportion of the total number of cases or deaths. (GLOBOCAN 2018. Global Cancer Observatory (http://gco.iarc.fr/) © International Agency for Research on Cancer 2019.)

with the recent increase in smoking prevalence in China, Indonesia, Eastern Europe, and the Northern and Southern parts of Africa.[5,7] Up to 80% of current smokers now live in low- or middle-income countries, and more than one-half of lung cancer deaths occur in less developed regions.[6–8] By contrast, lung cancer incidence is decreasing or expected to decrease in countries that "took up" smoking the earliest and are now successfully implementing smoking cessation and avoidance campaigns.[5] These countries are generally high-income and include the United States, the United Kingdom, the Nordic countries, Australia, New Zealand, Singapore, Germany, and Uruguay.[5,7]

Although the increasing lung cancer burden globally is driven by lung cancer cases in men, most countries are also observing an increasing incidence in women.[5] Although breast cancer is the leading cause of cancer-associated deaths in women globally,[7] lung cancer is the leading cause of cancer death in women in several areas, including North America, Northern/Western Europe, Australia, and New Zealand (see **Fig. 1**).[5] The higher mortality rates in these areas likely reflect local smoking patterns. The World Health Organization estimates that 48% of men and 10% of women globally are smokers.[8] Although smoking prevalence is similar between men in developed and developing countries, smoking prevalence is significantly lower in women in developing countries (**Fig. 2**).[2] In areas where tobacco smoking rates in women are low, nontobacco risk factors likely play a more significant role in lung cancer development. For example, despite a lower smoking prevalence in Chinese women, the incidence rate of lung cancer is similar to that of many European countries, which may be related to the inhalation of smoke from charcoal, heating, or cooking.[5]

Unfortunately, owing to the global increase in the number of smokers since 1980,[2] the burden of lung cancer will likely continue to increase in the coming years primarily in developing countries, where high-quality cancer registry data are unavailable.[5,7] These trends underscore 2 important points. First, the role of tobacco avoidance and cessation efforts cannot be underestimated, because a country's tobacco cessation efforts may not be recognized for many years after reductions in smoking rates. In the United States, for example, lung cancer incidence and mortality improved 20 to 30 years after smoking prevalence began to fall.[9,10] Second, more emphasis and

resources for high-quality data collection on tobacco smoking patterns, cancer development, and cancer outcomes in developing countries are needed to implement tobacco cessation and cancer control programs.

Lung Cancer Trends in the United States

In the United States, lung cancer remains the second most common cancer and the leading cause of cancer death (**Fig. 3**).[11,12] According to the Surveillance, Epidemiology, and End Results program, lung cancer currently accounts for approximately 12.9% of all new cancer cases in the United States and 538,243 people in the United States were estimated to be living with lung cancer in 2016.[10] Data from 2016 revealed deaths from lung cancer in men and women were 80,775 and 68,095, respectively,[12] which exceeded the combined number of deaths for breast cancer, prostate cancer, colon cancer, and leukemia.[12] For 2019, Siegel and colleagues[13] estimated 228,150 new cases of lung cancer and 142,670 deaths. There is a trend in both sexes of more lung cancer cases but fewer deaths.[11,12,14] When stratifying by sex, the estimated number of new cases and deaths in 2019 for men continues to exceed those values in women.[12]

Although lung cancer incidence and mortality were rising in women before 2000, both values are now steadily improving in males and females.[10] **Fig. 4** shows the overall incidence and mortality of lung cancer in the United States since 1975.[10,15] Owing to lung cancer's high case fatality rate, disease incidence is paralleled by disease mortality.[6] Although lung cancer incidence and

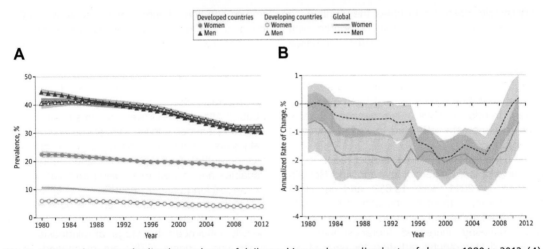

Fig. 2. Estimated age-standardized prevalence of daily smoking and annualized rate of change, 1980 to 2012. (*A*) Prevalence of smoking by year. (*B*) Annualized rate of change in the prevalence of daily smoking by year. (*From* Ng M, Freeman MK, Fleming TD, et al. Smoking prevalence and cigarette consumption in 187 countries, 1980-2012. JAMA 2014;311(2):183-192; with permission.)

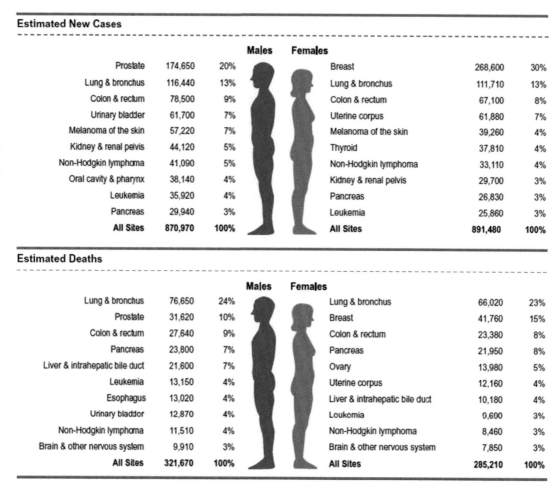

Fig. 3. Estimated new cancer cases and deaths by sex, United States, 2019. (*From* Siegel RL, Miller KD, Jemal A. Cancer statistics, 2019. CA Cancer J Clin 2019;69(1):7-34; with permission.)

mortality rates are higher in males, they continue to decrease more rapidly in men compared with women,[12] possibly attributed to earlier decreases in smoking prevalence among men and women's increased uptake of smoking around World War II. **Fig. 5** shows steady reduction in US smoking prevalence in both sexes since 1965; however, if current trends continue, lung cancer mortality rates in women are estimated to exceed those in men by 2045.[16]

The 5-year survival of lung cancer reported by the Surveillance, Epidemiology, and End Results program in 2011 was 15.6% and in 2019 19.4%.[10] Improvement in lung cancer survival is likely multifactorial and owing to decreases in tobacco smoking, increased thoracoscopic surgeries and stereotactic radiation for early stage disease, and better treatments for advanced stage disease (ie, targeted and immunologic therapies).[12,17] Tobacco smoking trends and broader

implementation of lung cancer screening (LCS) suggest that lung cancer survival will continue to improve. **Fig. 5** shows that tobacco smoking rates in the United States are improving in both sexes, and modeling studies estimate that if smoking rates continue to decline, age-adjusted lung cancer mortality may decrease by up to 79% by 2065.[16] Although improvements in smoking rates and lung cancer survival are encouraging, both values are not uniformly falling across the country. Demographic, socioeconomic, and geographic variables are related to smoking prevalence and (therefore) lung cancer rates.[18]

Despite modest improvements in outcomes in the United States, lung cancer survival remains heavily influenced by stage at diagnosis, and most lung cancers (57%) are diagnosed when the cancer has metastasized outside the lung (**Fig. 6**).[10,15] Although LCS efforts will likely "shift" the diagnosis of lung cancer to earlier stages,[19]

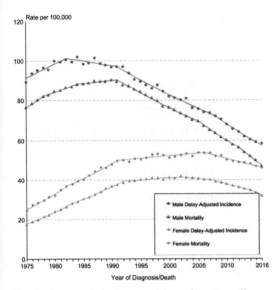

Fig. 4. Cancer of the lung and bronchus Surveillance, Epidemiology, and End Results delay-adjusted incidence and US death rates, 1975 to 2016, all races, by sex. (*From* Howlader N NA, Krapcho M, Miller D, Brest A, Yu M, Ruhl J, Tatalovich Z, Mariotto A, Lewis DR, Chen HS, Feuer EJ, Cronin KA (eds). SEER Cancer Statistics Review, 1975-2016. 2019; https://seer.cancer.gov/csr/1975_2016/. Accessed May 26, 2019; with permission.)

uptake has been slow with only 4% of eligible Americans undergoing low-dose computed tomography screening in 2015.[20] Continued implementation of LCS combined with therapeutic advances for early and advanced stage disease may help reverse our current trends of late-stage diagnosis and low overall survival.

Perhaps the greatest change in our understanding of lung cancer epidemiology in the United States is the recognition of the disease's "diversity." That is, lung cancer can no longer be stereotyped as a disease of older male smokers. **Fig. 4** demonstrates the meaningful change in lung cancer development and outcomes by gender in the last 50 years. Although smoking history and older age remain the predominant risk factors for lung cancer development, current estimates are that 10% to 20% of patients who develop lung cancer are never smokers,[21] and lung cancer incidence in women is approaching that in men. Also, although the overall trend in the United States is toward fewer lung cancer deaths and longer survival, many groups struggle with more lung cancer cases and worsening outcomes. Several demographic factors have been identified that influence lung cancer development and outcomes, including gender, age, race, geography, and socioeconomic status (SES).

Gender

Christina R. MacRosty and M. Patricia Rivera's article, "Lung Cancer in Women: A Modern Epidemic," in this issue, of this *Clinics* issue is dedicated to lung cancer in women. Owing to the significant changes in lung cancer epidemiology, we mention 3 points here. First, lung cancer incidence and mortality are consistently lower in women compared with men (see **Fig. 4**), although the gender "gap" is narrowing owing to both values falling more rapidly in men. If current trends continue, modeling studies suggest that the number of lung cancer deaths in women will exceed those in men in 2045.[16] Second, the demographics of women diagnosed with lung cancer are different than those in men. Specifically, women tend to be diagnosed with lung cancer at a younger age, are more likely to be nonsmokers, and are more likely to be diagnosed with an adenocarcinoma.[22] Finally, women have improved lung cancer survival across all disease stages than men.[23] In combination, these findings support unique biological and genetic mechanisms of lung cancer between men and women. Refer to Christina R. MacRosty and M. Patricia Rivera's article, "Lung Cancer in Women: A Modern Epidemic," in this issue, for a complete discussion of lung cancer in women.

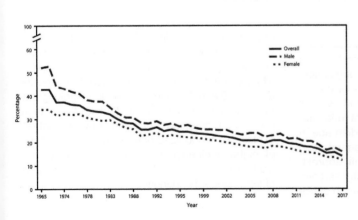

Fig. 5. Percentage of adults aged 18 years and older who were current cigarette smokers, overall and by sex; National Health Interview Survey, United States, 1965 to 2017. (*From* Wang TW, Asman K, Gentzke AS, et al. Tobacco Product Use Among Adults - United States, 2017. MMWR Morb Mortal Wkly Rep 2018;67(44):1225-1232; with permission.)

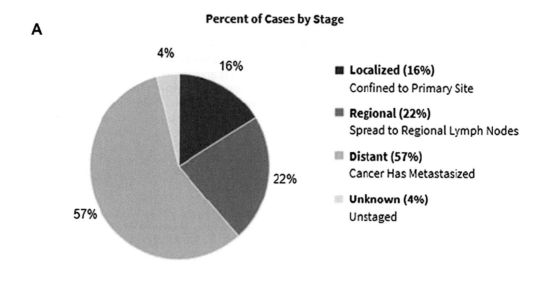

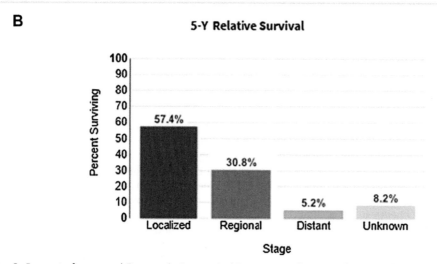

Fig. 6. Percent of cases and 5-year relative survival by stage at diagnosis: lung and bronchus cancer. (*A*) Surveillance, Epidemiology, and End Results 18 data (2009 to 2015), all races, both sexes by (*B*) Surveillance, Epidemiology, and End Results summary stage (2000). (*From* Howlader N NA, Krapcho M, Miller D, Brest A, Yu M, Ruhl J, Tatalovich Z, Mariotto A, Lewis DR, Chen HS, Feuer EJ, Cronin KA (eds). SEER Cancer Statistics Review, 1975-2016. 2019; https://seer.cancer.gov/csr/1975_2016/. Accessed May 26, 2019.)

Age

Lung cancer is most common in men and women 70 years of age and older[12] (**Fig. 7**).[10] Lung cancer has become the most common cause of cancer death in men ages 40 and older and women ages 60 and older.[12] The median age at lung cancer diagnosis is 70 years, and the median age at lung cancer death is 72 years.[6] In general, lung cancer mortality increases with age until approximately ages 80 to 85 (**Fig. 8**), after which heart disease exceeds cancer as the most common cause of death in both genders.[6,12] Interestingly, a recent study identified higher incidence rates of lung cancer among young Hispanic and non-Hispanic white women (compared with men) between the ages of 30 and 49 years.[24] Although smoking patterns likely contribute to this finding, the authors noted that smoking behaviors did not entirely explain the recognized differences. The discovery of higher incidence of lung cancer in younger women demonstrates how our "traditional" view of lung cancer is changing.

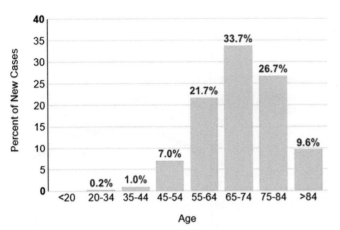

Lung and bronchus cancer is most frequently diagnosed among people aged 65-74.

Median Age At Diagnosis
70

Fig. 7. Percent of new cases by age group: lung and bronchus cancer. Surveillance, Epidemiology, and End Results 21 data (2012 to 2016), all races, both sexes. AI/AN, American Indian/Alaska Native; API, Asian/Pacific Islander. (*From* Howlader N NA, Krapcho M, Miller D, Brest A, Yu M, Ruhl J, Tatalovich Z, Mariotto A, Lewis DR, Chen HS, Feuer EJ, Cronin KA (eds). SEER Cancer Statistics Review, 1975-2016. 2019; https://seer.cancer.gov/csr/1975_2016/. Accessed May 26, 2019.)

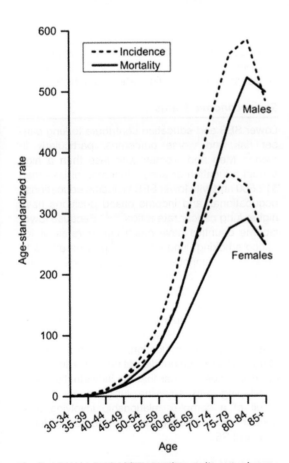

Fig. 8. Lung cancer incidence and mortality rates by sex and age, United States, 2006 to 2010. Rates are 100,000 and age-adjusted to the 2000 US standard population. (*From* Torre LA, Siegel RL, Jemal A. Lung Cancer Statistics. Adv Exp Med Biol 2016;893:1-19; with permission.)

Race

Overall, lung cancer incidence and mortality are highest in African American men and lowest in Hispanic women.[6] In data from 2008 to 2014, compared with Caucasians, African Americans had lower rates of localized disease at diagnosis (13% vs 17%) and worsened 5-year relative survival for localized (52% vs 56%), regional (27% vs 30%), and all-stage disease (16% vs 19%).[12] Higher lung cancer-associated mortality by race is likely multifactorial, including smoking prevalence, access to health insurance, and SES. American Indians/Alaska Natives currently have the highest overall smoking rate in the United States (21.9%).[25] Whereas lung cancer mortality has been decreasing in most races since the early 1990s, lung cancer mortality in American Indians and Alaska Natives did not start falling until approximately 2010 (**Fig. 9**).

There are significantly lower rates of surgical and chemotherapy treatments in African Americans.[26,27] Worse survival in Hispanics with early stage non small cell lung cancer has been noted, which was largely explained by lower resection rates.[28] Racial differences in lung cancer mortality have also been noted in screening efforts. In the National Lung Screening Trial, all-cause mortality was higher in black participants and low-dose computed tomography screening decreased lung cancer-associated mortality more in African Americans.[29] In combination, these reports suggest that racial differences in lung cancer therapy and screening persist and achieving equivalent outcomes will require a multifaceted approach including access to health care, smoking

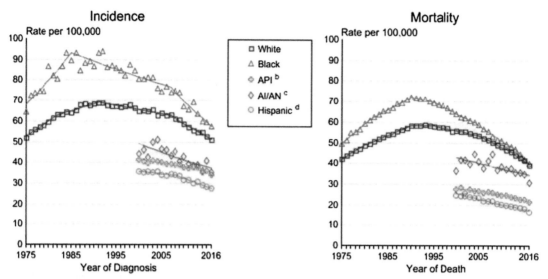

Fig. 9. Surveillance, Epidemiology, and End Results incidence and US death rates. Cancer of the lung and bronchus, both sexes. (Howlader N NA, Krapcho M, Miller D, Brest A, Yu M, Ruhl J, Tatalovich Z, Mariotto A, Lewis DR, Chen HS, Feuer EJ, Cronin KA (eds). SEER Cancer Statistics Review, 1975-2016. 2019; https://seer.cancer.gov/csr/1975_2016/. Accessed May 26, 2019.)

cessation, early diagnosis, and equivalent stage-appropriate treatments.

Geography

Much like trends globally, geography influences lung cancer epidemiology in the United States, and smoking patterns determine the higher and lower risk areas. Currently, the highest lung cancer incidence and mortality rates are in Kentucky, where the age-adjusted incidence per 100,000 people is 112.8 for men and 79.0 for women.[12] The age-adjusted mortality per 100,000 people is 84.5 in men and 52.2 in women.[12] In contrast, the lowest incidence and age-adjusted lung cancer death rates are in Utah, with incidences of 32.4 and 23.7 and mortality rates of 23.4 and 15.6 in men and women, respectively.[10–12] Although lung cancer incidence and mortality rates are decreasing nationally, several areas of the country with higher smoking prevalence have not observed the same improvements in lung cancer outcomes. Comparing the time periods 1990 to 1999 and 2006 to 2015, Ross and colleagues[30] used county-level data and identified 2 hotspots (Appalachia and the Midwest) where lung cancer death rates in women actually increased with time, which is consistent with prior work showing higher lung cancer rates for women living in southern and midwestern states.[31] Greater smoking cessation rates in western states and decline in smoking prevalence correlating with cigarette taxes and indoor air legislation has been reported.[32] Nationwide differences in lung cancer incidence and mortality are likely to persist until similar smoking cessation rates are achieved.

Socioeconomic Status

Lower SES and education contribute to lung cancer risk and worse outcomes, particularly in men.[33] Men and women with less than a high school education or annual incomes of less than $12,500 and with lower SES including educational, occupational, and income-based positions have higher lung cancer rate ratios.[34,35] Because lower income counties have much higher rates of tobacco smoking, lung cancer disparities owing to SES are analogous to those seen geographically.[12] In poor counties (compared with affluent counties), lung cancer mortality in men is more than 40% higher,[12] and low SES may increase the risk of death during hospitalization for a lung cancer resection.[36] However, studies have shown that controlling for education, SES,[33] and smoking status[37] decreased but did not normalize lung cancer risk. It seems clear that the individual's risk of developing and surviving lung cancer is the result of a complex relationship involving age, gender, race, smoking status, geographic location, and SES.

ETIOLOGY AND PREVENTION OF LUNG CANCER

With decreasing smoking prevalence and increasing cases of lung cancer in nonsmokers, there is heightened importance to better understand disease development. Although tobacco smoking remains the leading risk factor for lung cancer, risk is linked to other exposures and lung cancer prevention should focus on avoiding or decreasing exposure to known risk factors.

Tobacco Smoking

Tobacco use in the form of cigarettes has significantly increased with the average adult smoking fewer than 100 cigarettes per year in the 1900s to the estimated maximum of approximately 4400 cigarettes per person per year in the 1960s.[38,39] The seminal US Public Health Service report by the Surgeon General in 1964 was instrumental in highlighting the adverse effects of cigarette smoking on health,[40] concluding that cigarette smoking was associated with a 70% increase in the age-specific death rates for men, a lesser increase in the death rates for women, and that cigarette smoking was causally related to lung cancer. Moreover, cigarette smoking was believed to be more important than occupational exposures in the cause of lung cancer. Since the report, smoking has decreased from 20.8% of all US adults aged 18 years or older in 2005% to 14.0% in 2017.[14] The proportion of ever smokers that have quit has also increased.[14]

The effects of cigarette smoking outweigh all other factors that lead to lung cancer. In 1912, Adler[41] described 374 cases of primary lung cancer in autopsy cases from the United States and western Europe; this represented only 0.5% of all cancer cases at the time. Lung cancer constituted 1% of all cancers in the United States in 1920. In 1938, an association of cigarette smoking with increased risk of death was described in moderate and heavy white male smokers greater than 30 years of age.[42] A 1941 review of lung carcinoma reported that "the increase in the incidence of pulmonary carcinoma is due largely to the increase in smoking."[43] Two large landmark studies in 1950 established tobacco smoking as a causal factor in bronchogenic carcinoma and concluded that (1) excessive and prolonged use of tobacco was an important factor in lung cancer induction, (2) lung cancers in nonsmokers were rare (current experience show that this is not the case anymore), and (3) that there could be a lag of 10 or more years between smoking cessation and the clinical onset of carcinoma.[44,45] In 2004, the United States Surgeon General re-emphasized the message that "cigarette smoking is the major cause of lung cancer."[46] To this day, there is no question that tobacco smoking remains the most important modifiable risk factor for lung cancer

with about 90% of lung cancers arising owing to tobacco use.[47]

Tobacco Smoke Carcinogens

Tobacco cigarette smoke is a complex aerosol composed of gaseous and particulate compounds. The smoke consists of mainstream smoke and side stream smoke components. Mainstream smoke is produced by inhalation of air through the cigarette and is the primary source of smoke exposure for the smoker. Side stream smoke is produced from smoldering of the cigarette between puffs and is the major source of environmental tobacco smoke (ETS). The main determinant of tobacco addiction is nicotine, whereas the tar is the total particulate matter (PM) of cigarette smoke after nicotine and water have been removed. Cumulative exposure to tar seems to be a major component of lung cancer risk. There are more than 4000 chemical constituents of cigarette smoke.[48] The International Agency for Research on Cancer has identified at least 50 carcinogens in tobacco smoke.[49]

Mainstream smoke contains many potential carcinogens, including polycyclic aromatic hydrocarbons, aromatic amines, N-nitrosamines, and other organic and inorganic compounds, such as benzene, vinyl chloride, arsenic, and chromium. The polycyclic aromatic hydrocarbons and N-nitrosamines require metabolic activation to become carcinogenic. Metabolic detoxification of these compounds can also occur, and the balance between activation and detoxification likely affects individual cancer risk. Radioactive materials, such as radon and its decay products, bismuth, and polonium, are also present in tobacco smoke.

The agents of particular concern in lung cancer are the tobacco-specific N-nitrosamines formed by nitrosation of nicotine during tobacco processing and smoking. Of the tobacco-specific N-nitrosamines, 4-(methylnitrosamino)-1(3-pyridyl)-1-butanone seems to be the most important inducer of lung cancer. The mechanisms of carcinogenesis from tobacco also include formation of DNA adducts, their metabolites, and free radical damage.[50] The primary factor determining the intensity of cigarette use is the nicotine dependence of the smoker, and, although modern cigarettes contain less nicotine and tar, smokers tend to smoke more intensively with a greater number of puffs per minute and deeper inhalations to satisfy their nicotine need. Interestingly, low-yield filtered cigarettes might be a contributing factor to the increase in the incidence of adenocarcinoma of the lung.[51] With deeper inhalation, higher-order bronchi with more susceptible peripheral lung epithelium are exposed to carcinogen-containing smoke linked to the induction of adenocarcinoma.

The relative risk of lung cancer in long-term smokers has been estimated as 10-fold to 30-fold compared with lifetime nonsmokers. The cumulative lung cancer risk among heavy smokers can be as high as 30% compared with a lifetime risk of less than 1% in nonsmokers. One in 6 smokers eventually develops lung cancer.[47] The lung cancer risk is proportional to the quantity of cigarette consumption, and important factors include the number of packs per day smoked, the age of onset of smoking, the degree of inhalation, the tar and nicotine content of cigarettes, and use of unfiltered cigarettes.[52] Up to 20% of all cancer deaths worldwide could be prevented by the elimination of tobacco smoking.[53] Although more than 80% of lung cancers occur in persons with tobacco exposure, fewer than 20% of average smokers develop lung cancer. This variability in cancer susceptibility is likely affected by other environmental factors or by genetic predisposition.

Rate of Tobacco Use

In the United States, cigarette smoking prevalence is steadily decreasing in both sexes (see **Fig. 4**) and recent estimates show cigarette smoking at its lowest prevalence to date (14% or 34.3 million US adults).[14] Interestingly, analogous to the risk of lung cancer development, several demographic, social, and medical factors influence an individual's likelihood of smoking (**Table 1**).[14] The number of adult smokers in the United States is likely to continue decreasing. The Centers for Disease Control and Prevention reported increases in the proportion of smokers trying to quit, recently quitting, receiving advice to quit, and using proven cessation methods.[54] For additional details regarding tobacco cessation and treatment, we direct the reader to Hasmeena Kathuria and Enid Neptune's article, "Primary and Secondary Prevention of Lung Cancer: Tobacco Treatment," in this issue.

Environmental Tobacco Smoke

ETS or secondhand smoke is known to contribute to an increased risk for lung cancer. Longitudinal studies have shown this increased risk relationship between ETS and lung cancer in never smokers.[55,56] A recent meta-analysis evaluating cancer risk associated with ETS across all cancers found an increased risk of lung cancer (odds ratio [OR], 1.24) involving never smokers with tobacco smoke exposure compared with never smokers without such exposure with the association strongest in women.[57] At least 17% of lung cancers in nonsmokers are attributable to exposure to high levels of ETS during childhood and adolescence.[58] One large epidemiologic study found an excess

Table 1
Factors influencing likelihood of cigarette smoking

Factor	Those at Highest Risk of Smoking
Gender	Males
Age	Adults <65 y
Race	Non-Hispanic American Indians/Alaska Natives Whites Blacks Multiracial adults
Geography	South Midwest
Education	Those with a General Education Development certificate
Income	<$35,000/y
Sexual orientation	Lesbian, gay, or bisexual adults
Marital status	Divorced, separated, widowed Single, never married, or not living with a partner
Insurance	Uninsured Insured by Medicaid or other public insurance (not Medicare)
Comorbidities	Adults with a disability or serious psychological distress

From Wang TW, Asman K, Gentzke AS, et al. Tobacco Product Use Among Adults - United States, 2017. MMWR Morb Mortal Wkly Rep 2018;67(44):1225-1232.

risk for lung cancer of 24% in nonsmokers who lived with a smoker.[59] Nonsmoking women married to men who smoke have an increased risk of lung cancer.[60]

ETS consists of both mainstream (exhaled) smoke and side stream smoke (from burning end of cigarettes) and contains carcinogens that include benzene, benzo-a-pyrene, and 4-(methyl-nitrosamino)-1(3-pyridyl)-1-butanone. Nonsmokers exposed to side stream smoke generated by machine smoking of cigarettes had measurable carcinogenic metabolites in their urine.[61] Eighty-eight percent of nontobacco users had detectable levels of serum cotinine, a metabolite of nicotine, suggesting the exposure to ETS and the pervasive presence of ETS.[62] However, with 14% of the American adult population still smoking, ETS will continue to be a major public health issue until cigarette smoking altogether is eliminated.

The majority (80%–90%) of lung cancers develop in current or former tobacco smokers and could be avoided with tobacco smoking prevention and cessation.[63] If individuals are able to quit smoking before middle age, up to 90% of associated risk from tobacco smoking can be avoided.[64] Decreases in the number of smokers will also decrease the number of individuals exposed to ETS. If smoking cessation patterns in the United States continue, lung cancer mortality will be greatly reduced in the future.[16] Thus, the importance of smoking cessation in reducing risk of lung cancer cannot be over-estimated. Refer to Hasmeena Kathuria and Enid Neptune's article, "Primary and Secondary Prevention of Lung Cancer: Tobacco Treatment," in this issue on tobacco treatment.

Electronic Nicotine Delivery Systems and E-Cigarettes

The newest and most controversial products potentially influencing lung cancer risk are electronic nicotine delivery systems (ENDS) including electronic cigarettes (e-cigarettes), e-pens, e-pipes, e-hookah, and e-cigars.[65] These products are marketed as a safer alternative to tobacco smoking[66] by delivering nicotine without the other combustible exposures inherent to tobacco smoke and a mechanism of tobacco smoking cessation.[67] ENDS allow liquid to be heated to create an aerosol containing nicotine and substances such as flavorings, propylene glycol, vegetable glycerin, and other ingredients that the user inhales.[65] About 12.6% of adults in the United States have tried an e-cigarette at least once[68] and the overall prevalence of ENDS use in adults was

3.2% in 2016.[65] Almost one-half of current cigarette smokers (47.6%) and more than one-half of recent former cigarette smokers (55.4%) had ever tried an e-cigarette.[68] The use of e-cigarettes has become popular with teenagers and young adults, resulting in a 900% increase in e-cigarette use in high school students between 2011 and 2015, with more than 2 million middle and high school students using ENDS in 2016.[69] Although ENDS are advertised as a smoking cessation tool, previous nonsmokers of traditional cigarettes comprised a good proportion of ENDS users. E-cigarette use is associated with a greater risk for subsequent cigarette smoking initiation underscoring the urgency for strong regulation to curb use among youth and limit the future population-level burden of cigarette smoking.[70]

The alarming increased use of ENDS with unregulated multiple brands and flavorings have made it difficult to evaluate the safety of these devices. Although the components of e-cigarette vapor are different from those in traditional tobacco cigarettes, available data suggest that formaldehyde, acetaldehyde, and reactive oxygen species are present in sufficient concentrations to cause inflammatory damage to the airway and lung epithelium. Aerosols for ENDS can contain polycyclic aromatic hydrocarbons, nitrosamines, and trace metals, and their contribution to tumorigenesis is unclear.[71]

Presently, conclusive evidence regarding the safety of e-cigarettes overall or compared with tobacco smoking is unavailable. A position statement from the Forum of International Respiratory Societies suggest the devices should be restricted or banned until more convincing evidence is available.[67] Since Because -cigarette use is popular and growing in middle and high school students, and could actually promote tobacco use, underage use must be avoided.[65,69]

Marijuana and Other Recreational Drugs

The effects of inhaling smoke from recreational drugs, such as marijuana and cocaine, are less studied and there is no clear consensus on whether marijuana use is associated with cancer risk. The main psychoactive ingredient in cannabis, Δ9-tetrahydrocannabinol, is not known to be carcinogenic but, like nicotine, produces addiction. An association between marijuana smoking and initiation of tobacco use in young people has been described.[72] The number of marijuana users has increased given the legalization for nonmedical recreational use in some places. Marijuana continues to be the most commonly used illegal substance in the United States, with up to

12% of adolescents and adults admitting use.[73] Abnormal metaplastic histologic and molecular changes similar to premalignant alterations have been described in the bronchial epithelium in habitual smokers of marijuana or cocaine.[74] However, a clear association has not been fully established between such inhalant drug use and lung cancer. A case-control study reported an 8% increased risk for lung cancer for each joint-year of marijuana smoking after adjusting for tobacco cigarette smoking.[75] In fact, tar levels in marijuana smoke and carcinogenic polyaromatic hydrocarbon concentrations can be much higher than those in tobacco.[76] However, lung cancer studies largely seem not to support an association with marijuana use, possibly because of the smaller amounts of marijuana regularly smoked compared with tobacco, but more investigations are warranted.[77] The relationship between other inhalational recreational drug use such as cocaine and lung cancer are not well-studied.

Never Smokers

The term never smoker refers to persons who have smoked fewer than 100 cigarettes in their lifetime, including lifetime nonsmokers. The overall global statistics estimate that 15% of lung cancers in men and up to 53% in women are not attributable to smoking, highlighting a strong gender bias in never smokers.[78] In addition, never smokers account for up to 25% of all lung cancer cases worldwide. If lung cancer in never smokers was considered separately, it would rank as the seventh most common cause of cancer death worldwide before cervical, pancreatic, and prostate cancers. In the United States, 1 study estimated that 19% of lung cancer in women and 9% of lung cancer in men occurs in never smokers.[79] In South Asian countries, up to 80% of women with lung cancer are never smokers.[80] The proportion of never smokers with adenocarcinoma non small cell lung cancer increased from 8.0% to 14.9% from 1990 to 1995 to 2011 to 2013, which was not the case for never smokers with small cell lung cancer or squamous cell non small cell lung cancer.[81] With the decreasing smoking prevalence and increasing rate of lung cancer in nonsmokers, there is heightened urgency to better understand other etiologic factors contributing to lung cancer aside from smoking tobacco.

Biomass Burning

Wood is burned for cooking and heating purposes in many parts of the world, and approximately 3 billion people worldwide rely on solid fuels as their primary source of domestic energy.[82] Combustion of coal in homes has been linked with lung cancer in China.[83] A study of residents living who burn coal and unprocessed biomass (crop residues, wood, sticks, and twigs) for heating and cooking found increased lung cancer risk associated with coal use (OR, 1.29) after adjusting for smoking.[84] Indoor emissions from household coal combustion are classified by the International Agency for Research on Cancer as carcinogenic and emissions from biomass fuel primarily from wood as probable carcinogenic. Compared with nonsolid fuel users, predominant coal users (OR, 1.64; coal users in Asia with OR, 4.93), and wood users in North American and European countries (OR, 1.21) exhibited a higher risk for lung cancer.[85] It has been suggested that the lung cancer that arises from wood smoke may behave differently from lung cancer owing to tobacco smoke.

Air Pollution

Air pollution, a serious global problem owing to climate change and the staggering rate of industrialization, is worsening in many large populated cities across the globe where the highest concentrations of suspected particulates, sulfur dioxide, and smoke have been recorded. Epidemiologic studies suggest that air pollution, especially PM exposure, is associated with increased lung cancer risk and mortality independent of cigarette smoking.[86]

Early studies involving urban–rural comparisons showed that there was an "urban factor," which was associated with a 10% to 40% increase in lung cancer deaths.[87] Two large cohort studies suggest that there is an excess risk for lung cancer of approximately 19% per 10 mg/m^3 increment in the long-term average exposure to fine particulates.[88,89] Fine particulate and sulfur oxide-related pollution were associated with 8% increased risk for lung cancer mortality. Despite these studies, it is difficult to pinpoint the carcinogenic role played by single constituents of air pollution. There is a gradient range of relative risk for lung cancer associated with exposure to combustion products, from 7.0 to 22.0 in cigarette smokers, to 2.5 to 10.0 in coke oven workers, to 1.0 to 1.6 in residents of areas with high levels of air pollution, to 1.0 to 1.5 in nonsmokers exposed to ETS.[89,90] Diesel exhaust found in air pollution contain gaseous components, such as benzene, formaldehyde, and 1,3-butadiene has known carcinogenic effects. There is strong support that occupational exposures to diesel exhaust, especially those in the trucking industry, is associated with 30% to 50% increase in the relative risk for lung cancer.[91] Data linking gasoline engine exhaust and lung cancer are less clear. A meta-analysis of European cohort studies found statistically significant association between risk for lung cancer and PM10 (hazard ratio [HR], 1.22 per 10 $\mu g/m^3$) and PM2.5 (HR, 1.18 per 5 $\mu g/m^3$).[92] An increase in road traffic of 4000 vehicle-kilometers per day within 100 m of the residence was significantly associated with an HR for lung cancer of 1.09.[93] Significant associations were found with specific PM components (PM2.5 Cu, PM10 S, PM10 Ni, PM10 Zn, PM10 K) and lung cancer.[93]

Uranium, Radium, and Radon

The natural decay of uranium produces radium, which decays into radon gas when alpha particles are emitted. Uranium and radium are found in soil, rock, and mines with variable concentrations. Likely owing to these exposures, mining is the oldest occupation associated with lung cancer. Although the etiologic factors causing the increased lung cancer risk were originally speculated as dust-related pneumoconiosis, arsenic, or cobalt, the actual carcinogens have been identified as radioactive materials, primarily radon and its decay products. Alpha-radiation is highly damaging to tissues, including the respiratory epithelium. Inhalation of these radon decay products and subsequent alpha particle emission in the lung may cause damage to cells and genetic material. Ultimately, radon decay produces lead, which has a long half-life of 22 years. Radon is a well-established carcinogen with extensive data available both as an occupational hazard as well as exposure experienced by the general population.

A linear relationship between radon exposure and lung cancer risk is reported in underground miners,[94] and pooled data from 11 cohort studies showed that almost 40% of all lung cancer deaths (70% in never smokers and 39% in smokers) were likely due to radon exposure with potential synergistic effect with smoking.[95] The potential importance of radon as a carcinogen in the nonsmoking population was highlighted where nonsmoking miners had a higher relative risk for lung cancer compared with all types of miners.[96] Fortunately, uranium mining has now ceased in the United States; however, radon exposure continues to be an occupational concern in nonuranium mining and underground work and in uranium mines around the world. Occupational exposure to radon is legislatively controlled in the United States where individual exposure records are mandated for all workers with annual cumulative exposure limit. It has been estimated that a 40-year exposure at this level would increase a person's lifetime risk for lung cancer by approximately 2-fold.[97]

Radon, a ubiquitous indoor air pollutant in many homes, has been projected that to be the second leading cause of lung cancer after smoking, becoming a major concern for the general population. The primary factor determining radon gas concentration in homes is the concentration of radium in the soil and rock beneath those structures. Indoor-to-outdoor air exchange may also affect the radon concentration within the home. A meta-analysis of 8 studies that included 4263 patients with lung cancer and 6612 controls concluded that greater residential exposure levels were associated with an increased relative risk for lung cancer of 1.14.[98] Although there has been some initial question to the estimated lung cancer risk of indoor radon, recent systematic review of 16 studies from 12 different countries found the attributable fraction to range to be from 3% to 17%.[99]

Occupational Exposures (Asbestos)

Occupational exposures suggested or proven to be lung carcinogens include arsenic, asbestos, beryllium, cadmium, chloromethyl ethers, chromium, nickel, radon, silica, and vinyl chloride. It has been estimated that 10% of lung cancer deaths among men and 5% among women worldwide could be attributable to exposure to occupational carcinogens, namely asbestos, arsenic, beryllium, cadmium, chromium, nickel, silica, and diesel fumes.[100] Approximately 6800 to 17,000 lung cancers were a result of exposure to chemicals in the workplace in the United States.[101]

Asbestos is a naturally occurring fibrous mineral consisting primarily of 2 types: serpentine (chrysotile) and amphibole (amosite, crocidolite, and tremolites) and has for centuries been used commercially because of its strong and fire-retardant properties, making it useful for construction and insulation materials. There is a debate as to whether asbestos exposure alone and asbestosis (fibrosis related to asbestos exposure) contribute to actual risk for lung cancer. Some have argued that asbestosis is a necessary precursor to asbestos-attributable lung cancer.[102] Others report that asbestos can act as a carcinogen independent of the presence of asbestosis.[103]

Although the risk for lung cancer from nonoccupational asbestos exposure in the general environment is extremely low, occupational exposure is associated with a relative risk for lung cancer of 3.5 after adjusting for age, smoking, and vitamin use.[104] The risk is dose dependent, but varied with the type of asbestos fiber exposure, with a higher risk for workers exposed to amphibole fibers than for those exposed to chrysotile fibers, after adjusting for similar exposure level.[105] In the United States, chrysotile has been by far the most commonly used type of asbestos.

The interaction between asbestos and smoking regarding lung cancer risk has been described to be between additive and multiplicative.[106] The relative risk for lung cancer with asbestos exposure alone is 6-fold, with cigarette smoking alone it is 11-fold, but with exposure to both asbestos and cigarette smoke, the increase may be as high as 59-fold.[106] Smoking cessation should be the most important goal of cancer prevention programs in this population, with targeting of the subgroup of workers with asbestosis. Fortunately, with recognition of the harmful health risks related to asbestos, its use has precipitously decreased in the United States since the 1970s.

Prevention of Environmental and Occupational Exposures

In the United States, the Occupational Safety and Health Administration defines standards for exposure and worker production in the construction industry and associated employment sectors.[107] From an environmental perspective, radon and environmental and household air pollution (ie, smoke from warming or cooking houses) are the predominant exposures. Because radon is diluted to low concentrations outdoors, the most worrisome exposures are in homes. Prevention via testing for radon in both newly built and existing homes is recommended.[108] Decreasing exposure to air pollution is a particular problem in developing and industrializing nations. Household exposure may be decreased via alternative heating/cooking methods or wearing a mask to avoid direct lung exposure. Toward this end, the World Health Organization is developing a Clean Household Energy Solution Toolkit, which may be implemented to decrease the risks of household fuel combustion.[109] Decreases in environmental air pollution will require national and international efforts to improve air quality.

Genetic Predisposition and History of Cancer

There is a genetic component to the pathogenesis of lung cancer, whether it relates to host susceptibility to lung cancer (with or without exposure to cigarette smoke and to the development of certain types of lung cancer) or to an individual's responsiveness to therapies. The importance of a family history of cancer, especially for family members with early onset lung cancer, has been highlighted by the incorporation into several lung cancer risk prediction algorithms.[110,111] A lot has been learned about the molecular epidemiology of lung cancer and on host susceptibility genetic markers to lung carcinogens (see Ramin Salehi-Rad and colleagues' article, "The Biology of Lung Cancer: Development of More Effective Methods for Prevention, Diagnosis and Treatment," in this issue). The susceptibility genetic factors include high-penetrance, low-frequency genes; low-penetrance, high-frequency genes; and acquired epigenetic polymorphisms. Familial association approaches such as those in rare mendelian cancer syndromes (Bloom and Werner syndromes) have been used to discover high-penetrance, low-frequency genes. There is a 2-fold increased risk for lung cancer in smokers with a family history of lung cancer with an increased risk also present in nonsmokers.[112] Large-effect genome-wide associations for squamous lung cancer with the rare variants BRCA2 and CHEK2 has recently been described in a European cohort.[113]

Many candidate susceptibility genes that are of low penetrance and high frequency have been reported. There have been more than 1000 candidate gene association studies on genetic susceptibility to lung cancer in the past 2 decades but without clear consensus. One study reported 22 of 21 genes (including ATM, CXCR2, CYP1A1, CYP2E1, ERCC1, ERCC2, FGFR4, SOD2, TERT, and TP53) exhibiting significant associations with lung cancer susceptibility.[114] Genotypic analysis combined with existing data for an aggregated genome-wide association study analysis of lung cancer identified 18 (including 10 new) susceptibility loci that highlighted striking heterogeneity in genetic susceptibility across the histologic subtypes of lung cancer.[115] This work highlighted RNASET2, SECISBP2L, and NRG1 as candidate genes, as well as cholinergic nicotinic receptor, CHRNA2, and the telomere-related genes OFBC1 and RTEL1.[115] High-depth, high-accuracy microsatellite genotyping revealed 2 genes (ARID1B and REL) and 2 significantly enriched pathways (chromatin organization and cellular stress response), suggesting lung carcinogenesis to be linked to chromatin remodeling, inflammation, and tumor microenvironment restructuring.[116]

Susceptibility to carcinogenic agents may also be affected by individual differences in mutagen sensitivity as noted by studies of DNA repair and lung cancer risks.[117] Polymorphisms in DNA repair enzymes active in base excision repair (XRCC1 and OGG1), nucleotide excision repair (ERCC1, XPD, and XPA), and double-strand break repair (XRCC3), and different mismatch repair pathways have been linked to lung cancer risks. Chronic inflammation in response to repetitive tobacco exposure has been theorized as being involved in lung tumorigenesis. Genes encoding for the interleukins or cyclo-oxygenase involved in inflammation, or the metalloproteases involve in repair during inflammation have been associated with lung cancer risk.[116] Several cell cycle–related genes have been implicated in lung cancer susceptibility, including tumor suppressor genes p53 and p73, and apoptosis genes FAS and FASL. DNA adducts can be measured as biomarkers to represent the degree of carcinogenesis and lung cancer susceptibility. Acquired or epigenetic changes to DNA chromosome can also lead to increased lung cancer susceptibility. These events include DNA methylation, histone deacetylation, and phosphorylation, all of which can affect gene expression.

Lung cancer susceptibility is determined at least in part by host genetic factors. Persons with genetic susceptibility might therefore be at higher risk if they smoke tobacco. As more is being discovered about genetic risks to lung cancer, it may be possible to target high-risk subgroups for lung cancer for specific interventions, including intensive efforts at smoking cessation, screening, and prevention programs.

Chronic Lung Diseases

Chronic lung diseases have been associated with an increased risk for lung cancer, the strongest association being with chronic obstructive pulmonary disease (COPD), especially in men.[118] The prevalence of COPD in newly diagnosed lung cancer in 1 study was 6-fold greater than matched smokers, suggesting that COPD itself is an important independent risk factor.[118] COPD is characterized by chronic inflammation and a study found that the likelihood of developing lung cancer was increased if C-reactive protein, a nonspecific measure of inflammation, was greater than 3 mg/L compared with patients with lower levels (<1 mg/L).[119] A large retrospective study of patients with COPD found that the risk for lung cancer was lower among patients who took high-dose inhaled corticosteroids (ICS) compared with patients taking lower doses or none at all.[120] A recent study using population-based linked administrative data in Canada showed that ICS exposure was associated with a 30% reduced risk of lung cancer with a HR of 0.70.[121] These results highlight the use of ICS as a potential chemoprevention in lung cancer among patients with COPD. However, this finding must be tempered, given that other investigators have shown that patients with COPD with post-ICS tuberculosis or pneumonia had increased risk of lung cancers.[122]

Alpha1-antitrypsin deficiency carriers have a higher risk for lung cancer (2-fold), after adjusting for tobacco smoke and COPD.[123] The incidence of lung cancer in patients with interstitial fibrosis is reported to be markedly increased with an OR for lung cancer of 8.25 compared with control subjects, even after adjustment for smoking.[124] The risk of development of lung cancer in idiopathic pulmonary fibrosis or usual interstitial fibrosis is higher for older male smokers and significantly higher in those with combined usual interstitial fibrosis and emphysema syndrome compared with fibrosis only.[125] Other fibrosing diseases, including asbestosis and scleroderma-related lung disease, also have an increased association with lung cancer. Although the mechanisms by which pulmonary interstitial disease may predispose to lung malignancy are not clear, various hypotheses have been raised, including malignant transformation related to chronic inflammation, epithelial hyperplasia, impaired clearance of carcinogens, and infections.

Infections

Infection as a causative factor in lung cancer remains debatable. A potential role for human papillomavirus (HPV) has been suggested in lung cancer because it has been detected in bronchial squamous cell lesions.[105] A high incidence of HPV DNA in lung cancer has been reported in Asian cohorts, especially in nonsmokers; however, studies in Western Europe failed to show an etiologic role of HPV in lung cancer.[126] HPV serotypes 16 and 18 have been associated with lung cancer more than other serotypes. E6 and E7 oncogenes from these HPV serotypes have been shown to immortalize human tracheal epithelial cells, which themselves are highly prone to genetic damage.[127] It will take time to see if an HPV-directed vaccine for cervical cancer has any impact on the incidence of lung cancer.

Bioinformatic analyses of The Cancer Genome Atlas data found that viral sequences can be identified in 21% of the lung cancer samples compared with paired adjacent normal tissues.[128] Viral sequences from only 8 viruses were found in lung cancer and these include HPV16, HPV18, HPV30, HPV33, human herpesvirus 4 (or Epstein-Barr virus), human herpesvirus 5 (or cytomegalovirus CMV), human herpesvirus 6 and hepatitis B virus. Epstein-Barr virus, which is associated with Burkitt lymphoma and nasopharyngeal carcinoma, has been strongly associated with lymphoepithelioma-like carcinoma, a rare form of lung cancer, in Asian patients, but this association has not been observed in the Western population.[129] Other viruses suggested as etiologic for lung cancer include BK virus, JC virus, the human cytomegalovirus, simian virus 40, measles virus, and Torque tenovirus; however, the results have remained inconclusive.[130–132]

Chlamydia (*Chlamydophila*) *pneumonia* is a common cause of respiratory infection, especially in smokers and might have a role in lung cancer.[133] Although not known as an oncogenic pathogen, the inflammation resulting from Chlamydia infection and or *C pneumoniae* proteins can lead to DNA damage and cellular injury conferring selective advantages for tumorigenesis.[134] A cohort study of tuberculosis patients showed an increased risk for lung cancer in these patients with hazard ratio of 3.3 after adjusting for COPD.[135] Another study found that tuberculosis was significantly associated with increased risk for lung cancer (HR, 1.37) and mortality (HR, 1.43).[136] Interestingly, there was no evidence for synergism between a history of tuberculosis and smoking. It has been speculated that the tuberculosis-related inflammation and scarring contribute to lung cancer pathogenesis.[137]

Patients infected with the human immunodeficiency virus (HIV) are living longer owing to antiretroviral treatments; however, there is an increase in the proportion of deaths attributable to non–AIDS-defining tumors, especially lung cancer, which has become a leading cause of death among people living with HIV.[138,139] More than 40% of people living with HIV in the United States smoke cigarettes and HIV itself independently increases the risk of lung cancer.[140] Tobacco use and HIV together may accelerate the development of lung cancer. The risk of lung cancer is increased by the presence of HIV through mechanisms likely involving chronic inflammation, immunomodulation, and other infections. HIV was associated with a hazard ratio of 3.6 for lung cancer after controlling for smoking.[141] An increased risk of lung cancer in veteran patients with HIV was associated with low CD4 cell count, high viral load, and more bacterial pneumonia episodes.[142] Other factors that could contribute to the higher incidence of lung cancer in patients with HIV include the greater prevalence of co-infection with oncogenic viruses (HPV, Epstein-Barr virus, and Kaposi sarcoma virus), the potential direct effects of the HIV virus, and the consequences of long-term immunosuppression.[143] Certain lung microbiota dysbiosis has recently been correlated with development of lung cancer.[144] For example, the lower airways of patients with lung cancer were enriched for oral taxa *Streptococcus* and *Veillonella*, which was associated with an up-regulation of the ERK and PI3K inflammatory signaling pathways.[145] Overall, evidence suggests that infection could play a role in lung cancer; however, definite proof of a causal relationship remains lacking.

Diet

Certain dietary items such as red meat, dairy products, saturated fats, and lipids have been suggested to increase the risk for lung cancer. A meta-analysis found a significant (24%) increased risk of lung cancer for high consumption of red meat (relative risk, 1.24) among never smokers and nonsmokers[146] but not for high consumption of other types of meat or fish or for heterocyclic amines. A pooled analysis of 10 prospective cohort studies showed that high intakes of total and saturated fat were associated with increased risk of lung cancer (HR, 1.07 and 1.14, respectively) where the positive association was greater in current smokers than former/never smokers, whereas a high intake of polyunsaturated fat was associated with a decreased risk of lung cancer (HR, 0.92).[147] Moreover, a 5% energy substitution of saturated fat with polyunsaturated fat was associated with a 16% to 17% lower risk of small cell and squamous cell carcinoma, respectively. Other foods with an adverse effect on lung cancer include food that contain nitrosodimethylamines and nitrites (found in salted and smoked meat products).[148]

Many large-scale studies of vitamin supplementation have yielded disappointingly negative results.[149,150] Because of the large body of epidemiologic literature pointing to the benefits of fruits and vegetables, most health authorities continue to recommend a balanced dietary intake incorporating fruits and vegetables.[151] Vitamin A has both an animal (retinol) and a vegetable (carotenoid) source; the vegetable component may have protective effects against lung cancer. In particular, studies have shown beta-carotene (a prominent carotenoid) and vitamins C and E (alpha-tocopherol) may have some protective effect against lung cancer.[152,153] However, large trials such as The Alpha-Tocopherol, Beta Carotene Cancer Prevention (ATBC) Study and the Beta-Carotene and Retinol Efficacy Trial (CARET) not only did not find benefit of dietary supplementation, but they found higher than expected mortality in the group that received beta-carotene and or vitamin A.[150,154] As a result of these studies, among others, the use of supplemental beta-carotene and vitamin A is discouraged. There have also been suggestions that low dietary intake of certain minerals, including magnesium, zinc, copper, and iron, is associated with increased lung cancer risk; however, later prospective cohort studies observed no associations between total mineral intake and lung cancer.[155,156] Overall, dietary supplementation in lung cancer prevention is unclear and these studies should serve as a reminder that indiscreet and excessive intake of vitamins or other chemicals can be potentially harmful.

Fruits and vegetables that contain carotenoids and other antioxidants have been hypothesized to decrease lung cancer risk. Comparing the highest with the lowest intakes incorporating a large number of independent studies, the summary relative risk estimates were 0.92 for vegetables and 0.82 for fruits.[157] Significant inverse dose–response associations were observed for each 100 g/d increase for fruits and vegetables with no additional benefit when increasing consumption more than 400 g/d. A meta-analysis of 37 studies showed similar significant associations between vegetables and fruits intake and lung cancer risk with effects stronger in females than in males.[158] Although these studies showed that any types of vegetables and fruits have beneficial effects with lung cancer, the consumption of vegetables described as cruciferous, such as broccoli and cabbage, which are rich in isothiocyanates, has protective effect against lung cancer.[159] Low or no intake of fruits or vegetables has been associated with up to a 3-fold risk for lung cancer.[160] Furthermore, consuming fruits or vegetables raw rather than cooked is associated with a further decrease in the risk for lung cancer because important carotenoids can be destroyed with cooking.[161]

Flavonoid plant metabolites have antioxidant and antiproliferative properties and can be found in foods, such as berries, citrus fruits, tea, dark chocolate, and red wine. A prospective study showed the risk for lung cancer was lower in men with high total flavonoid intake.[162] Consumption of vegetables, tea, and wine, all of which are rich sources of flavonoids, was associated inversely with lung cancer among tobacco smokers.

A pooled analysis of the International Lung Cancer Consortium and the SYNERGY study found an inverse association between overall risk of lung cancer and consumption of alcoholic beverages compared with nondrinkers.[163] The lowest risk was observed for persons who consumed 10.0 to 19.9 g/d of alcoholic beverage where 1 drink is approximately 12 to 15 g. There is an inverse association found between the consumption of wine and liquor, but not beer, and lung cancer.[164]

Epidemiologic studies investigating the association between coffee consumption and lung cancer risk have yielded inconsistent results, although recent studies have consistently indicated a significantly increased risk by 47% in the population with the highest category intake of coffee compared with the lowest category of intake.[165]

Obesity and Exercise

Globally, more than 1.9 billion adults are overweight and of these 650 million are obese. Although a meta-analysis showed an inverse association between body mass index (BMI) and lung cancer risk, and obesity may even have a protective role,[166] the association between BMI and lung cancer was not significant in the absence of cigarette smoking. The observed BMI and cancer association may be related to residual strong confounding effects of smoking because smokers tend to have a lower BMI than their matched nonsmokers with some gaining weight upon smoking cessation.[167] A meta-analysis of 29 studies showed, that compared with normal weight, the relative risk for lung cancer was 0.77 for excess body weight with a BMI of 25 kg/m^2 or greater.[168] Underweight has also been associated with lower lung cancer risk, with a nonlinear, inverted U-shaped relationship.[169] Waist circumference has been found to be positively associated with lung cancer risk in smokers.[170]

The role of physical activity and lung cancer risk has been mixed. Physical activity has been associated with lower lung cancer risk with estimates, ranging from a 20% to a 50% lower risk in the most active study participants.[171] A prospective study found that, in middle-aged men with no history of lung cancer, increasing levels of cardiorespiratory fitness serve as a protective factor against lung cancer.[172] Using a large database of subjects in a cancer prevention study, physical activity was not associated with lung cancer risk within any of the smoking strata except in former smokers less than 10 years since quitting (relative risk, 0.77).[169] Favorable lifestyle including good cardiorespiratory fitness, healthy dietary habits and nonsmoking lifestyle considerably reduces the risk of cancer, especially lung cancer in men.[173]

Lung Cancer Risk Predictive Models

With a better understanding of the risk factors for lung cancer, predictive models have improved. The implementation of LCS has heightened the importance of predicting individual lung cancer risk. Updated lung cancer risk prediction models have built on prior findings and several are currently available.[174] For example, the PLCO$_{M2012}$ model using patients from the Prostate, Lung, Colorectal and Ovarian (PLCO) Cancer Screening Trial and the National Lung Screening Trial who were current or former smokers incorporated age, race, education, BMI, smoking history, family history of lung cancer, personal history of cancer, and COPD.[175] When compared with established LCS criteria (including age and smoking history; Nina A. Thomas and Nichole T. Tanner's article, "Lung Cancer Screening: Patient Selection and Implementation," in this issue), PLCO$_{M2012}$ had a higher sensitivity and positive predictive value for determining individual risk of developing lung cancers. Risk-based selection of patients for LCS may be associated with a lower number needed to screen.[176] Trials are underway comparing lung cancer predictive models with current LCS criteria.[177]

Chemopreventive Agents

Although multiple potential chemopreventive agents, including beta-carotene supplementation, vitamin E, retinoids, *N*-acetylcysteine, isotretinoin, aspirin, selenium, prostacyclin analogues, cyclooxygenase-2 inhibitors, anethole dithiolethione, inhaled steroids, pioglitazone, myoinositol, tea extract, and metformin have been studied; however, to date none have been identified as effective.[178] Decreasing inflammation is a purported mechanism for reducing lung cancer risk and large retrospective studies have reported lower lung cancer risk in patients receiving cholesterol-lowering statin medications[179] and in patients with COPD treated with ICS.[120,121] Unfortunately, conflicting results have been reported for both medication classes, showing no effects on lung cancer risk reduction.[147,180]

SUMMARY

Lung cancer remains a major problem in the United States and globally. Despite recent advances, the disease remains the number one cause of cancer death and portends one of the lowest 5-year survival rates among all cancer types. In the United States, incidence and mortality are improving, whereas globally the number of lung cancer cases is still increasing likely due to rising tobacco use in developing and lower- and middle-income countries. The primary risk factor for lung cancer is cigarette smoking, and smoking cessation is an imperative component of cancer prevention. Effective smoking cessation in the United States is changing traditional patterns of lung cancer development; in fact, some have estimated that 25% of all lung cancer cases are observed in never

smokers and this number is likely to increase in the future. Understanding the role of nontobacco risk factors will be increasingly important. Future preventive efforts and research needs to prioritize non–tobacco-related modifiable risk factors and provide more clarity with regard to modern exposures, such as noncigarette tobacco smoking products. There is likely benefit to maintaining a healthy body weight, increased physical activity, and healthy eating with a diet rich in whole grains, fruit, and vegetables. From a population health perspective, continued measures to promote tobacco smoking avoidance or cessation, protect workers from known inhaled carcinogens, and maintain clean air are needed to facilitate a decreased risk of lung cancer. The challenge in the future will be to modify the impact of all risk factors while continuing to expand our knowledge of the genetic and molecular basis of carcinogenesis.

CONFLICTS OF INTEREST

None.

REFERENCES

1. World Health Organization. Cancer. 2018. Available at: http://www.who.int/news-room/fact-sheets/detail/cancer. Accessed 24 November, 2018.
2. Ng M, Freeman MK, Fleming TD, et al. Smoking prevalence and cigarette consumption in 187 countries, 1980-2012. JAMA 2014;311(2):183–92.
3. Dela Cruz CS, Tanoue LT, Matthay RA. Lung cancer: epidemiology, etiology, and prevention. Clin Chest Med 2011;32(4):605–44.
4. World Health Organization. Cancer fact sheets, lung cancer. 2018. Available at: http://gco.iarc.fr/today/fact-sheets-cancers. Accessed December 2, 2018.
5. Bray F, Ferlay J, Soerjomataram I, et al. Global cancer statistics 2018: GLOBOCAN estimates of incidence and mortality worldwide for 36 cancers in 185 countries. CA Cancer J Clin 2018;68(6): 394–424.
6. Torre LA, Siegel RL, Jemal A. Lung cancer statistics. Adv Exp Med Biol 2016;893:1–19.
7. Torre LA, Bray F, Siegel RL, et al. Global cancer statistics, 2012. CA Cancer J Clin 2015;65(2):87–108.
8. American Lung Association. Trends in tobacco use. 2011. Available at: https://www.lung.org/assets/documents/research/tobacco-trend-report.pdf. Accessed November 30, 2018.
9. American Lung Association Research and Program Services. Trends in tobacco use. 2011. Available at: https://www.lung.org/assets/documents/research/tobacco-trend-report.pdf. Accessed 24 November, 2018.

10. Howlader N, NA, Krapcho M, et al, editors. SEER cancer statistics review, 1975-2016. 2019. Available at: https://seer.cancer.gov/csr/1975_2016/2019. Accessed May 26, 2019.

11. Siegel R, Ward E, Brawley O, et al. Cancer statistics, 2011: the impact of eliminating socioeconomic and racial disparities on premature cancer deaths. CA Cancer J Clin 2011;61(4):212–36.

12. Siegel RL, Miller KD, Jemal A. Cancer statistics, 2019. CA Cancer J Clin 2019;69(1):7–34.

13. Siegel RL, Miller KD, Jemal A. Cancer statistics, 2017. CA Cancer J Clin 2017;67(1):7–30.

14. Wang TW, Asman K, Gentzke AS, et al. Tobacco product use among adults - United States, 2017. MMWR Morb Mortal Wkly Rep 2018;67(44):1225–32.

15. Cronin KA, Lake AJ, Scott S, et al. Annual report to the nation on the status of cancer, part I: national cancer statistics. Cancer 2018;124(13):2785–800.

16. Jeon J, Holford TR, Levy DT, et al. Smoking and lung cancer mortality in the United States from 2015 to 2065: a comparative modeling approach. Ann Intern Med 2018;169(10):684–93.

17. Boyer MJ, Williams CD, Harpole DH, et al. Improved survival of stage I non-small cell lung cancer: a VA Central cancer registry analysis. J Thorac Oncol 2017;12(12):1814–23.

18. Silvestri GA, Carpenter MJ. Smoking trends and lung cancer mortality: the good, the bad, and the ugly. Ann Intern Med 2018;169(10):721–2.

19. National Lung Screening Trial Research Team, Aberle DR, Adams AM, Berg CD, et al. Reduced lung-cancer mortality with low-dose computed tomographic screening. N Engl J Med 2011;365(5):395–409.

20. Jemal A, Fedewa SA. Lung cancer screening with low-dose computed tomography in the United States-2010 to 2015. JAMA Oncol 2017;3(9):1278–81.

21. Reck M, Rabe KF. Precision diagnosis and treatment for advanced non-small-cell lung cancer. N Engl J Med 2017;377(9):849–61.

22. Donington JS, Colson YL. Sex and gender differences in non-small cell lung cancer. Semin Thorac Cardiovasc Surg 2011;23(2):137–45.

23. Kligerman S, White C. Epidemiology of lung cancer in women: risk factors, survival, and screening. AJR Am J Roentgenol 2011;196(2):287–95.

24. Jemal A, Miller KD, Ma J, et al. Higher lung cancer incidence in young women than young men in the United States. N Engl J Med 2018;378(21):1999–2009.

25. American Lung Association. Tobacco use in racial and ethnic populations. 2018. Available at: https://www.lung.org/stop-smoking/smoking-facts/tobacco-use-racial-and-ethnic.html. Accessed October 28, 2018.

26. Bach PB, Cramer LD, Warren JL, et al. Racial differences in the treatment of early-stage lung cancer. N Engl J Med 1999;341(16):1198–205.

27. Hardy D, Liu CC, Xia R, et al. Racial disparities and treatment trends in a large cohort of elderly black and white patients with nonsmall cell lung cancer. Cancer 2009;115(10):2199–211.

28. Wisnivesky JP, McGinn T, Henschke C, et al. Ethnic disparities in the treatment of stage I non-small cell lung cancer. Am J Respir Crit Care Med 2005;171(10):1158–63.

29. Tanner NT, Gebregziabher M, Hughes Halbert C, et al. Racial differences in outcomes within the national lung screening trial. Implications for widespread implementation. Am J Respir Crit Care Med 2015;192(2):200–8.

30. Ross K, Kramer MR, Jemal A. Geographic inequalities in progress against lung cancer among women in the United States, 1990-2015. Cancer Epidemiol Biomarkers Prev 2018;27(11):1261–4.

31. Jemal A, Ma J, Rosenberg PS, et al. Increasing lung cancer death rates among young women in southern and midwestern States. J Clin Oncol 2012;30(22):2739–44.

32. Jemal A, Thun M, Yu XQ, et al. Changes in smoking prevalence among U.S. Adults by state and region: estimates from the tobacco use supplement to the current population Survey, 1992-2007. BMC Public Health 2011;11:512.

33. Hastert TA, Beresford SA, Sheppard L, et al. Disparities in cancer incidence and mortality by area-level socioeconomic status: a multilevel analysis. J Epidemiol Community Health 2015;69(2):168–76.

34. Clegg LX, Reichman ME, Miller BA, et al. Impact of socioeconomic status on cancer incidence and stage at diagnosis: selected findings from the surveillance, epidemiology, and end results: national Longitudinal Mortality Study. Cancer Causes Control 2009;20(4):417–35.

35. Sidorchuk A, Agardh EE, Aremu O, et al. Socioeconomic differences in lung cancer incidence: a systematic review and meta-analysis. Cancer Causes Control 2009;20(4):459–71.

36. LaPar DJ, Bhamidipati CM, Harris DA, et al. Gender, race, and socioeconomic status affects outcomes after lung cancer resections in the United States. Ann Thorac Surg 2011;92(2):434–9.

37. Hovanec J, Siemiatycki J, Conway DI, et al. Lung cancer and socioeconomic status in a pooled analysis of case-control studies. PLoS One 2018;13(2):e0192999.

38. Warner KE, Mendez D. Tobacco control policy in developed countries: yesterday, today, and tomorrow. Nicotine Tob Res 2010;12(9):876–87.

39. Wynder EL, Graham EA. Tobacco smoking as a possible etiologic factor in bronchiogenic

carcinoma; a study of 684 proved cases. J Am Med Assoc 1950;143(4):329–36.

40. U.S. Public Health Service, Office of the Surgeon General: the health consequences of smoking. 72-7516 PNH. Washington, DC: National Clearinghouse for Smoking Health.; 1972.

41. Adler I. Primary malignant growth of the lung and bronchi. New York: Longman, Green, Company.; 1912.

42. Pear R. Tobacco smoking and longevity. Science 1938;87:216.

43. Ochsner A, DeBakey M. Primary pulmonary malignancy: treatment of total pneumonectomy. Analysis of seventy-nine collected cases and presentation of seven personal cases. Surg Gynecol Obstet 1939;68:435.

44. Doll R, Hill AB. Smoking and carcinoma of the lung; preliminary report. Br Med J 1950;2(4682):739–48.

45. Wynder EL, Graham EA. Etiologic factors in bronchiogenic carcinoma with special reference to industrial exposures; report of eight hundred fifty-seven proved cases. AMA Arch Ind Hyg Occup Med 1951;4(3):221–35.

46. US Department of Health, Education, and Welfare. Smoking and health report of the advisory committee to the surgeon general of the public health service. Washington: US Department of Health, Education, and Welfare, Public Health Service; 1964. PHS Publication No. 1103.

47. US Department of Health and Human Services. The health consequences of smoking: 50 Years of progress. A report of the surgeon general. Atlanta (GA): US Department of Health and Human Services, Centers for Disease Control and Prevention, National Center for Chronic Disease Prevention and Health Promotion, Office on Smoking and Health; 2014.

48. Hoffmann D, Hoffmann I. The changing cigarette, 1950-1995. J Toxicol Environ Health 1997;50(4):307–64.

49. Smith CJ, Perfetti TA, Mullens MA, et al. "IARC group 2B Carcinogens" reported in cigarette mainstream smoke. Food Chem Toxicol 2000;38(9):825–48.

50. Akopyan G, Bonavida B. Understanding tobacco smoke carcinogen NNK and lung tumorigenesis. Int J Oncol 2006;29(4):745–52.

51. Wynder EL, Hoffmann D. Smoking and lung cancer: scientific challenges and opportunities. Cancer Res 1994;54(20):5284–95.

52. Harris JE, Thun MJ, Mondul AM, et al. Cigarette tar yields in relation to mortality from lung cancer in the cancer prevention study II prospective cohort, 1982-8. BMJ 2004;328(7431):72.

53. Pisani P, Bray F, Parkin DM. Estimates of the worldwide prevalence of cancer for 25 sites in the adult population. Int J Cancer 2002;97(1):72–81.

54. Babb S, Malarcher A, Schauer G, et al. Quitting smoking among adults - United States, 2000-2015. MMWR Morb Mortal Wkly Rep 2017;65(52):1457–64.

55. Johnson KC, Hu J, Mao Y, et al. Lifetime residential and workplace exposure to environmental tobacco smoke and lung cancer in never-smoking women, Canada 1994-97. Int J Cancer 2001;93(6):902–6.

56. Lee CH, Ko YC, Goggins W, et al. Lifetime environmental exposure to tobacco smoke and primary lung cancer of non-smoking Taiwanese women. Int J Epidemiol 2000;29(2):224–31.

57. Kim AS, Ko HJ, Kwon JH, et al. Exposure to secondhand smoke and risk of cancer in never smokers: a meta-analysis of epidemiologic studies. Int J Environ Res Public Health 2018;15(9) [pii: E1981].

58. Janerich DT, Thompson WD, Varela LR, et al. Lung cancer and exposure to tobacco smoke in the household. N Engl J Med 1990;323(10):632–6.

59. Hackshaw AK, Law MR, Wald NJ. The accumulated evidence on lung cancer and environmental tobacco smoke. BMJ 1997;315(7114):980–8.

60. Cardenas VM, Thun MJ, Austin H, et al. Environmental tobacco smoke and lung cancer mortality in the American Cancer Society's Cancer Prevention Study. II. Cancer Causes Control 1997;8(1):57–64.

61. Hecht SS, Carmella SG, Murphy SE, et al. A tobacco-specific lung carcinogen in the urine of men exposed to cigarette smoke. N Engl J Med 1993;329(21):1543–6.

62. Pirkle JL, Flegal KM, Bernert JT, et al. Exposure of the US population to environmental tobacco smoke: the third national health and Nutrition Examination Survey, 1988 to 1991. JAMA 1996;275(16):1233–40.

63. Jemal A, Bray F, Center MM, et al. Global cancer statistics. CA Cancer J Clin 2011;61(2):69–90.

64. Jha P, Ramasundarahettige C, Landsman V, et al. 21st-century hazards of smoking and benefits of cessation in the United States. N Engl J Med 2013;368(4):341–50.

65. Dinakar C, O'Connor GT. The health effects of electronic cigarettes. N Engl J Med 2016;375(14):1372–81.

66. Meo SA, Al Asiri SA. Effects of electronic cigarette smoking on human health. Eur Rev Med Pharmacol Sci 2014;18(21):3315–9.

67. Schraufnagel DE, Blasi F, Drummond MB, et al. Electronic cigarettes. A position statement of the forum of international respiratory societies. Am J Respir Crit Care Med 2014;190(6):611–8.

68. Schoenborn CA, Gindi RM. Electronic cigarette use among adults: United States, 2014. NCHS Data Brief 2015;(217):1–8.

69. Jamal A, Gentzke A, Hu SS, et al. Tobacco use among middle and high school students-United States, 2011-2016. MMWR-Morbid Mortal W 2017;66(23):597–603.

70. Soneji S, Barrington-Trimis JL, Wills TA, et al. Association between initial use of e-cigarettes and subsequent cigarette smoking among adolescents and young adults: a systematic review and meta-analysis. JAMA Pediatr 2017;171(8):788–97.

71. Tegin G, Mekala HM, Sarai SK, et al. E-cigarette toxicity? South Med J 2018;111(1):35–8.

72. Ramo DE, Liu H, Prochaska JJ. Tobacco and marijuana use among adolescents and young adults: a systematic review of their co-use. Clin Psychol Rev 2012;32(2):105–21.

73. Volkow ND, Baler RD, Compton WM, et al. Adverse health effects of marijuana use. N Engl J Med 2014; 370(23):2219–27.

74. Barsky SH, Roth MD, Kleerup EC, et al. Histopathologic and molecular alterations in bronchial epithelium in habitual smokers of marijuana, cocaine, and/or tobacco. J Natl Cancer Inst 1998; 90(16):1198–205.

75. Aldington S, Harwood M, Cox B, et al. Cannabis use and risk of lung cancer: a case-control study. Eur Respir J 2008;31(2):280–6.

76. Tashkin DP. Effects of marijuana smoking on the lung. Ann Am Thorac Soc 2013;10(3):239–47.

77. Huang YH, Zhang ZF, Tashkin DP, et al. An epidemiologic review of marijuana and cancer: an update. Cancer Epidemiol Biomarkers Prev 2015; 24(1):15–31.

78. Parkin DM, Bray F, Ferlay J, et al. Global cancer statistics, 2002. CA Cancer J Clin 2005;55(2): 74–108.

79. Wakelee HA, Chang ET, Gomez SL, et al. Lung cancer incidence in never smokers. J Clin Oncol 2007;25(5):472–8.

80. Sun S, Schiller JH, Gazdar AF. Lung cancer in never smokers–a different disease. Nat Rev Cancer 2007;7(10):778–90.

81. Pelosof L, Ahn C, Gao A, et al. Proportion of never-smoker non-small cell lung cancer patients at three diverse institutions. J Natl Cancer Inst 2017;109(7).

82. Bonjour S, Adair-Rohani H, Wolf J, et al. Solid fuel use for household cooking: country and regional estimates for 1980-2010. Environ Health Perspect 2013;121(7):784–90.

83. Luo RX, Wu B, Yi YN, et al. Indoor burning coal air pollution and lung cancer–a case-control study in Fuzhou, China. Lung Cancer 1996;14(Suppl 1): S113–9.

84. Kleinerman RA, Wang Z, Wang L, et al. Lung cancer and indoor exposure to coal and biomass in rural China. J Occup Environ Med 2002;44(4): 338–44.

85. Hosgood HD, Boffetta P, Greenland S, et al. In-home coal and wood use and lung cancer risk: a pooled analysis of the International Lung Cancer Consortium. Environ Health Perspect 2010; 118(12):1743–7.

86. Li J, Li WX, Bai C, et al. Particulate matter-induced epigenetic changes and lung cancer. Clin Respir J 2017;11(5):539–46.

87. Pershagen G. Air pollution and cancer. IARC Sci Publ 1990;(104):240–51.

88. Dockery DW, Pope CA, Xu X, et al. An association between air pollution and mortality in six U.S. cities. N Engl J Med 1993;329(24):1753–9.

89. Pope CA, Burnett RT, Thun MJ, et al. Lung cancer, cardiopulmonary mortality, and long-term exposure to fine particulate air pollution. JAMA 2002;287(9): 1132–41.

90. Cohen AJ, Brauer M, Burnett R, et al. Estimates and 25-year trends of the global burden of disease attributable to ambient air pollution: an analysis of data from the Global Burden of Diseases Study 2015. Lancet 2017;389(10082):1907–18.

91. Lipsett M, Campleman S. Occupational exposure to diesel exhaust and lung cancer: a meta-analysis. Am J Public Health 1999;89(7):1009–17.

92. Raaschou-Nielsen O, Pedersen M, Stafoggia M, et al. Outdoor air pollution and risk for kidney parenchyma cancer in 14 European cohorts. Int J Cancer 2017;140(7):1528–37.

93. Raaschou-Nielsen O, Beelen R, Wang M, et al. Particulate matter air pollution components and risk for lung cancer. Environ Int 2016;87:66–73.

94. Samet JM. Residential radon and lung cancer: end of the story? J Toxicol Environ Health A 2006;69(7): 527–31.

95. Lubin JH, Boice JD, Edling C, et al. Lung cancer in radon-exposed miners and estimation of risk from indoor exposure. J Natl Cancer Inst 1995;87(11): 817–27.

96. Saccomanno G, Huth GC, Auerbach O, et al. Relationship of radioactive radon daughters and cigarette smoking in the genesis of lung cancer in uranium miners. Cancer 1988;62(7):1402–8.

97. Fabrikant JI. Radon and lung cancer: the BEIR IV Report. Health Phys 1990;59(1):89–97.

98. Lubin JH, Boice JD. Lung cancer risk from residential radon: meta-analysis of eight epidemiologic studies. J Natl Cancer Inst 1997;89(1): 49–57.

99. Ajrouche R, Ielsch G, Cléro E, et al. Quantitative health risk assessment of indoor radon: a systematic review. Radiat Prot Dosimetry 2017;177(1–2): 69–77.

100. Fingerhut M, Nelson DI, Driscoll T, et al. The contribution of occupational risks to the global burden of disease: summary and next steps. Med Lav 2006; 97(2):313–21.

101. Steenland K, Burnett C, Lalich N, et al. Dying for work: the magnitude of US mortality from selected causes of death associated with occupation. Am J Ind Med 2003;43(5):461–82.

102. Jones RN, Hughes JM, Weill H. Asbestos exposure, asbestosis, and asbestos-attributable lung cancer. Thorax 1996;51(Suppl 2):S9–15.

103. Egilman D, Reinert A. Lung cancer and asbestos exposure: asbestosis is not necessary. Am J Ind Med 1996;30(4):398–406.

104. Weiss W. Asbestosis: a marker for the increased risk of lung cancer among workers exposed to asbestos. Chest 1999;115(2):536–49.

105. Syrjänen KJ. Bronchial squamous cell carcinomas associated with epithelial changes identical to condylomatous lesions of the uterine cervix. Lung 1980;158(3):131–42.

106. Nielsen LS, Bælum J, Rasmussen J, et al. Occupational asbestos exposure and lung cancer–a systematic review of the literature. Arch Environ Occup Health 2014;69(4):191–206.

107. United States Department of Labor. Occupational safety and health administration. 2019. Available at: https://www.osha.gov/. Accessed January 6, 2019.

108. World Health Organization. Radon and health. 2016. Available at: https://www.who.int/en/news-room/factsheets/detail/radon-and-health. Accessed January 6, 2019.

109. World Health Organization. Air pollution. 2018. Available at: https://www.who.int/airpollution/household/en/. Accessed January 6, 2019.

110. Spitz MR, Etzel CJ, Dong Q, et al. An expanded risk prediction model for lung cancer. Cancer Prev Res (Phila) 2008;1(4):250–4.

111. Cassidy A, Myles JP, van Tongeren M, et al. The LLP risk model: an individual risk prediction model for lung cancer. Br J Cancer 2008;98(2):270–6.

112. Matakidou A, Eisen T, Houlston RS. Systematic review of the relationship between family history and lung cancer risk. Br J Cancer 2005;93(7):825–33.

113. Wang Y, McKay JD, Rafnar T, et al. Rare variants of large effect in BRCA2 and CHEK2 affect risk of lung cancer. Nat Genet 2014;46(7):736–41.

114. Wang J, Liu Q, Yuan S, et al. Genetic predisposition to lung cancer: comprehensive literature integration, meta-analysis, and multiple evidence assessment of candidate-gene association studies. Sci Rep 2017;7(1):8371.

115. McKay JD, Hung RJ, Han Y, et al. Large-scale association analysis identifies new lung cancer susceptibility loci and heterogeneity in genetic susceptibility across histological subtypes. Nat Genet 2017;49(7):1126–32.

116. Velmurugan KR, Varghese RT, Fonville NC, et al. High-depth, high-accuracy microsatellite genotyping enables precision lung cancer risk classification. Oncogene 2017;36(46):6383–90.

117. Spitz MR, Wei Q, Dong Q, et al. Genetic susceptibility to lung cancer: the role of DNA damage and repair. Cancer Epidemiol Biomarkers Prev 2003;12(8):689–98.

118. Turner MC, Chen Y, Krewski D, et al. Chronic obstructive pulmonary disease is associated with lung cancer mortality in a prospective study of never smokers. Am J Respir Crit Care Med 2007;176(3):285–90.

119. Siemes C, Visser LE, Coebergh JW, et al. C-reactive protein levels, variation in the C-reactive protein gene, and cancer risk: the Rotterdam Study. J Clin Oncol 2006;24(33):5216–22.

120. Parimon T, Chien JW, Bryson CL, et al. Inhaled corticosteroids and risk of lung cancer among patients with chronic obstructive pulmonary disease. Am J Respir Crit Care Med 2007;175(7):712–9.

121. Raymakers AJN, Sadatsafavi M, Sin DD, et al. Inhaled corticosteroids and the risk of lung cancer in COPD: a population-based cohort study. Eur Respir J 2019;53(6) [pii:1801257].

122. Wu MF, Jian ZH, Huang JY, et al. Post-inhaled corticosteroid pulmonary tuberculosis and pneumonia increases lung cancer in patients with COPD. BMC Cancer 2016;16(1):778.

123. Yang P, Sun Z, Krowka MJ, et al. Alpha1-antitrypsin deficiency carriers, tobacco smoke, chronic obstructive pulmonary disease, and lung cancer risk. Arch Intern Med 2008;168(10):1097–103.

124. Hubbard R, Venn A, Lewis S, et al. Lung cancer and cryptogenic fibrosing alveolitis. A population-based cohort study. Am J Respir Crit Care Med 2000;161(1):5–8.

125. Antoniou KM, Tomassetti S, Tsitoura E, et al. Idiopathic pulmonary fibrosis and lung cancer: a clinical and pathogenesis update. Curr Opin Pulm Med 2015;21(6):626–33.

126. de Freitas AC, Gurgel AP, de Lima EG, et al. Human papillomavirus and lung carcinogenesis: an overview. J Cancer Res Clin Oncol 2016;142(12):2415–27.

127. Willey JC, Broussoud A, Sleemi A, et al. Immortalization of normal human bronchial epithelial cells by human papillomaviruses 16 or 18. Cancer Res 1991;51(19):5370–7.

128. Cao S, Wendl MC, Wyczalkowski MA, et al. Divergent viral presentation among human tumors and adjacent normal tissues. Sci Rep 2016;6:28294.

129. Castro CY, Ostrowski ML, Barrios R, et al. Relationship between Epstein-Barr virus and lymphoepithelioma-like carcinoma of the lung: a clinicopathologic study of 6 cases and review of the literature. Hum Pathol 2001;32(8):863–72.

130. Bando M, Takahashi M, Ohno S, et al. Torque teno virus DNA titre elevated in idiopathic pulmonary fibrosis with primary lung cancer. Respirology 2008;13(2):263–9.

131. Giuliani L, Jaxmar T, Casadio C, et al. Detection of oncogenic viruses SV40, BKV, JCV, HCMV, HPV and p53 codon 72 polymorphism in lung carcinoma. Lung Cancer 2007;57(3):273–81.

132. Sion-Vardy N, Lasarov I, Delgado B, et al. Measles virus: evidence for association with lung cancer. Exp Lung Res 2009;35(8):701–12.

133. Littman AJ, Jackson LA, Vaughan TL. Chlamydia pneumoniae and lung cancer: epidemiologic evidence. Cancer Epidemiol Biomarkers Prev 2005; 14(4):773–8.

134. Khan S, Imran A, Khan AA, et al. Systems Biology approaches for the prediction of possible role of Chlamydia pneumoniae proteins in the etiology of lung cancer. PLoS One 2016;11(2):e0148530.

135. Yu YH, Liao CC, Hsu WH, et al. Increased lung cancer risk among patients with pulmonary tuberculosis: a population cohort study. J Thorac Oncol 2011;6(1):32–7.

136. Hong S, Mok Y, Jeon C, et al. Tuberculosis, smoking and risk for lung cancer incidence and mortality. Int J Cancer 2016;139(11):2447–55.

137. Engels EA, Shen M, Chapman RS, et al. Tuberculosis and subsequent risk of lung cancer in Xuanwei, China. Int J Cancer 2009;124(5):1183–7.

138. Morris A, Crothers K, Beck JM, et al. An official ATS workshop report: emerging issues and current controversies in HIV-associated pulmonary diseases. Proc Am Thorac Soc 2011;8(1):17–26.

139. Reddy KP, Kong CY, Hyle EP, et al. Lung cancer mortality associated with smoking and smoking cessation among people living with HIV in the United States. JAMA Intern Med 2017;177(11):1613–21.

140. Sigel K, Wisnivesky J, Gordon K, et al. HIV as an independent risk factor for incident lung cancer. AIDS 2012;26(8):1017–25.

141. Kirk GD, Merlo C, O' Driscoll P, et al. HIV infection is associated with an increased risk for lung cancer, independent of smoking. Clin Infect Dis 2007; 45(1):103–10.

142. Sigel K, Wisnivesky J, Crothers K, et al. Immunological and infectious risk factors for lung cancer in US veterans with HIV: a longitudinal cohort study. Lancet HIV 2017;4(2):e67–73.

143. Mitsuyasu RT. Non–AIDS-defining malignancies in HIV. Top HIV Med 2008;16(4):117–21.

144. Mao Q, Jiang F, Yin R, et al. Interplay between the lung microbiome and lung cancer. Cancer Lett 2018;415:40–8.

145. Tsay JJ, Wu BG, Badri MH, et al. Airway microbiota is associated with upregulation of the PI3K pathway in lung cancer. Am J Respir Crit Care Med 2018;198(9):1188–98.

146. Gnagnarella P, Caini S, Maisonneuve P, et al. Carcinogenicity of high consumption of meat and lung cancer risk among non-smokers: a comprehensive meta-analysis. Nutr Cancer 2018;70(1):1–13.

147. Jacobs EJ, Newton CC, Thun MJ, et al. Long-term use of cholesterol-lowering drugs and cancer incidence in a large United States cohort. Cancer Res 2011;71(5):1763–71.

148. Hecht SS. Approaches to cancer prevention based on an understanding of N-nitrosamine carcinogenesis. Proc Soc Exp Biol Med 1997;216(2):181–91.

149. Boone CW, Kelloff GJ, Malone WE. Identification of candidate cancer chemopreventive agents and their evaluation in animal models and human clinical trials: a review. Cancer Res 1990;50(1):2–9.

150. Goodman GE, Thornquist MD, Balmes J, et al. The Beta-Carotene and Retinol Efficacy Trial: incidence of lung cancer and cardiovascular disease mortality during 6-year follow-up after stopping beta-carotene and retinol supplements. J Natl Cancer Inst 2004;96(23):1743–50.

151. Wright ME, Park Y, Subar AF, et al. Intakes of fruit, vegetables, and specific botanical groups in relation to lung cancer risk in the NIH-AARP Diet and Health Study. Am J Epidemiol 2008;168(9): 1024–34.

152. Buring JE, Hennekens CH. beta-carotene and cancer chemoprevention. J Cell Biochem Suppl 1995; 22:226–30.

153. Yong LC, Brown CC, Schatzkin A, et al. Intake of vitamins E, C, and A and risk of lung cancer. The NHANES I epidemiologic followup study. First National Health and Nutrition Examination Survey. Am J Epidemiol 1997;146(3):231–43.

154. Omenn GS, Goodman GE, Thornquist MD, et al. Effects of a combination of beta carotene and vitamin A on lung cancer and cardiovascular disease. N Engl J Med 1996;334(18):1150–5.

155. Mahabir S, Spitz MR, Barrera SL, et al. Dietary zinc, copper and selenium, and risk of lung cancer. Int J Cancer 2007;120(5):1108–15.

156. Mahabir S, Forman MR, Dong YQ, et al. Mineral intake and lung cancer risk in the NIH-American association of retired persons diet and health study. Cancer Epidemiol Biomarkers Prev 2010; 19(8):1976–83.

157. Vieira AR, Abar L, Vingeliene S, et al. Fruits, vegetables and lung cancer risk: a systematic review and meta-analysis. Ann Oncol 2016;27(1):81–96.

158. Wang M, Qin S, Zhang T, et al. The effect of fruit and vegetable intake on the development of lung cancer: a meta-analysis of 32 publications and 20,414 cases. Eur J Clin Nutr 2015;69(11): 1184–92.

159. Brennan P, Hsu CC, Moullan N, et al. Effect of cruciferous vegetables on lung cancer in patients stratified by genetic status: a mendelian randomisation approach. Lancet 2005;366(9496): 1558–60.

160. Fontham ET. Protective dietary factors and lung cancer. Int J Epidemiol 1990;19(Suppl 1):S32–42.

161. Cooper DA, Eldridge AL, Peters JC. Dietary carotenoids and lung cancer: a review of recent research. Nutr Rev 1999;57(5 Pt 1):133–45.

162. Mursu J, Nurmi T, Tuomainen TP, et al. Intake of flavonoids and risk of cancer in Finnish men: the Kuopio Ischaemic heart disease risk factor study. Int J Cancer 2008;123(3):660–3.

163. Brenner DR, Fehringer G, Zhang ZF, et al. Alcohol consumption and lung cancer risk: a pooled analysis from the International Lung Cancer Consortium and the SYNERGY study. Cancer Epidemiol 2019; 58:25–32.

164. Fehringer G, Brenner DR, Zhang ZF, et al. Alcohol and lung cancer risk among never smokers: a pooled analysis from the international lung cancer consortium and the SYNERGY study. Int J Cancer 2017;140(9):1976–84.

165. Xie Y, Qin J, Nan G, et al. Coffee consumption and the risk of lung cancer: an updated meta-analysis of epidemiological studies. Eur J Clin Nutr 2016; 70(2):199–206.

166. Renehan AG, Tyson M, Egger M, et al. Body-mass index and incidence of cancer: a systematic review and meta-analysis of prospective observational studies. Lancet 2008;371(9612):569–78.

167. Renehan AG, Soerjomataram I, Leitzmann MF. Interpreting the epidemiological evidence linking obesity and cancer: a framework for population-attributable risk estimations in Europe. Eur J Cancer 2010;46(14):2581–92.

168. Zhu H, Zhang S. Body mass index and lung cancer risk in never smokers: a meta-analysis. BMC Cancer 2018;18(1):635.

169. Patel AV, Carter BD, Stevens VL, et al. The relationship between physical activity, obesity, and lung cancer risk by smoking status in a large prospective cohort of US adults. Cancer Causes Control 2017;28(12):1357–68.

170. Kabat GC, Kim M, Hunt JR, et al. Body mass index and waist circumference in relation to lung cancer risk in the Women's Health Initiative. Am J Epidemiol 2008;168(2):158–69.

171. Friedenreich CM, Orenstein MR. Physical activity and cancer prevention: etiologic evidence and biological mechanisms. J Nutr 2002;132(11 Suppl): 3456S–64S.

172. Pletnikoff PP, Tuomainen TP, Laukkanen JA, et al. Cardiorespiratory fitness and lung cancer risk: a prospective population-based cohort study. J Sci Med Sport 2016;19(2):98–102.

173. Laukkanen JA, Pukkala E, Rauramaa R, et al. Cardiorespiratory fitness, lifestyle factors and cancer risk and mortality in Finnish men. Eur J Cancer 2010;46(2):355–63.

174. Katki HA, Kovalchik SA, Petito LC, et al. Implications of nine risk prediction models for selecting ever-smokers for computed tomography lung cancer screening. Ann Intern Med 2018;169(1):10–9.

175. Tammemagi MC, Katki HA, Hocking WG, et al. Selection criteria for lung-cancer screening. N Engl J Med 2013;368(8):728–36.

176. Katki HA, Kovalchik SA, Berg CD, et al. Development and validation of risk models to select ever-smokers for CT lung cancer screening. JAMA 2016;315(21):2300–11.

177. Tammemagi MC. Selecting lung cancer screenees using risk prediction models-where do we go from here. Transl Lung Cancer Res 2018;7(3):243–53.

178. Szabo E, Mao JT, Lam S, et al. Chemoprevention of lung cancer: diagnosis and management of lung cancer, 3rd ed: American College of Chest Physicians evidence-based clinical practice guidelines. Chest 2013;143(5 Suppl):e40S–60S.

179. Khurana V, Bejjanki HR, Caldito G, et al. Statins reduce the risk of lung cancer in humans: a large case-control study of US veterans. Chest 2007; 131(5):1282–8.

180. Sorli K, Thorvaldsen SM, Hatlen P. Use of inhaled corticosteroids and the risk of lung cancer, the HUNT study. Lung 2018;196(2):179–84.

The Biology of Lung Cancer
Development of More Effective Methods for Prevention, Diagnosis, and Treatment

Ramin Salehi-Rad, MD, PhD[a,b], Rui Li, MD, PhD[a], Manash K. Paul, PhD[a], Steven M. Dubinett, MD[a,b,c,d,e],*, Bin Liu, PhD[a],*

KEYWORDS

- Biology of lung cancer • NSCLC and SCLC • Genomic alterations • Tumor microenvironment
- Lung cancer prevention • Lung cancer early detection • Targeted therapy • Immunotherapy

KEY POINTS

- Lung tumorigenesis is a multistage process defined by the progressive accumulation of mutations in oncogenes and tumor suppressor genes, resulting in perturbation of multiple cellular pathways.
- Chronic airway inflammation contributes to pathologic alteration of the lung microenvironment and promotes carcinogenesis.
- Host immunosurveillance imposes selective pressure on tumor cells during the evolutionary course of lung cancer.
- Advances in genomic profiling of lung cancer have facilitated the development of targeted therapies.
- Enhanced understanding of critical immunologic pathways within the tumor microenvironment have led to the discovery of immunotherapies that have revolutionized the treatment of lung cancer.

INTRODUCTION: THE BIOLOGY OF LUNG CANCER

Lung cancer is the leading cause of cancer-related death worldwide. Approximately 15% of lung cancers have the histologic subtype of small cell lung cancer (SCLC) and the remaining 85% are classified as non–small cell lung cancer (NSCLC). The most common subtypes of NSCLC are lung adenocarcinoma (LUAD) and lung squamous cell carcinoma (LUSC). Lung cancer, most often associated with tobacco smoking, is a heterogeneous disease with an abundance of genetic and epigenetic alterations. These genetic changes result in activation of oncogenic pathways and/or inhibition of tumor suppressor genes that are critical for malignant transformation of tumor precursor cells. However, the pathophysiology of lung cancer cannot be fully understood by enumeration of dysregulated pathways in the tumor cells but instead must encompass the contributions of the tumor microenvironment (TME) and host immune responses, which are intimately intertwined during every step of tumorigenesis. Enhanced understanding of the genomic landscape of lung cancer and the biology of the TME and host immune cells

[a] Department of Medicine, David Geffen School of Medicine at UCLA, 10833 Le Conte Avenue, 43-22 CHS, Los Angeles, CA 90095-1690, USA; [b] Department of Medicine, VA Greater Los Angeles Healthcare System, 11301 Wilshire Boulevard, Los Angeles, CA 90073, USA; [c] Department of Pathology and Laboratory Medicine, David Geffen School of Medicine at UCLA, 757 Westwood Plaza, Los Angeles, CA 90095, USA; [d] Jonsson Comprehensive Cancer Center, University of California Los Angeles, 8-684 Factor Building, Box 951781, Los Angeles, CA 90095-1781, USA; [e] Department of Molecular and Medical Pharmacology, David Geffen School of Medicine at UCLA, 650 Charles E Young Dr S, 23-120 CHS, Los Angeles, CA 90095, USA

* Corresponding authors. 10833 Le Conte Avenue, 43-229 CHS, Los Angeles, CA 90095-1690, USA.

E-mail addresses: SDubinett@mednet.ucla.edu (S.M.D.); bliu@mednet.ucla.edu (B.L.)

Clin Chest Med 41 (2020) 25–38
https://doi.org/10.1016/j.ccm.2019.10.003

has led to the development of novel targeted therapeutics and immunotherapies that have revolutionized the treatment of lung cancer.

Genomic Landscape of Lung Cancer

The multistage process of lung tumorigenesis, from dysplasia and preneoplasia through carcinoma in situ to metastatic cancer, is defined by the progressive accumulation of mutations in oncogenes with dominant gain of function and tumor suppressor genes with recessive loss of function.[1] Genomic alterations can originate from somatic mutations, homozygous gene deletions, gene amplifications and translocations, or epigenetic silencing. These genomic alterations, in turn, result in dysregulated cellular pathways that enable premalignant cells to become tumorigenic. Detailed genomic profiling of lung cancer has revealed significant heterogeneity among patients.[2–4] Many oncogenes and tumor suppressor genes have been identified, paving the way for the development of novel targeted therapeutics (**Fig. 1**).

The genomic landscape of lung cancer in an individual is not static but is spatially and temporally heterogeneous. During carcinogenesis, genomic instability within the bulk tumor results in divergent evolution of tumor cell clones with distinct genomic profiles and molecular signatures.[5] This intratumoral heterogeneity has important clinical implications in cancer genome evolution and acquired resistance to therapy. A recent study using whole-exome sequencing (WES) of multiple regions of individual tumors from patients with NSCLC revealed significant intratumoral heterogeneity in somatic mutations and copy-number alterations, which was associated with an increased risk of recurrence and death.[6]

Genetic and molecular alterations of non–small cell lung cancer

Large-scale sequencing studies have revealed distinct genomic differences between LUAD and LUSC.[7–9] The most commonly mutated oncogenes in LUAD are kristen rat sarcoma (KRAS) and epidermal growth factor receptor (EGFR), which are implicated in the initiation of tumorigenesis. Although KRAS and EGFR mutations are usually mutually exclusive, when they coexist, the KRAS mutation drives resistance to EGFR inhibitors.[10] Other targetable oncogenes in LUAD

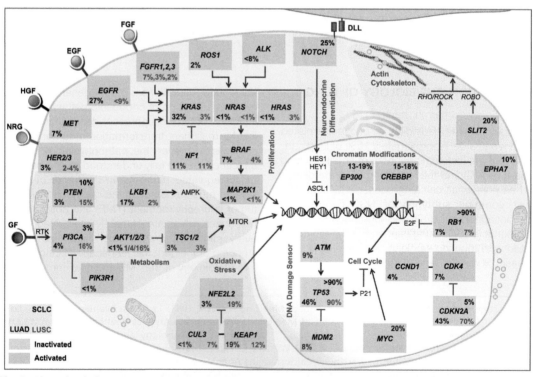

Fig. 1. Alteration in key genes and oncogenic pathways in SCLC, LUAD, and LUSC. The numbers in each box indicate the frequencies of genomic alterations based on the sum of somatic mutations, homozygous deletions, focal amplifications, and significant alterations in gene expression. Other integral proteins mediating the pathways are also presented. DLL, deltalike; EGF, epidermal growth factor; FGF, fibroblast growth factor; GF, growth factor; HGF, hepatocyte growth factor; NRG, neuregulin; RTK, receptor tyrosine kinase. (*Data from* Refs.[3,4,8,9,17])

include human epidermal growth factor receptor 2 (*HER2*), MET proto-oncogene (*MET*), and ret proto-oncogene (*RET*). Fusion oncogenes involving anaplastic lymphoma kinase (*ALK*), and reactive oxygen species proto-oncogene 1 (*ROS1*) are also observed in LUAD.[2] In contrast, actionable driver mutations are not prevalent in LUSC.

The most commonly mutated tumor suppressor genes in LUAD include tumor protein p53 (*TP53*), kelch-like ECH-associated protein 1 (*KEAP1*), liver kinase B1 (*LKB1*), and neurofibromin 1 (*NF1*). *TP53* mutation is also present in more than 90% of LUSC. TP53, which is an integral sensor of genomic damage and suppressor of proliferation, is implicated in tumor progression. Cyclin-dependent kinase inhibitor 2a (CDKN2A), a tumor suppressor that regulates the cell cycle, is also inactivated in 70% of LUSC.

Although smoking is implicated in the pathogenesis of NSCLC, approximately 10% of cases occur in never-smokers. Studies reveal that the genomic landscape in NSCLC is distinct between smokers and nonsmokers. NSCLCs from smokers have among the highest tumor mutational burdens (TMBs) of all malignancies, and frequently contain the tobacco exposure signature of cytosine to adenine (C>A) transversions.[8,9,11,12] In contrast, NSCLCs in never-smokers generally have a 10-fold lower number of point mutations compared with smokers, and predominantly contain transition of cytosine to thymine (C>T).[13] Furthermore, the prevalence of oncogene-addicted NSCLC with *EGFR* mutations and/or *ALK* and *ROS1* translocations is higher in never-smokers, whereas *KRAS* and *TP53* mutations are more commonly found in smokers.

Genetic and molecular alterations of small cell lung cancer

SCLC is a high-grade neuroendocrine (NE) tumor. Approximately 75% of SCLCs express the transcription factor achaete-scute complex–like 1 (ASCL1) and 15% express neurogenic differentiation factor 1 (NEUROD1), which are master regulators of neuronal and NE differentiation.[3] However, approximately 15% of SCLC tumors lack these transcription factors and do not express the NE program. Although SCLC has been regarded as a homogeneous disease, recent studies reveal considerable intertumoral heterogeneity in the genomic landscape of SCLC.[3,14]

The dominant genetic alteration in more than 90% of SCLCs is the loss of function of *TP53* and retinoblastoma protein (*RB1*), which are essential for tumor initiation.[15] These two canonical tumor suppressors are critical sensors that

integrate intracellular and extracellular signals to regulate cell proliferation and apoptosis.[1] The *MYC* family of oncogenes are also frequently overexpressed or amplified in SCLC, and are associated with genomic instability and shortened survival.[16,17] Notch signaling, which can have oncogenic and tumor-suppressive effects, is also altered in SCLC. As a tumor suppressor in SCLC, Notch pathway negatively regulates NE differentiation. This pathway is inactivated in most SCLCs by either inactivating mutations or overexpression of nonfunctional Notch ligand delta–like protein 3 (DLL3).[15]

Similar to NSCLC in smokers, SCLCs possess high TMB with the tobacco exposure signature of C>A transversions.[11,12,18] In contrast with NSCLC, mutations in kinase genes in SCLCs are modest, and mutations in *EGFR* or *KRAS* are extremely rare.[15] There is currently no US Food and Drug Administration (FDA)–approved targeted therapy for SCLC.

The Tumor Microenvironment

The TME contains extracellular matrix, vascular and lymphatic networks, cancer-associated fibroblasts, and infiltrating host immune cells, which are intimately intertwined with tumorigenesis.[19] Studies reveal that intrinsic genomic alterations within premalignant or neoplastic cells can reprogram the composition of the TME to facilitate carcinogenesis. In contrast, chronic inflammation caused by extrinsic factors, such as unresolved infections or exposure to carcinogens, can orchestrate the lung TME to promote cancer progression.[20]

Host immune cells are a critical component of the TME, and studies reveal that immune cells are present within the TME of nearly all premalignant and neoplastic lung lesions.[21–24] The composition and function of these infiltrating immune cells have been a subject of intense investigation in the past decade.[19] It is now understood that host immune cells play a dichotomous role throughout the evolution of lung cancer, and can either facilitate the eradication of malignancy or promote an immunosuppressive TME favoring tumor progression.

The immune tumor microenvironment: tumor-promoting chronic inflammation

Evidence suggests that chronic airway inflammation contributes to pathologic alterations of the lung microenvironment to facilitate cancer initiation and progression.[20] Epidemiologic studies reveal that patients with chronic microbial colonization have an increased risk of lung cancer.[25] Patients with chronic obstructive pulmonary disease, which is a chronic inflammatory disorder, also possess increased risk of lung cancer even after correction for the risk associated with cigarette exposure.[26]

Chronic inflammation may contribute to tumorigenesis via several mechanisms. Inflammation-induced leukocyte infiltration into the lung can induce DNA damage through the generation of reactive oxygen species (ROS). Dysregulated chronic inflammation can also foster aberrant expression of growth factors and cytokines, such as transforming growth factor beta (TGF-β), interleukin (IL)-1β, IL-4, IL-6, IL-8, IL-10, and IL-22, which activate multiple tumorigenic pathways, such as nuclear factor kappa B subunit (NF-κB) and cyclooxygenase 2 (COX-2) to promote tumorigenesis.[20]

The transcription factor NF-κB operates as a lynchpin by exerting oncogenic effects within the tumor cells through suppression of apoptosis and stimulation of proliferation, and concomitantly activating protumorigenic inflammatory genes in the TME.[27] In addition, NF-κB regulates the expression of various inducible protumorigenic enzymes, such as matrix metalloproteinases (MMPs), inducible nitric oxide synthase (iNOS), and COX-2, which generate mutagenic molecules and growth factors that promote lung cancer progression.[28]

COX-2 has been implicated in the pathogenesis of inflammation-associated lung cancer, and its increased expression is associated with poor outcomes.[29] COX-2 is the rate-limiting enzyme in the conversion of arachidonic acid into prostaglandin H2 (PGH2), which is a substrate for prostaglandin and thromboxane synthases. Induction of COX-2 activity by inflammatory mediators, such as TGF-β and IL-1β, or by cigarette smoke results in increased production of prostaglandin E2 (PGE2). PGE2 is a potent growth-promoting and inflammatory metabolite that activates multiple downstream signaling pathways associated with proliferation, epithelial-to-mesenchymal transition, and apoptosis resistance.[20]

The immune tumor microenvironment: antitumor immunity

Immune surveillance Immunosurveillance by host immune effectors imposes continuous selective pressure on tumor cells throughout the evolution of lung cancer. Although both innate and adaptive immune responses are involved in antitumor immunity, host T cell recognition of tumor antigens represents the central tenet of immunosurveillance and immunoediting.[30]

Specificity is the hallmark of adaptive T-cell immunity against tumor. Genomic mutations in lung cancer can give rise to mutant proteins that, when processed, result in the generation of neoantigens. Appropriate presentation of tumor antigens by professional antigen-presenting cells (APCs), namely dendritic cells (DCs), within the major histocompatibility complex (MHC) molecules (signal 1), along with positive costimulatory signal cluster of differentiation 80 (CD80) or CD86 (signal 2) and proinflammatory cytokines (signal 3) primes naive host T cells against specific tumor antigens. Following priming and activation, effector T cells no longer require costimulatory signals and can eliminate tumor cells after recognition of MHC-bound cancer antigens. Indeed, a recent study in patients with early-stage NSCLC identified CD8[+] tumor-infiltrating lymphocytes (TILs) that are reactive to tumor clonal neoantigens.[31] Furthermore, the presence of mature DCs, tertiary lymphoid structures, and cytolytic CD8[+] T cells within the TME has been implicated as a positive prognostic indicator in patients with lung cancer.[32-34]

Immune escape Most lung cancers escape host immune surveillance through a variety of mechanisms. Tumors can directly suppress host immune responses by activating negative regulatory pathways known as immune checkpoints. Two checkpoints, cytotoxic T-lymphocyte protein 4 (CTLA-4) and programmed cell death-1 (PD-1) have generated much attention recently.[35] The coinhibitory receptor CTLA-4 is upregulated on T cells following activation and initiates negative regulation by competing with the CD28 receptor for binding of costimulatory CD80 and CD86 molecules expressed by APCs (**Fig. 2**A). In contrast, PD-1 is primarily expressed by exhausted T effector cells during long-term antigen exposure, such as chronic viral infection or malignancy.[36] Adaptive expression of programmed cell death ligand-1 (PD-L1) within the TME by tumor cells or the myeloid compartment, in response to inflammatory signals such as interferon (IFN)-γ, can significantly attenuate the antitumor activity of PD-1–expressing TILs that recognize tumor-specific antigens (**Fig. 2**B).[37] Immune checkpoint blockade with antibodies targeting PD-1 or PD-L1 results in preferential activation of exhausted tumor-specific T cells and is generally associated with lower toxicity profile compared with CTLA-4 inhibitors.

Lung tumors also restrict host immunosurveillance through suppression of functional antigen presentation. Loss of heterozygosity in human

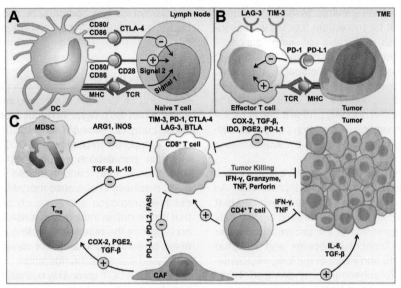

Fig. 2. Interactions between the tumor and host immune cells. (*A*) Negative regulation of T cell priming by CTLA-4 in the lymph node. Naive T cells recognize tumor antigens presented by MHC the surface of DCs through their TCR (signal 1). This signal is not sufficient to activate naive T cells. A costimulatory signal (signal 2) is required for activation, which is provided by DCs through binding of CD80 and CD86 to CD28 receptor on T cells. CTLA-4 is upregulated on T cells shortly after activation and provides inhibitory signal on binding to CD80 and CD86. (*B*) Negative regulation of effector T cell function by PD-1 in the TME. PD-1 is expressed on effector T cells during prolonged antigen exposure. Binding of PD-1 to programmed cell death ligand-1 (PD-L1) expressed on tumor cells and myeloid cells within the TME provides a negative signal for effector T cell function, and results in T cell exhaustion. Other immune checkpoints that limit activated T cell responses within the TME include T cell immunoglobulin mucin receptor 3 (TIM-3) and Lymphocyte activation gene 3 (LAG-3). (*C*) Interactions between tumor cells and different cell types in the TME. MDSC, myeloid-derived suppressor cell; T$_{reg}$, regulatory T cell; TCR, T cell receptor.

leukocyte antigen (HLA) was found to occur in 40% of patients with NSCLC, which was associated with a high burden of subclonal neoantigens.[38] Genomic variation within MHC class I has also been implicated in hindering host immune responses against certain epitopes.[39] Recently, a study revealed that tumors evade immune recognition by epigenetic repression of neoantigen transcription through promoter hypermethylation.[23]

Lung cancers can also alter the composition of the TME to establish an immunosuppressive milieu characterized by an abundance of inhibitory molecules, such as TGF-β, IL-6, PGE2, and vascular endothelial growth factor (VEGF), and an accumulation of immunosuppressive cells, such as regulatory T cell (T$_{reg}$) and myeloid-derived suppressor cells (MDSCs) (**Fig. 2**C). T$_{reg}$ and MDSCs limit tumor-specific T cell responses via multiple mechanisms. Tumor-infiltrating T$_{reg}$ in NSCLC correlates with COX-2 expression within the TME and portends a poor prognosis.[40] MDSC infiltration into the TME is also associated with negative clinical outcomes.[41]

DEVELOPMENT OF MORE EFFECTIVE METHODS FOR PREVENTION, DIAGNOSIS, AND TREATMENT

Targeting Inflammation for Lung Cancer Prevention

Although the prevalence of smoking has decreased, it remains the most important risk factor for the development of lung cancer. Lung cancer prevention strategies have largely focused on tobacco cessation and are reviewed elsewhere in this issue. Significant efforts are also directed at developing chemoprevention strategies, which encompass the use of agents to prevent, delay, or reverse carcinogenic progression in high-risk populations.

Given the strong association between chronic inflammation and carcinogenesis, studies have evaluated the role of antiinflammatory drugs in cancer prevention. Evidence suggests that long-term use of aspirin is associated with reduction in cancer death. However, the chemopreventive efficacy of aspirin to mitigate lung cancer risk is equivocal according to recent meta-analyses.[42,43] Recently, a nationwide retrospective study evaluating 13 million patients revealed that low-dose aspirin use for more than 5 years was associated with risk reduction of lung cancer.[44] Although the overall effect is modest, a subgroup analysis revealed enhanced efficacy in patients older than 65 years. Future studies are needed to identify patient populations that would derive the greatest benefit. An ongoing phase II trial is evaluating chemoprevention with aspirin compared with placebo in high-risk patients with subsolid lung nodules.

Selective inhibition of COX-2 with celecoxib has also been evaluated for lung cancer prevention. An early-phase study in active smokers revealed that treatment with celecoxib for 6 months significantly reduced the expression of the proliferation maker Ki-67 in serial bronchial biopsies and inhibited secretion of IL-10 and PGE2 in the lung microenvironment.[45] In 2 subsequent randomized trials, treatment of current and former smokers with celecoxib also resulted in significant reduction of Ki-67 in post-treatment biopsies compared with placebo.[46,47] Similarly, a chemoprevention trial in lung cancer evaluating the effect of inhaled iloprost, an analogue of prostaglandin I2 (PGI2), revealed significant improvement of endobronchial histology in former smokers, but not current smokers, which highlights the importance of smoking cessation in lung cancer prevention.[48]

Recently, IL-1β, a critical mediator of inflammation-driven carcinogenesis, has emerged as a potential target for lung cancer prevention. In the CANTOS trial, canakinumab, a monoclonal antibody targeting IL-1β, was associated with a significantly lower rate of recurrent cardiovascular events than placebo in patients with prior myocardial infarction.[49] Remarkably Canakinumab resulted in significant dose-dependent reduction of lung cancer incidence and mortality compared with placebo. Further analysis revealed that patients with the greatest reductions in biomarkers of inflammation, namely high-sensitivity C-reactive protein and IL-6, benefited the most from canakinumab, highlighting the antiinflammatory role of canakinumab in lung cancer prevention. Ongoing trials are evaluating canakinumab as monotherapy or in combination with checkpoint inhibitors as adjuvant or neoadjuvant therapy in early-stage NSCLC.

Strategies designed to enhance host immune responses against premalignant lesions are also being used for lung cancer immunoprevention. A phase I study is evaluating the potential of vaccination with Mucin 1, a common cancer-associated antigen, in cancer prevention in current and former smokers with high risk of lung cancer. An ongoing phase II study is evaluating the checkpoint inhibitor, pembrolizumab, a PD-1 antibody, in patients with high-risk pulmonary nodules.

Early Detection of Lung Cancer

Most lung cancers are diagnosed at an advanced stage, when the prognosis remains poor. In the National Lung Screening Trial (NSLT), annual low-dose computed tomography (LDCT) screening in high-risk populations resulted in 20% relative reduction in lung cancer–related mortality and 6.7% decrease in all-cause mortality.[50] Lung cancer risk prediction scores, such as $PLCO_{m2012}$, that better define individuals at risk of lung cancer and improve the receiver operating characteristics of this screening tool have been developed, and are discussed elsewhere in this issue.

Although LDCT screening has led to progress in early lung cancer detection, improvement in patient outcomes has been incremental. Recently, a transformative cancer interception strategy has been proposed that aims to shift the paradigm of diagnosis and treatment to the earliest phase of the disease in order to block the progression of premalignancy to invasive cancer.[51] These efforts have been facilitated by the PreCancer Atlas (PCA) initiative, introduced by the National Cancer Institute (NCI), which uses a comprehensive multiomic strategy to establish detailed molecular and cellular characteristics of premalignant lesions and their evolution to invasive cancer.[52] Technological advances such as autofluorescence bronchoscopy (AFB), which allows serial sampling of preinvasive lesions within the proximal airways, as well as laser capture microscopy and multiplex immunofluorescence (MIF), which permit in-depth genomic interrogation and immunophenotyping of paraffin-imbedded tissue, have expedited these efforts in early detection and characterization of pulmonary premalignancy. Recent advances in the development of pulmonary PCA are highlighted below.

Studies in lung cancer have highlighted a field cancerization phenomenon, in which histologically normal-appearing tissues adjacent to lung cancer share common genomic abnormalities with the tumor.[53] These molecular changes likely represent early alterations in normal tissue, which undergo positive selection and clonal expansion during progression to NSCLC. Consistently, a study utilizing targeted deep DNA and RNA sequencing of LUAD and tumor-adjacent atypical adenomatous hyperplasia (AAH) lesions, which are known precursors of LUAD, revealed presence of common driver mutations, such as *BRAF* and *KRAS*, in AAH lesions.[54]

A clearer picture of the immune contexture associated with pulmonary premalignancy has also emerged recently. A study evaluated paraffin-imbedded lung cancer specimens at various stages, including premalignant AAH, adenocarcinomas in situ, and invasive LUAD, by WES and MIF, and identified somatic mutations in both premalignancy and the associated tumor as progression-associated mutations.[21] Predicted neoantigens from these shared mutations were highly correlated with T cell infiltration and PD-L1 upregulation in premalignant lesions, suggesting an adaptive immune response to these neoantigens. These results provide evidence for mutational heterogeneity and immune recognition in pulmonary premalignancy.

Researchers are beginning to define the genomic evolution of premalignancy throughout the course of tumorigenesis. Although histologically identical, half of lung carcinoma in situ (CIS) lesions, which are precursors of LUSC, progress to invasive cancer, whereas the other half regress or remain static. Recently, an elegant study used multiple approaches to decipher the genomic, transcriptomic, and epigenomic landscape of CIS from serial samples obtained with the guidance of AFB in a longitudinally monitored patient cohort, and identified predictive models of progressive lesions with remarkable accuracy.[55] Moreover, characteristic mutations, copy-number changes, and epigenomic modifications associated with lung cancer were observed in premalignant lesions, offering a window into early carcinogenesis.

A similar study using RNA sequencing to determine the transcriptome profile of serial endobronchial biopsies from high-risk smokers identified 4 molecular subtypes associated with clinical phenotypes in bronchial premalignant lesions (PMLs), which are precursors of LUSC.[56] A proliferative gene signature was identified with specificity for clinical progression of PMLs. Notably, this proliferative gene signature was present even in uninvolved large airway brushings of subjects with progressive PMLs. Furthermore, the investigators observed decreased gene expression in IFN signaling, antigen processing and presentation, and T cell–mediated immunity among progressive and persistent proliferative lesions compared with regressive lesions, and these pathways correlated with decreases in immune cell types.

These studies have significantly enhanced our understanding of the early molecular, cellular, and immunologic properties that fuel the progression of PMLs to invasive cancer. Further studies are ongoing to improve early detection and risk stratification strategies, and develop personalized preventive therapies.

Lung Cancer Treatment

Identification of driver mutations in lung cancer, along with characterization of critical molecular, cellular, and immunologic pathways within the TME, has led to the discovery of multiple targeted therapeutics and immunotherapies that have revolutionized lung cancer treatment. The seminal trials that led to the approval of these drugs, and ongoing efforts to develop novel therapies, are discussed next.

Targeted therapy

Non–small cell lung cancer Screening for driver mutations is a critical part of diagnostic work-up of lung cancer. In a recent French study, oncogenic drivers were observed in 50% of patients with NSCLC, and targeted therapy was associated with improved overall survival (OS).[57] Similarly, the multicenter Lung Cancer Mutation Consortium in the United States identified targetable driver mutations in 64% of patients with LUAD.[58] The patients with an oncogenic driver who received genotype-directed therapy had improved survival compared with those without targeted therapy.

Multiple tyrosine kinase inhibitors (TKIs) are FDA approved for NSCLC treatment, and these have been reviewed extensively elsewhere.[4] EGFR and ALK alterations are the most prevalent targetable mutations in NSCLC and occur more frequently in nonsmokers and women. Osimertinib is a third-generation EGFR TKI with activity against the T780M mutation that is the most common cause of acquired resistance to the first-generation TKIs. In a randomized phase III trial comparing first-line osimertinib with either erlotinib or gefitinib in patients with EGFR-mutated advanced-stage NSCLC, osimertinib was associated with significantly improved progression-free survival (PFS), establishing osimertinib as the standard of care.[59] The second-generation ALK inhibitor, alectinib, is currently the first-line TKI for patients with ALK-positive NSCLC because of its enhanced efficacy compared with first-generation inhibitors in 2 randomized trials.[60,61]

ROS1 gene rearrangements are observed in approximately 2% of LUADs. Because of a high degree of homology between the tyrosine kinase domains of ROS1 and ALK, many TKIs approved for ALK-positive NSCLC have shown activity in ROS1-positive tumors. Crizotinib is currently the standard of care for the treatment of ROS1-positive NSCLC.[62] Mutations in v-raf murine sarcoma viral oncogene homolog B1 (BRAF) gene are observed in approximately 7% of LUADs and 4% of LUSCs. BRAF belongs to the mitogen-activated protein kinase (MAPK) pathway, which includes RAS-RAF-MEK-ERK. Although NSCLC patients with *BRAF*-V600E mutation respond to single-agent BRAF TKIs, combination therapy with BRAF and MEK inhibitors is preferred because of the enhanced efficacy.[63]

Significant efforts have been devoted to extending the scope of targeted therapies in NSCLC. Alterations in MET signaling are present in 7% of LUADs and are associated with acquired resistance to EGFR TKI.[64] Several ongoing trials are evaluating the efficacy of selective inhibitors as single agents in advanced NSCLC with *MET* mutation, and in combination with EGFR TKIs in EGFR TKI-resistant NSCLC with acquired *MET* amplification. Targeted therapy with anti–c-MET antibody-drug conjugate, telisotuzumab vedotin, has also shown promising results in early-phase clinical trials for patients with *MET*-amplified NSCLC.[65]

Other potentially targetable alterations in NSCLC include rearrangement of the proto-oncogene *RET*, which is present in 1% to 2% of patients.[9] Treatment of patients with *RET*-rearranged lung cancer with multikinase inhibitors has shown limited efficacy.[66] Ongoing early clinical trials are evaluating the efficacy of highly selective inhibitors of RET, BLU-667, and LOXO-299 in *RET*-altered NSCLC. Mutations in *HER2*, which is an EGFR family receptor tyrosine kinase (RTK), are detected in 3% of LUADs.[67] However, targeting HER2 in lung cancer has resulted in modest efficacy.[68,69]

Small cell lung cancer There is currently no FDA-approved targeted therapy for SCLC. In 2012, the US Congress recognized SCLC as a recalcitrant cancer based on its 5-year survival rate of less than 7%. In the past several years, renewed effort has led to the identification of multiple therapeutic targets.[3]

Genomic abnormalities in the *MYC* family of transcription factors are observed in 20% of SCLCs.[16] In a phase II clinical trial in patients with progressive or recurrent SCLC, alisertib, a selective inhibitor of aurora kinase A that is regulated by MYC, showed a 21% objective response rate (ORR), although the genomic status of *MYC* was unknown in these patients.[70]

Notch ligand DLL3 has been a target for the development of novel strategies in SCLC with promising initial results. However, a phase III study of rovalpituzumab tesirine (ROVA-T), a DLL3-targeting antibody-drug conjugate, as a second-line treatment of patients with advanced SCLC was recently placed on hold because of shortened OS. An ongoing phase III trial is evaluating ROVA-T as a maintenance therapy following frontline treatment in patients with extensive-stage SCLC (ES-SCLC).

Immunotherapy

Advances in immunotherapy have changed the treatment landscape of lung cancer. To date, 4 immune checkpoint inhibitors (ICIs) have FDA approval for NSCLC treatment: nivolumab and pembrolizumab targeting PD-1, as well as atezolizumab and durvalumab targeting PD-L1.[71] Four immunohistochemistry (IHC)-based diagnostic assays measuring PD-L1 expression within the TME have also been approved by the FDA to aid with patient selection. Recently, atezolizumab, nivolumab, and pembrolizumab obtained FDA approval, and durvalumab was granted orphan drug designation (ODD) for the treatment of ES-SCLC.

Non-small cell lung cancer

Immune checkpoint inhibitors for metastatic non–small cell lung cancer Three ICIs, namely nivolumab, pembrolizumab, and atezolizumab, are approved as single agents for the treatment of advanced NSCLC with disease progression on chemotherapy.[72] Pembrolizumab is the only ICI with FDA approval as single-agent first-line treatment of advanced NSCLC. This approval is based on the results of the KEYNOTE-024 trial, which revealed superior OS with pembrolizumab compared with platinum-based chemotherapy in patients with NSCLC with PD-L1 expression greater than or equal to 50% and without *EGFR/ALK* alterations.[73] Prolonged follow-up data showed persistent median OS (30.0 vs 14.2 months) benefit with pembrolizumab compared with chemotherapy.[74]

Several trials have evaluated combinations of ICIs with platinum chemotherapy as first-line regimens in NSCLC irrespective of PD-L1 expression. In the phase III KEYNOTE-189 study, first-line pembrolizumab plus pemetrexed and platinum in patients with nonsquamous metastatic NSCLC showed significant improvement in 12-month OS (69.2% vs 49.4%), with similar toxicity profile, compared with placebo plus chemotherapy irrespective of PD-L1 tumor expression.[75] Similarly, in the phase III KEYNOTE-407, first-line pembrolizumab in combination with carboplatin and taxane in patients with metastatic LUSC irrespective of PD-L1 tumor expression resulted in improved median OS (15.9 vs 11.3 months) compared with placebo plus chemotherapy.[76] As a result, pembrolizumab in combination with platinum chemotherapy is now an FDA-approved first-line treatment regimen for all patients with advanced NSCLC without *EGFR/ALK* alterations, irrespective of PD-L1 tumor expression.

In the phase III Impower 150 trial, atezolizumab and anti-VEGF antibody bevacizumab combined with carboplatin and paclitaxel in patients with metastatic nonsquamous NSCLC without *EGFR/ALK* alterations improved median OS (19.2 vs 14.7 months) compared with bevacizumab, carboplatin, and paclitaxel combination, regardless of PD-L1 expression.[77] These data led to the FDA approval of atezolizumab, bevacizumab, carboplatin, and paclitaxel as first-line treatment of this patient population. An ongoing trial is evaluating this first-line regimen in metastatic LUSC.

Immune checkpoint inhibitors for locally advanced and early-stage non–small cell lung cancer Until recently, the standard of care for unresectable stage III NSCLC consisted of concurrent chemoradiation, which was associated with poor long-term outcome, with 5-year survival of approximately 15%.[78] In the PACIFIC trial, which compared durvalumab (anti–PD-L1) with placebo in patients with stage III NSCLC who had completed definitive chemoradiation, durvalumab significantly improved PFS, establishing durvalumab as the standard of care in this setting.[79] Follow-up survival results revealed that durvalumab significantly improved 24-month OS (66.3% vs 55.6%) compared with placebo.[80] Ongoing phase III trials are evaluating the efficacy of PD-1/PD-L1 blockade following surgical resection and adjuvant chemotherapy in patients with locally advanced NSCLC.

Neoadjuvant trials of ICIs in early-stage (stage I–IIIA) NSCLC also hold promise. Although surgical resection with curative intent is the standard of care for early-stage NSCLC, relapse rates are high despite adjuvant and neoadjuvant platinum-based chemotherapy for selected patients.[78] In a pilot study, neoadjuvant nivolumab in patients with surgically resectable early NSCLC induced a major pathologic response in 45% of resected tumors.[81] Importantly, there were no treatment-related delays to definitive surgery. Several ongoing trials are evaluating the combination of neoadjuvant chemotherapy or radiation therapy with PD-1/PD-L1 blockade in early-stage NSCLC with promising initial and interim results.[78]

Primary and acquired resistance to immune checkpoint inhibitors Despite advances in cancer immunotherapy, many patients with NSCLC do not respond to ICIs (primary resistance), and others develop resistance after an initial response (acquired resistance). Significant effort has been devoted to identifying the biomarkers of response and the underlying molecular mechanisms of resistance.

PD-L1 expression by IHC is the only FDA-approved biomarker for patient selection. However, predictive potential of this test is limited, because many patients with PD-L1 expression do not respond to ICIs, whereas others with low PD-L1 levels benefit from ICIs.[72] Increased tumor T cell infiltration before treatment is also associated with favorable responses to ICIs, consistent with the proposed mechanism that the PD-1/PD-L1 checkpoint primarily constrains the effector function of the exhausted tumor-specific TILs within the TME.[82–84] Increased TMB has also been implicated in improved likelihood of response to ICIs, which supports the hypothesis that tumors with high somatic mutations likely possess neoepitopes that can be recognized by TILs.[85,86] Recent studies have identified tumor clonal neoantigen burden as a factor associated with improved responses to ICIs.[31,83] In contrast, *LKB1* inactivating mutations have been implicated in driving primary resistance to anti–PD-1 therapy in *KRAS*-mutant LUADs.[87]

Although mechanisms of acquired resistance in NSCLC remain obscure, several immune escape mechanisms discussed earlier, such as defective antigen presentation, immunosuppressive TME, and upregulation of other checkpoint inhibitors, may be involved. Mutations in the IFN pathways, such as *JAK1/2*, have also been implicated in acquired resistance to ICIs in melanoma.[88] Efforts are ongoing to develop synergistic combination therapies to enhance the efficacy of ICIs in patients with unfavorable genomic and immune profiles that derive primary or acquired resistance to immunotherapy.

Overcoming resistance to immune checkpoint inhibitors One approach to overcome resistance is to enhance immune responses by combining ICIs that target nonredundant pathways of T cell inhibition. Preliminary results from the phase III CheckMate 227 trial in treatment-naive patients with stage IV or recurrent NSCLC reveals that combination of nivolumab and anti–CTLA-4 antibody ipilimumab is associated with higher PFS compared with chemotherapy in patients with high TMB, regardless of PD-L1 expression.[89] Other synergistic checkpoints, such as LAG-3, B7-H4, and B7-H3, are also currently being evaluated in combination with ICIs targeting the PD-1 axis.[72]

Another promising strategy involves combining ICIs with tumor vaccines, which can potentially restore tumor antigen presentation and enhance tumor-specific T cell responses. In a phase I trial in previously treated patients with advanced NSCLC, intratumoral injection of autologous DCs expressing chemoattractant CCL21 (CCL21-DC) showed local and systemic immune responses, including enhanced CD8[+] T cell infiltration and PD-L1 upregulation in the TME, as well as systemic recognition of autologous tumor antigens.[90] Expanding on these results, an ongoing trial is evaluating the combination therapy for intratumoral CCL21-DC plus pembrolizumab in advanced NSCLC. Other early-phase studies are evaluating the use of personalized neoantigen cancer vaccines in combination with ICIs.

Radiotherapy is also being evaluated in combination with ICIs to enhance immune responses. A phase II trial, PEMBRO-RT, recently evaluated whether stereotactic body radiotherapy to a single tumor site preceding pembrolizumab could enhance responses to ICI in patients with metastatic NSCLC.[91] A doubling of ORR in the pembrolizumab plus radiotherapy group was observed compared with pembrolizumab alone. The largest clinical benefit was observed in patients with no baseline PD-L1 expression, suggesting that radiotherapy may enhance immune responses in immunosuppressed tumors.

Combination of ICIs with epigenetic modulators such as inhibitors of histone deacetylase and DNA methyltransferases (DNMTs), which may increase the tumor immunogenicity, are also being evaluated in early-phase trials.

Small cell lung cancer Multiple ICIs have been evaluated in SCLC with promising results over the past year. Based on the results of early-phase studies, nivolumab and pembrolizumab have recently been granted accelerated FDA approval for the treatment of metastatic SCLC with disease progression after platinum-based chemotherapy and at least 1 other line of therapy.

ICIs have also been evaluated as frontline therapy for SCLC. In the phase III Impower133 trial, frontline regimen with atezolizumab in combination with carboplatin and etoposide in patients with ES-SCLC improved median OS (12.3 vs 10.3 months) compared with chemotherapy plus placebo, leading to FDA approval of this frontline regimen in ES-SCLC.[92] Similarly, according to the results of a planned interim analysis of the phase III CASPIAN trial, frontline therapy with durvalumab in combination with etoposide and platinum-based chemotherapy in patients with ES-SCLC led to significant improvement in OS and PFS.[93] Based on these results, durvalumab was recently granted ODD by the FDA for the treatment of ES-SCLC. Multiple ongoing trials are evaluating the efficacy of frontline pembrolizumab in combination with platinum/etoposide for patients with ES-SCLC.

Several other synergistic strategies are being investigated for their potential to enhance the efficacy of ICIs in SCLC. A phase I/II study is evaluating ROVA-T in combination with nivolumab or nivolumab and ipilimumab in patients with ES-SCLC. An early-phase trial is exploring tumor vaccination with TP53-DC vaccine in combination with nivolumab and ipilimumab in SCLC. Other strategies designed to increase tumor immunogenicity with targeted therapies, such as DNMT or PARP (poly-ADP ribose polymerase) inhibitors, in combination with ICIs are also being evaluated in early-phase studies.

SUMMARY

In the past 2 decades, unprecedented advances in the understanding of the biology of lung cancer have revolutionized the diagnosis and treatment landscape of the disease, and ushered an exciting era of personalized medicine. TKIs and ICIs have changed the paradigm of treatment of advanced lung cancer with improved survival for a subset of patients. However, many patients do not respond and others develop resistance after an initial response. Comprehensive data including genomic, epigenomic, and cellular profiles of PMLs, primary and metastatic tumors, along with composition of the TME and host immune responses are being gathered throughout the course of the disease. Integration of this information will provide further insight into the mechanisms of tumorigenesis and resistance to therapy and establish a foundation for rational selection of personalized therapeutics. Furthermore, it is anticipated that the application of this comprehensive and integrative immunogenomic approach in pulmonary premalignancy will lead to the development of interventions that can potentially intercept cancer progression at the earliest stage of the disease.

DISCLOSURE

S.M. Dubinett reports receiving a commercial research grant from Johnson & Johnson and is a consultant/advisory board member for LungLifeAI, Early Dx, Inc, the Johnson & Johnson Lung Cancer Initiative, and T-Cure Biosciences, Inc.

REFERENCES

1. Hanahan D, Weinberg RA. Hallmarks of cancer: the next generation. Cell 2011;144(5):646–74.
2. Chen Z, Fillmore CM, Hammerman PS, et al. Non-small-cell lung cancers: a heterogeneous set of diseases. Nat Rev Cancer 2014;14(8):535–46.

3. Gazdar AF, Bunn PA, Minna JD. Small-cell lung cancer: what we know, what we need to know and the path forward. Nat Rev Cancer 2017;17(12):765.

4. Herbst RS, Morgensztern D, Boshoff C. The biology and management of non-small cell lung cancer. Nature 2018;553(7689):446–54.

5. Dagogo-Jack I, Shaw AT. Tumour heterogeneity and resistance to cancer therapies. Nat Rev Clin Oncol 2018;15(2):81–94.

6. Jamal-Hanjani M, Wilson GA, McGranahan N, et al. Tracking the evolution of non-small-cell lung cancer. N Engl J Med 2017;376(22):2109–21.

7. Campbell JD, Alexandrov A, Kim J, et al. Distinct patterns of somatic genome alterations in lung adenocarcinomas and squamous cell carcinomas. Nat Genet 2016;48(6):607–16.

8. Cancer Genome Atlas Research Network. Comprehensive genomic characterization of squamous cell lung cancers. Nature 2012;489(7417):519–25.

9. Cancer Genome Atlas Research Network. Comprehensive molecular profiling of lung adenocarcinoma. Nature 2014;511(7511):543–50.

10. Pao W, Wang TY, Riely GJ, et al. KRAS mutations and primary resistance of lung adenocarcinomas to gefitinib or erlotinib. PLoS Med 2005;2(1):e17.

11. Alexandrov LB, Nik-Zainal S, Wedge DC, et al. Signatures of mutational processes in human cancer. Nature 2013;500(7463):415–21.

12. Lawrence MS, Stojanov P, Polak P, et al. Mutational heterogeneity in cancer and the search for new cancer-associated genes. Nature 2013;499(7457):214–8.

13. Govindan R, Ding L, Griffith M, et al. Genomic landscape of non-small cell lung cancer in smokers and never-smokers. Cell 2012;150(6):1121–34.

14. Bunn PA Jr, Minna JD, Augustyn A, et al. Small cell lung cancer: can recent advances in biology and molecular biology be translated into improved outcomes? J Thorac Oncol 2016;11(4):453–74.

15. George J, Lim JS, Jang SJ, et al. Comprehensive genomic profiles of small cell lung cancer. Nature 2015;524(7563):47–53.

16. Alves Rde C, Meurer RT, Roehe AV. MYC amplification is associated with poor survival in small cell lung cancer: a chromogenic in situ hybridization study. J Cancer Res Clin Oncol 2014;140(12):2021–5.

17. Peifer M, Fernandez-Cuesta L, Sos ML, et al. Integrative genome analyses identify key somatic driver mutations of small-cell lung cancer. Nat Genet 2012; 44(10):1104–10.

18. Pleasance ED, Stephens PJ, O'Meara S, et al. A small-cell lung cancer genome with complex signatures of tobacco exposure. Nature 2010; 463(7278):184–90.

19. Altorki NK, Markowitz GJ, Gao D, et al. The lung microenvironment: an important regulator of tumour growth and metastasis. Nat Rev Cancer 2019; 19(1):9–31.

20. Dubinett SM. Inflammation and lung cancer. New York: Springer; 2015.

21. Krysan K, Tran LM, Grimes BS, et al. The immune contexture associates with the genomic landscape in lung adenomatous premalignancy. Cancer Res 2019;79(19):5022–33.

22. Lavin Y, Kobayashi S, Leader A, et al. Innate immune landscape in early lung adenocarcinoma by paired single-cell analyses. Cell 2017;169(4):750–65.e17.

23. Rosenthal R, Cadieux EL, Salgado R, et al. Neoantigen-directed immune escape in lung cancer evolution. Nature 2019;567(7749):479–85.

24. Mascaux C, Angelova M, Vasaturo A, et al. Immune evasion before tumour invasion in early lung squamous carcinogenesis. Nature 2019;571(7766):570–5.

25. Engels EA. Inflammation in the development of lung cancer: epidemiological evidence. Expert Rev Anticancer Ther 2008;8(4):605–15.

26. Punturieri A, Szabo E, Croxton TL, et al. Lung cancer and chronic obstructive pulmonary disease: needs and opportunities for integrated research. J Natl Cancer Inst 2009;101(8):554–9.

27. DiDonato JA, Mercurio F, Karin M. NF-kappaB and the link between inflammation and cancer. Immunol Rev 2012;246(1):379–400.

28. Wistuba II. Genetics of preneoplasia: lessons from lung cancer. Curr Mol Med 2007;7(1):3–14.

29. Khuri FR, Wu H, Lee JJ, et al. Cyclooxygenase-2 overexpression is a marker of poor prognosis in stage I non-small cell lung cancer. Clin Cancer Res 2001;7(4):861–7.

30. Mittal D, Gubin MM, Schreiber RD, et al. New insights into cancer immunoediting and its three component phases–elimination, equilibrium and escape. Curr Opin Immunol 2014;27:16–25.

31. McGranahan N, Furness AJ, Rosenthal R, et al. Clonal neoantigens elicit T cell immunoreactivity and sensitivity to immune checkpoint blockade. Science 2016;351(6280):1463–9.

32. Dieu-Nosjean MC, Antoine M, Danel C, et al. Long-term survival for patients with non-small-cell lung cancer with intratumoral lymphoid structures. J Clin Oncol 2008;26(27):4410–7.

33. Fucikova J, Becht E, Iribarren K, et al. Calreticulin expression in human non-small cell lung cancers correlates with increased accumulation of antitumor immune cells and favorable prognosis. Cancer Res 2016;76(7):1746–56.

34. Goc J, Germain C, Vo-Bourgais TKD, et al. Dendritic cells in tumor-associated tertiary lymphoid structures signal a Th1 cytotoxic immune contexture and license the positive prognostic value of infiltrating CD8+ T cells. Cancer Res 2014;74(3):705–15.

35. Chen DS, Mellman I. Elements of cancer immunity and the cancer-immune set point. Nature 2017; 541(7637):321–30.

36. Wherry EJ. T cell exhaustion. Nat Immunol 2011; 12(6):492–9.

37. Sanmamed MF, Chen L. A paradigm shift in cancer immunotherapy: from enhancement to normalization. Cell 2018;175(2):313–26.

38. McGranahan N, Rosenthal R, Hiley CT, et al. Allele-specific HLA loss and immune escape in lung cancer evolution. Cell 2017;171(6):1259–71.e11.

39. Marty R, Kaabinejadian S, Rossell D, et al. MHC-I genotype restricts the oncogenic mutational landscape. Cell 2017;171(6):1272–83.e15.

40. Shimizu K, Nakata M, Hirami Y, et al. Tumor-infiltrating Foxp3+ regulatory T cells are correlated with cyclooxygenase-2 expression and are associated with recurrence in resected non-small cell lung cancer. J Thorac Oncol 2010;5(5):585–90.

41. Messmer MN, Netherby CS, Banik D, et al. Tumor-induced myeloid dysfunction and its implications for cancer immunotherapy. Cancer Immunol Immunother 2015;64(1):1–13.

42. Hochmuth F, Jochem M, Schlattmann P. Meta-analysis of aspirin use and risk of lung cancer shows notable results. Eur J Cancer Prev 2016;25(4):259–68.

43. Jiang HY, Huang TB, Xu L, et al. Aspirin use and lung cancer risk: a possible relationship? Evidence from an updated meta-analysis. PLoS One 2015;10(4):e0122962.

44. Ye S, Lee M, Lee D, et al. Association of long-term use of low-dose aspirin as chemoprevention with risk of lung cancer. JAMA Netw Open 2019;2(3):e190185.

45. Mao JT, Fishbein MC, Adams B, et al. Celecoxib decreases Ki-67 proliferative index in active smokers. Clin Cancer Res 2006;12(1):314–20.

46. Mao JT, Roth MD, Fishbein MC, et al. Lung cancer chemoprevention with celecoxib in former smokers. Cancer Prev Res (Phila) 2011;4(7):984–93.

47. Kim ES, Hong WK, Lee JJ, et al. Biological activity of celecoxib in the bronchial epithelium of current and former smokers. Cancer Prev Res (Phila) 2010;3(2):148–59.

48. Keith RL, Blatchford PJ, Kittelson J, et al. Oral iloprost improves endobronchial dysplasia in former smokers. Cancer Prev Res (Phila) 2011;4(6):793–802.

49. Ridker PM, MacFadyen JG, Thuren T, et al. Effect of interleukin-1beta inhibition with canakinumab on incident lung cancer in patients with atherosclerosis: exploratory results from a randomised, double-blind, placebo-controlled trial. Lancet 2017;390(10105):1833–42.

50. National Lung Screening Trial Research Team, Aberle DR, Adams AM, et al. Reduced lung-cancer mortality with low-dose computed tomographic screening. N Engl J Med 2011;365(5):395–409.

51. Blackburn EH. Cancer interception. Cancer Prev Res (Phila) 2011;4(6):787–92.

52. Srivastava S, Ghosh S, Kagan J, et al, National Cancer Institute's HI. The making of a precancer atlas: promises, challenges, and opportunities. Trends Cancer 2018;4(8):523–36.

53. Kadara H, Wistuba II. Field cancerization in non-small cell lung cancer: implications in disease pathogenesis. Proc Am Thorac Soc 2012;9(2):38–42.

54. Sivakumar S, Lucas FAS, McDowell TL, et al. Genomic landscape of atypical adenomatous hyperplasia reveals divergent modes to lung adenocarcinoma. Cancer Res 2017;77(22):6119–30.

55. Teixeira VH, Pipinikas CP, Pennycuick A, et al. Deciphering the genomic, epigenomic, and transcriptomic landscapes of pre-invasive lung cancer lesions. Nat Med 2019;25(3):517–25.

56. Beane JE, Mazzilli SA, Campbell JD, et al. Molecular subtyping reveals immune alterations associated with progression of bronchial premalignant lesions. Nat Commun 2019;10(1):1856.

57. Barlesi F, Mazieres J, Merlio JP, et al. Routine molecular profiling of patients with advanced non-small-cell lung cancer: results of a 1-year nationwide programme of the French Cooperative Thoracic Intergroup (IFCT). Lancet 2016;387(10026):1415–26.

58. Kris MG, Johnson BE, Berry LD, et al. Using multiplexed assays of oncogenic drivers in lung cancers to select targeted drugs. JAMA 2014;311(19):1998–2006.

59. Soria JC, Ohe Y, Vansteenkiste J, et al. Osimertinib in untreated EGFR-mutated advanced non-small-cell lung cancer. N Engl J Med 2018;378(2):113–25.

60. Hida T, Nokihara H, Kondo M, et al. Alectinib versus crizotinib in patients with ALK-positive non-small-cell lung cancer (J-ALEX): an open-label, randomised phase 3 trial. Lancet 2017;390(10089):29–39.

61. Peters S, Camidge DR, Shaw AT, et al. Alectinib versus crizotinib in untreated ALK-positive non-small-cell lung cancer. N Engl J Med 2017;377(9):829–38.

62. Shaw AT, Ou SH, Bang YJ, et al. Crizotinib in ROS1-rearranged non-small-cell lung cancer. N Engl J Med 2014;371(21):1963–71.

63. Planchard D, Smit EF, Groen HJM, et al. Dabrafenib plus trametinib in patients with previously untreated BRAF(V600E)-mutant metastatic non-small-cell lung cancer: an open-label, phase 2 trial. Lancet Oncol 2017;18(10):1307–16.

64. Sequist LV, Waltman BA, Dias-Santagata D, et al. Genotypic and histological evolution of lung cancers acquiring resistance to EGFR inhibitors. Sci Transl Med 2011;3(75):75ra26.

65. Strickler JH, Weekes CD, Nemunaitis J, et al. First-in-human phase i, dose-escalation and -expansion study of telisotuzumab vedotin, an antibody-drug

conjugate targeting c-Met, in patients with advanced solid tumors. J Clin Oncol 2018;36(33): 3298–306.

66. Gautschi O, Milia J, Filleron T, et al. Targeting RET in patients with RET-rearranged lung cancers: results from the global, multicenter RET registry. J Clin Oncol 2017;35(13):1403–10.

67. Pillai RN, Behera M, Berry LD, et al. HER2 mutations in lung adenocarcinomas: a report from the Lung Cancer Mutation Consortium. Cancer 2017; 123(21):4099–105.

68. Mazieres J, Barlesi F, Filleron T, et al. Lung cancer patients with HER2 mutations treated with chemotherapy and HER2-targeted drugs: results from the European EUHER2 cohort. Ann Oncol 2016;27(2): 281–6.

69. Li BT, Shen R, Buonocore D, et al. Ado-trastuzumab emtansine for patients with HER2-mutant lung cancers: results from a phase II basket trial. J Clin Oncol 2018;36(24):2532–7.

70. Melichar B, Adenis A, Lockhart AC, et al. Safety and activity of alisertib, an investigational aurora kinase A inhibitor, in patients with breast cancer, small-cell lung cancer, non-small-cell lung cancer, head and neck squamous-cell carcinoma, and gastro-oesophageal adenocarcinoma: a five-arm phase 2 study. Lancet Oncol 2015;16(4):395–405.

71. Brahmer JR, Govindan R, Anders RA, et al. The Society for Immunotherapy of Cancer consensus statement on immunotherapy for the treatment of non-small cell lung cancer (NSCLC). J Immunother Cancer 2018;6(1):75.

72. Doroshow DB, Sanmamed MF, Hastings K, et al. Immunotherapy in non-small cell lung cancer: facts and hopes. Clin Cancer Res 2019;25(15): 4592–602.

73. Reck M, Rodriguez-Abreu D, Robinson AG, et al. Pembrolizumab versus chemotherapy for PD-L1-positive non-small-cell lung cancer. N Engl J Med 2016;375(19):1823–33.

74. Reck M, Rodriguez-Abreu D, Robinson AG, et al. Updated analysis of KEYNOTE-024: pembrolizumab versus platinum-based chemotherapy for advanced non-small-cell lung cancer with PD-L1 tumor proportion score of 50% or greater. J Clin Oncol 2019; 37(7):537–46.

75. Gandhi L, Garassino MC. Pembrolizumab plus chemotherapy in lung cancer. N Engl J Med 2018; 379(11):e18.

76. Paz-Ares L, Luft A, Vicente D, et al. Pembrolizumab plus chemotherapy for squamous non-small-cell lung cancer. N Engl J Med 2018;379(21): 2040–51.

77. Socinski MA, Jotte RM, Cappuzzo F, et al. Atezolizumab for first-line treatment of metastatic nonsquamous NSCLC. N Engl J Med 2018;378(24): 2288–301.

78. Rosner S, Reuss JE, Forde PM. PD-1 blockade in early-stage lung cancer. Annu Rev Med 2019;70: 425–35.

79. Antonia SJ, Villegas A, Daniel D, et al. Durvalumab after chemoradiotherapy in stage III non-small-cell lung cancer. N Engl J Med 2017; 377(20):1919–29.

80. Antonia SJ, Villegas A, Daniel D, et al. Overall survival with durvalumab after chemoradiotherapy in stage III NSCLC. N Engl J Med 2018;379(24): 2342–50.

81. Forde PM, Chaft JE, Smith KN, et al. Neoadjuvant PD-1 blockade in resectable lung cancer. N Engl J Med 2018;378(21):1976–86.

82. Tumeh PC, Harview CL, Yearley JH, et al. PD-1 blockade induces responses by inhibiting adaptive immune resistance. Nature 2014;515(7528):568–71.

83. Gettinger SN, Choi J, Mani N, et al. A dormant TIL phenotype defines non-small cell lung carcinomas sensitive to immune checkpoint blockers. Nat Commun 2018;9(1):3196.

84. Fumet JD, Richard C, Ledys F, et al. Prognostic and predictive role of CD8 and PD-L1 determination in lung tumor tissue of patients under anti-PD-1 therapy. Br J Cancer 2018;119(8):950–60.

85. Rizvi H, Sanchez-Vega F, La K, et al. Molecular determinants of response to anti-programmed cell death (PD)-1 and anti-programmed death-ligand 1 (PD-L1) blockade in patients with non-small-cell lung cancer profiled with targeted next-generation sequencing. J Clin Oncol 2018;36(7):633–41.

86. Rizvi NA, Hellmann MD, Snyder A, et al. Cancer immunology. Mutational landscape determines sensitivity to PD-1 blockade in non-small cell lung cancer. Science 2015;348(6230):124–8.

87. Skoulidis F, Goldberg ME, Greenawalt DM, et al. STK11/LKB1 mutations and PD-1 inhibitor resistance in KRAS-mutant lung adenocarcinoma. Cancer Discov 2018;8(7):822–35.

88. Zaretsky JM, Garcia-Diaz A, Shin DS, et al. Mutations associated with acquired resistance to PD-1 blockade in melanoma. N Engl J Med 2016;375(9): 819–29.

89. Hellmann MD, Ciuleanu TE, Pluzanski A, et al. Nivolumab plus ipilimumab in lung cancer with a high tumor mutational burden. N Engl J Med 2018;378(22): 2093–104.

90. Lee JM, Lee MH, Garon E, et al. Phase I trial of intratumoral injection of CCL21 gene-modified dendritic cells in lung cancer elicits tumor-specific immune responses and CD8(+) T-cell infiltration. Clin Cancer Res 2017;23(16):4556–68.

91. Theelen W, Peulen HMU, Lalezari F, et al. Effect of pembrolizumab after stereotactic body radiotherapy vs pembrolizumab alone on tumor response in patients with advanced non-small cell lung cancer: results of the PEMBRO-RT phase 2 randomized

clinical trial. JAMA Oncol 2019. https://doi.org/10.1001/jamaoncol.2019.1478.

92. Horn L, Mansfield AS, Szczesna A, et al. First-line atezolizumab plus chemotherapy in extensive-stage small-cell lung cancer. N Engl J Med 2018; 379(23):2220–9.

93. Paz-Ares L, Chen Y, Reinmuth N, et al. Overall survival with durvalumab plus etoposide-platinum in first-line extensive-stage SCLC: results from the CASPIAN study. Presented at: IASLC 20th World Conference on Lung Cancer. Barcelona, Spain. September 7–10, 2019. Abstract PL02.11.

Primary and Secondary Prevention of Lung Cancer: Tobacco Treatment

Hasmeena Kathuria, MD[a], Enid Neptune, MD[b],*

KEYWORDS

- Tobacco dependence treatment • Nicotine addiction • Teachable moment • Lung cancer stigma
- Opt-out approaches • Lung cancer screening

KEY POINTS

- Achieving smoking abstinence in the lung cancer screening setting or after cancer diagnosis improves health outcomes.
- Clinicians should actively engage in efforts to minimize stigma associated with continued smoking, especially after the diagnosis of cancer.
- Proactive approaches to offering tobacco treatment to all smokers regardless of readiness to quit can increase smoking abstinence.
- Varenicline is more effective than placebo, bupropion, and nicotine patches in helping smokers achieve abstinence.

INTRODUCTION

Tobacco dependence accounts for 1 in 5 deaths and is the number 1 preventable cause of disease and death in the United States,[1] including the cause of about ~120,000 deaths from lung cancer per year and a contributor to more than 25% of all deaths from cancer.[2,3] The overall prevalence of smoking cigarettes has decreased in the United States, yet remains high among the lowest-income individuals, those with substance use disorders and mental health issues, communities of color, and the LGBTQ community.[4,5] These are the same groups for which tobacco dependence interventions are less available, and medical misinformation widespread.[6] Compared with other ethnic groups, African American smokers have the highest lung cancer mortality but show the lowest levels of cumulative smoke exposure, an observation often termed the "smoking paradox."[7] Persons with mental illness are challenged due to

poor engagement and agency within a complex medical system and stigma about their ability to comply with a treatment plan. When diagnosed with lung cancer, low socioeconomic status (SES) groups frequently show worse outcomes with treatment and are almost twice as likely to die from lung cancer reflecting both economic and infrastructural factors.[8]

These data suggest that the risk of lung cancer among smokers, especially in these populations with high tobacco use, is early, durable, and potent. Tobacco dependence is the most accessible and consequential target to reduce the burden of lung cancer worldwide. Smoking cessation after a lung cancer diagnosis improves survival and quality of life (QOL) and outreach efforts to direct lung cancer screening (LCS) to smokers in highly tobacco-encumbered but less medically accessible groups would likely yield tremendous health benefits. It remains unclear, however, whether the widespread incorporation of LCS will

a The Pulmonary Center, Boston University Medical Center, Boston University, 72 East Concord Street R304, Boston, MA 02118, USA; b Department of Internal Medicine, Division of Pulmonary and Critical Care Medicine, Johns Hopkins School of Medicine, 1830 East Monument Street, Room 549, Baltimore, MD 21287, USA
* Corresponding author.
E-mail address: eneptune@jhmi.edu

Clin Chest Med 41 (2020) 39–51
https://doi.org/10.1016/j.ccm.2019.10.002
0272-5231/20/© 2019 Elsevier Inc. All rights reserved.

reach full potential of improving outcomes for smokers or former smokers in low SES tobacco-burdened subpopulations, because these individuals are under-represented among participants undergoing LCS.[9] From a tobacco dependence treatment perspective, the most cost-effective strategy to reduce lung cancer mortality is to reduce initiation of tobacco use, enable aggressive multimodality tobacco dependence treatment for all smokers, and implement an LCS protocol that is anchored on tobacco dependence treatment. The ability to customize this 3-pronged approach to increase uptake in select populations is challenging and should be a priority for all health care providers. In this review, we describe the current state of tobacco dependence treatment, focusing on new paradigms and approaches and their particular relevance for persons at risk for or on treatment of lung cancer.

BENEFITS TO INCORPORATING TOBACCO TREATMENT INTO THE LUNG CANCER CARE CONTINUUM

In 2014, the Surgeon General's report highlighted that continued smoking after a cancer diagnosis adversely affects health outcomes and overall survival, but quitting after a cancer diagnosis can improve prognosis, overall health, and QOL.[10] Studies show that continuing to smoke cigarettes after a lung cancer diagnosis is associated with increased risk of recurrence, a second primary lung cancer, treatment-related complications, and worse survival among those with non-small cell lung cancer (NSCLC), including early-stage NSCLC, as well as those with small-cell lung cancer.[11–14] Furthermore, patients with lung cancer who smoke report lower QOL scores than those who do not smoke.[15] Clinical benefits of smoking cessation may differ by stage of lung cancer. Although a large single-center study showed smoking cessation after the diagnosis of NSCLC improves survival, a multivariate analysis incorporating stage of disease and previous surgery yielded a trend toward survival without statistical significance.[16] A larger meta-analysis, by contrast, of smoking cessation after diagnosis with early-stage lung cancer showed improved outcomes partially attributable to reduced cancer progression.[11] Several oncology professional organizations (the National Comprehensive Cancer Network and the American Society of Clinical Oncology) issued guidelines stressing the importance of smoking cessation and tobacco treatment of patients with cancer.[17,18]

Providing tobacco treatment in the context of LCS is another opportunity to reduce death from lung cancer and all-cause mortality of individuals with a substantial history of tobacco use. The National Lung Screening Trial (NLST) and the NELSON trial both demonstrated a reduction in lung cancer mortality with low-dose computed tomography (LDCT) screening of people at high risk of lung cancer.[19,20] Furthermore, in the NLST, current smokers, those with less than a high school education, and African Americans had a higher risk of death.[21] Current smokers who underwent annual LDCT and achieved smoking abstinence had the greatest mortality reduction.[22] Several guidelines recommend, and the Centers for Medicare and Medicaid Services require, that clinicians offer tobacco treatment with LCS.[23,24] An estimated half of individuals undergoing LCS will be current smokers[25]; thus LCS presents an opportunity to combine 2 interventions known to reduce smoking-related morbidity and mortality.[24,26] The Society for Research on Nicotine and Tobacco[27] and the American Thoracic Society[26,28] have prioritized identifying effective approaches to tobacco treatment in the context of LCS.

BARRIERS TO TOBACCO TREATMENT IN THE LUNG CANCER CARE CONTINUUM

A systematic review found that 30% of patients with lung cancer continue to smoke cigarettes after a cancer diagnosis.[29] Furthermore, among smokers undergoing LCS, quit rates are estimated to be only 11%, in part due to a lack of delivery of guideline-recommended tobacco treatment provided by screening programs.[30,31] It is critical to recognize and address how stigma, social factors associated with low SES populations, and clinician and system barriers contribute to critical gaps between recommended evidence-based tobacco treatment guidelines and actual delivery of tobacco cessation treatment in the lung cancer care continuum.

Stigma, Guilt, and Shame

Stigma, implicit bias, and nihilism are corrupting influences which reduce an active smoker's interest in the pursuit of tobacco dependence treatment across the entire lung cancer care spectrum. In fact, the stigma associated with lung cancer differentiates LCS process from all other screening. Many smokers blame themselves and also accept the blame of others for their smoking-related cancer diagnosis or their elevated risk. Studies have identified that patients with lung cancer often feel stigmatized because lung cancer tends to be associated with previous smoking.[32]

Among patients diagnosed with lung cancer, internalized stigma such as self-blame, guilt, and regret, has been associated with increased depressive symptoms, delays in medical help-seeking, and lower QOL.[32,33] These factors can lead to unnecessary delay in enrolling in screening programs and diagnosis, engagement in clinical trials, and reluctance to comply with tobacco dependence treatment.[33,34] Recognizing the importance of identifying lung cancer stigma, Ostroff and colleagues[33] developed the Lung Cancer Stigma Inventory, a reliable and valid assessment of 3 facets of stigma in lung cancer care settings: internalized stigma (directing negative societal attitudes toward oneself), perceived stigma (negative appraisal and devaluation from others), and constrained disclosure (discomfort in sharing one's lung cancer status with others).

Acceptance and Commitment Therapy for Lung Cancer Stigma, a patient-focused cognitive behavioral intervention to reduce the self-blame, guilt, and inhibited disclosure is currently being studied.[35] An urgent need exists for development and testing of additional psychosocial interventions that target lung cancer stigma as well as educational materials for clinicians and the general public to address stigma and implicit bias toward smokers. These materials should include information on how common smoking was in the days when many of those eligible for screening started smoking, describe the aggressive media campaigns by the tobacco industry to white-wash the attendant health risks, and delineate how tobacco control policies, in an effort to reduce the social acceptability of smoking, denormalized smoking and stigmatized smokers through positioning smoking as an environmental health issue (secondhand smoke), legislating smoke-free public areas and workplaces, and portraying smoking as a personal choice ultimately leading to a horrible death. Clinicians should approach smokers with sensitivity when discussing smoking status and actively engage in efforts to minimize the stigma associated with continued smoking, especially after the diagnosis of cancer.

Low Socioeconomic Status Barriers

SES is strongly associated with smoking status,[36] the most important risk factor for lung cancer. Smoking prevalence in low SES and other vulnerable populations such as those with mental health illness and substance use disorders has declined at negligible rates compared with the general population.[37] Low SES remains a risk factor for lung cancer diagnosis and mortality even after adjustment for smoking behavior[38] and area-level measures of SES are associated with lung cancer risk in current and shorter-term former smokers only in this population.[39] Conversely, an increase in SES over time was related to a decrease in mortality from respiratory disease, but not from lung cancer.[40] The lack of financial resources or the ability to make healthy financial choices directly undermine the goals of early detection of lung cancer. Patients with lung cancer who do not receive therapy are more likely to be older, not white, male, and unmarried, to have no insurance or public insurance other than Medicare, to live in a low SES neighborhood, to have been seen at a non-National Cancer Institute cancer center hospital or hospital serving lower SES patients, and to have larger tumors.[41] Therefore, SES significantly mediates racial/ethnic cancer survival disparities for several cancers including lung cancer.

Studies demonstrate that patient navigators, laypersons from the community who guide patients through the health care system to connect them with services they may have difficulty accessing,[42] are a promising approach to promote smoking cessation[43] and reduce disparities in cancer screening, diagnosis, and treatment.[44] Among smokers residing in public housing, a smoking cessation intervention delivered by peer health advocates trained in motivation interviewing, basic tobacco treatment skills, and patient navigation increased tobacco abstinence at 12 months.[45] In the LCS setting, a patient navigation program implemented in community health centers increased LDCT screening among high-risk current smokers.[46]

Financial incentives promotes tobacco treatment engagement and smoking cessation in low SES populations.[47] A randomized trial of low income smokers in the primary care setting showed that patient navigation combined with financial incentives increased 12-month tobacco abstinence.[48] Incentives for stopping smoking has not been tested among patients undergoing LCS. A clinical trial in the LCS setting is underway to test the effectiveness of 4 approaches to help patients stop smoking, including an approach that delivers payments for successfully quitting.[49]

Clinician and System Barriers

Clinicians' experiences and views on smoking cessation services and perceived organizational constraints in settings considered teachable moments (LCS programs and cancer diagnosis) influence change in smoking behavior.[50,51] In the LCS setting, studies suggest that smokers with a screen-detected pulmonary nodule are more likely to quit smoking than those with normal results, and that discussing a screen-detected nodule is an opportunity to initiate a conversation about the desire to quit smoking.[30,52] Yet research suggests that physicians often missed this opportunity, expressing concern about overwhelming patients by discussing smoking cessation during delivery of abnormal results.[51] Similarly, in the cancer diagnosis context, clinicians avoid talking about smoking because of competing priorities and concerns of implying and/or exacerbating patients' guilt of smoking, even though patients often expected some conversation on smoking cessation.[50] Barriers include time constraints, lack of awareness about smoking cessation services, and perceptions of responsibility for talking about smoking cessation. Thus, despite improved survival in patients with cancer who quit cigarettes,[11,53] many opportunities to promote smoking cessation are missed.[50,51]

Tobacco cessation treatment pathways for patients with cancer have been developed that outline individualized treatment plans.[54] However, within the lung cancer care continuum, tobacco treatment needs to be a team effort. Whether patients are interacting with a provider in the LCS setting, pulmonologists during diagnosis, and/or medical, radiation, and surgical oncologists during treatment, the unique challenges including stigma and cancer-related distress should be addressed. Strategies should include providing clinical evidence on the adverse effects of smoking on treatment outcomes and informing patients about the benefits of stopping smoking on side effects, treatment outcomes, and reduction in likelihood of recurrence.[51] In addition, system-level changes are needed to promote tobacco treatment across lung cancer care. Such changes include incorporating reminders into practice systems, allocating resources for the development of tobacco treatment programs embedded in the cancer care setting, and gaining competency in treating tobacco dependence either online (https://www.cdc.gov/tobacco/campaign/tips/partners/health/index.html) or by attending specialized training in tobacco treatment (http://ctttp.org/accredited-programs/).

A recently recognized systemic barrier to tobacco treatment is the issue of structural stigma.[55] The unintended effects of public policies and social norms aimed to reduce smoking can sometimes have adverse effects on health care access and availability of tobacco dependence treatment. For example, the recent United States Department of Housing and Urban Development policy to expand smoke-free public housing needs to be intimately tethered to reliable tobacco treatment services to avoid homelessness and destabilization of families. Clinicians need to be cognizant of the upstream social determinants of health that affect a smoker's engagement with the health system and how stigmatization of smoking validates discrimination by potential employers (eg, employers absorb a higher net cost of more than $6000 per year when they hire a smoker rather than a nonsmoker,[56] reinforcing a low SES status and reducing access to medical care). There has been a call for medical education to include training in "structural competency," in which knowledge about diseases is combined with analysis of social systems so that the structural determinants of stigma and health can be addressed.[55]

GUIDELINE-RECOMMENDED PHARMACOTHERAPY AND COUNSELING
Understanding Nicotine Addiction

Tobacco dependence is a chronic relapsing disease that is sustained by nicotine addiction.[57] Exogenous nicotine acts on nicotinic acetylcholine receptors (nAChRs) to activate brain dopamine release resulting in the rewarding effects of smoking cigarettes.[58] By engaging with nicotinic receptors in distinct locations (ventral tegmental area [VTA]), nicotine generates a powerful, but incorrect survival signal. In addition, nicotine promotes learned associations (eg, exposure to people, places, or things previously associated with smoking cigarettes) that become persistent over time, placing people at risk for lifelong relapse.

Opt-Out Approaches

Studies suggest that only about 30% of current smokers are ready to quit within the next 30 days.[59] Proactive approaches to offering guideline-recommended tobacco treatment to all smokers regardless of readiness to quit and allowing patients to refuse treatment ("opt-out") have been shown to have both a high acceptance rate and to increase smoking abstinence.[60–62] Among participants who quit smoking cigarettes, almost half stated that during initial assessment they were not ready to stop smoking cigarettes,[63] underscoring the importance of engaging all smokers with tobacco treatment, regardless of motivation to quit smoking.

Pharmacotherapy

Pharmacotherapy effectively reduces withdrawal symptoms,[64] and the combination of medication with counseling is more effective than either intervention alone in promoting smoking abstinence.[65] The 7 US Food and Drug

Administration (FDA)-approved medications for tobacco treatment include: (1) 5 types of nicotine replacement therapy (NRT) (over the counter: nicotine lozenges, gum and patches; prescription only: nicotine inhalers and nasal spray); (2) bupropion; and (3) varenicline.

Nicotine replacement therapy

NRT, an agonist at the nicotinic cholinergic receptors, delivers nicotine safely and prevents withdrawal symptoms.[66] NRT is a nonaddictive, safe alternative to smoking because there is a much slower release and absorption of nicotine into the blood compared with the immediate nicotine peaks produced by cigarettes.[64] Combination therapy with a transdermal nicotine patch (which delivers continuous dosing to provide steady levels of nicotine with peak blood levels of nicotine at 2–4 hours) and the nasal spray, inhaler, gum, or lozenge (delivers "as-needed" dosing in response to acute cravings; blood levels of nicotine peak 5 to 10 minutes after taking the nasal spray or inhaler and 20 minutes after using the gum or lozenge) is more effective in promoting prolonged abstinence, with a risk ratio of 1.34 compared with use of any single product.[65] The FDA recommends 12 weeks of treatment with NRT, although treatment specialists often extend duration based on patient factors such as cigarette cravings and confidence to remain quit (**Table 1**). No harm was reported in a randomized clinical trial with extended NRT use.[67]

Bupropion SR

Bupropion SR is a nontricyclic antidepressant that acts in part by blocking neuronal reuptake of dopamine.[68] Bupropion SR is most effective at promoting tobacco abstinence and relieving withdrawal symptoms when combined with NRT and counseling.[65] For patients who successfully quit after 12 weeks with bupropion SR, clinicians should consider an additional 12-week course based on a study that extended treatment for up to 1 year reduced relapse rate after initial cessation.[69] Bupropion lowers the seizure threshold and should not be used in patients who have risk factors for seizures (**Table 2**). A large clinical trial demonstrated the neuropsychiatric safety of Buprorion[70] resulting in removal of the Boxed Warning for serious mental health side effects from the drug label.

Varenicline

Varenicline, an agonist-antagonist of the α4β2 nicotinic cholinergic receptors in the VTA, works by partially mediating brain dopamine release while limiting receptor binding by nicotine from cigarettes.[66,71] A recent clinical trial demonstrated that varenicline is more effective than bupropion or single NRT in promoting smoking cessation.[70] A systematic review shows that combination NRT and varenicline achieved the greatest smoking cessation rates.[72] The FDA has approved extending varenicline for 6 months to prevent relapse.[73] Varenicline preloading with a flexible quit date and varenicline-assisted gradual reduction in cigarettes over 3 months (**Table 3**), rather than the FDA-recommended 1 week pretreatment period, are promising approaches to assist in stopping smoking.[74,75] Pooled clinical trial data, several large observational studies, and a large randomized trial (EAGLES)[70] assuaged concerns of the neuropsychiatric safety of varenicline and the FDA removed the Boxed Warning for serious mental health side effects in December 2016.

Counseling

Counseling, either group or individual, is effective in motivating smoking cessation, especially when it includes practical help focusing on problem solving skills and social support. Counseling is most effective when it is intensive rather than brief and accompanied by pharmacotherapy.[76] Mobile health, such as Quitlines (free telephone-based help lines that offer tobacco cessation counseling such as 1-800-QUIT NOW), interactive texting services, and interactive voice recognition interventions have been shown to be effective at improving smoking abstinence.[77,78] Quitlines may be an especially helpful resource for programs that have time and resource constraints. In cancer settings, however, studies have reported low cessation rates with Quitlines.[79] The addition of financial incentives to increase engagement with Quitline programs in the general population was shown to increase smoking cessation rates.[80] Such novel and more resource-intensive interventions may be efficacious in cancer survivors and should be tested in future studies.

Strategies for smokers unmotivated to quit smoking

Motivational interviewing Motivational interviewing (MI) is a method to improve a patient's motivation to quit by minimizing obstacles to change, resolving ambivalence, and building self-motivation.[81] MI focuses on asking questions instead of giving answers and avoids challenging resistance to change head-on. Shortened versions of MI, termed the 5 Rs, have been shown to increase smoking quit rates.[82,83] In the 5 Rs approach, clinicians engage patients to explore the personal "Relevance" of smoking cessation, the perceived

"Risks" of continuing to smoke cigarettes, the "Rewards" of quitting, and the "Roadblocks" to quitting. Clinicians need to "Repeat" these conversations as needed to facilitate change.[84]

Precessation pharmacotherapy and support to promote eventual abstinence In patients not motivated to quit, studies show that, although sampling nicotine replacement and practice quit

---

Table 1
FDA-approved pharmacotherapy to treat tobacco dependence: nicotine replacement therapy

Nicotine transdermal patch

Standard dosage	Dosing modifications	Adverse events
• >10 cigs/d: 21 mg/d × 4–6 wk 14 mg/d × 2 wk 7 mg/d × 2 wk • ≤10 cigs/d: 14 mg/d × 6 wk 7 mg/d × 2 wk Duration: 8–10 wk	• Pretreatment: Consider precessation treatment with nicotine patch before quit date • Higher dosage: >40 cigs/d: consider 42 mg/d • Combination + extended therapy: Consider >13 wk nicotine patch + short acting NRT as needed	• Sleep disturbances, local skin reactions, and headache Precautions • Recent MI within 2 wk, serious arrhythmias, unstable angina • Adolescents <18 y • Pregnancy and breastfeeding

Nicotine lozenge: blood levels of nicotine peak at 20 min

Standard dosage	Dosing modifications	Adverse events
• 1st cig <30 min after waking: 4 mg • 1st cig >30 min after waking: 2 mg Weeks 1–6: 1 lozenge q 1–2 h Weeks 7–9: 1 lozenge q 2–4 h Weeks 10–12: 1 lozenge q 4–8 h • Max = 20 lozenges/d Duration: up to 12 wk	• Combination + extended therapy: consider >13 wk transdermal patch + gum as needed	• Cough, nausea, hiccups, heartburn, flatulence, insomnia, and headache Precautions • Recent MI within 2 wk, serious arrhythmias, unstable angina • Adolescents <18 y Pregnancy and breastfeeding

Nicotine gum: blood levels of nicotine peak at 20 min

Standard dosage	Dosing modifications	Adverse events
• 1st cig <30 min after waking: 4 mg • 1st cig >30 min after waking: 2 mg Weeks 1–6: 1-piece q 1–2 h Weeks 7–9: 1-piece q 2–4 h Weeks 10–12: 1-piece q 4–8 h • Max = 24 pieces/d • Duration: up to 12 wk	• Combination + extended therapy: consider >13 wk transdermal patch + gum as needed	• Hiccups, dyspepsia, excess salivation; side effects from incorrect chewing (mouth and jaw soreness, nausea/vomiting) Precautions • Recent MI within 2 wk, serious arrhythmias, unstable angina • Adolescents <18 y • Pregnancy and breastfeeding

Nicotine inhaler blood: levels of nicotine peak at 5–10 min

Standard dosage	Dosing modifications	Adverse events
• 6–16 cartridges/d Initially use 1 cartridge q 1–2 h as needed and at least 6 cartridges per day • Max = 16 cartridges/d • Prescription only • Duration 3–6 mo	• Combination + extended therapy: consider >13 wk transdermal patch + ad lib inhaler	• Rhinitis, mouth/throat irritation, cough, dyspepsia, hiccups, and headaches Precautions • Recent MI within 2 wk, serious arrhythmias, unstable angina • Adolescents <18 y • Pregnancy and breastfeeding

Nicotine spray: blood levels of nicotine peak at 5–10 min

Standard dosage	Dosing modifications	Adverse events

• 8–40 doses/d
    One dose = 2 sprays (1 spray in each nostril)
    Initially use 1–2 doses/h and at least 8 doses/d
• Max = 5 doses/h or 40 doses (80 sprays)/d
• Prescription only
• Duration 3–6 mo
	• Combination + extended therapy:
	    consider >13 wk transdermal patch + nasal spray as needed
		• Rhinitis, sneezing, nasal/throat irritation, cough, and headache
		Precautions
		• Recent MI within 2 wk, serious arrhythmias, unstable angina
		• Adolescents <18 y
		• Pregnancy and breastfeeding

Abbreviations: cigs, cigarettes; MI, motivational interviewing; NRT, nicotine replacement therapy.

attempts leads to greater attempts to quit smoking, it does not increase smoking abstinence at 6 months.[85] Pretreatment with FDA-approved pharmacotherapy before a patient is ready to quit increases eventual abstinence.[86] Initial therapy with varenicline longer than the FDA-recommended 1 week pretreatment period may be needed to exert its maximum effect.[87] Among patients with no intention to stop smoking, reduction support plus medication was shown to increase smoking abstinence compared with no intervention or reduction support alone.[88]

ROLE OF HARM REDUCTION APPROACHES IN TOBACCO DEPENDENCE TREATMENT
Electronic Cigarettes

The explosive increase of modified risk tobacco product systems over the past decade has sustained a clinical debate as to whether these devices could be used as tobacco cessation devices through a harm reduction mechanism. The devices range from third- and fourth-generation electronic cigarettes (including JUUL) to hookahs to IQOS (I quit original smoking) products. Although reduced use of combustible tobacco products without quitting is a more achievable outcome than durable cessation with any nicotine delivery system, clinical benefits with respect to serious long-term outcomes such as mortality, lung cancer, chronic obstructive pulmonary disease, and heart disease are minimal or nonexistent.[89,90] A large prospective cohort study reported that, compared with never smokers, active smokers of fewer than 1 cigarette per day (CPD) (hazard ratio [HR] = 1.64; 95% CI, 1.07–2.51) or 1 to 10 CPD (HR = 1.87; 95% CI, 1.64–2.13) had a higher all-cause mortality risk.[91] Thus, only harm reduction

---

Table 2
FDA-approved pharmacotherapy to treat tobacco dependence

Bupropion SR

Standard dosage	Dosing modifications	Adverse events

• Start treatment 1–2 wk before quit date
    150 mg q am × 3 d, then 150 mg bid (max 300 mg/d)
• Duration: 12 wk, with maintenance for up to 6 mo in selected patients
• Decrease dose with renal or hepatic disease
Contraindications
• Anorexia nervosa or bulimia
• Seizure disorder
• Abruptly stopping alcohol or sedatives/benzodiazepines
• MAO inhibitors in preceding 14 d or concurrently taking reversible MAO inhibitors
	• Combination therapy:
	    Consider transdermal nicotine patch + bupropion
	• Extended duration:
	    consider additional 12 wk of treatment after quitting
		• Insomnia, seizures; difficulty concentrating; rare neuropsychiatric events (warning for serious mental health side effects removed in December 2016)
		Precautions
		• Medications and conditions that lower seizure threshold
		• Adolescents
		• Pregnancy (C)* and breastfeeding
		• Hepatic impairment

Abbreviation: MAO, monoamine oxidase.

* Adverse effect on the fetus and there are no adequate and well-controlled studies in humans, but potential benefits may warrant use of the drug in pregnant women despite potential risks.

Table 3
FDA-approved pharmacotherapy to treat tobacco dependence

Varenicline		
Standard dose	Dosing modification	Adverse effects

• Start 1 wk before quit date
    Days 1–3: 0.5 mg q am
    Days 4–7: 0.5 mg bid
    Weeks 2–12: 1 mg bid
• Decrease dose in renal disease
    CrCl <30: initial 0.5 mg, max dose 0.5 mg bid
    HD: max 0.5 mg daily
• Duration: 12 wk
	• Pretreatment:
	    Consider initiating 30 d before quit date OR decreasing smoking over a 12-wk period of treatment before quitting.
	• Extended duration:
	    Consider additional 12 wk of treatment after quitting
		• Insomnia, nausea, headache; rare neuropsychiatric events (warning for serious mental health side effects removed in December 2016)
		Precautions
		• Renal disease (see dose adjustment)
		• Pregnancy (C)* and breastfeeding
		• Adolescents

Abbreviations: CrCl, creatinine clearance; HD, hemodialysis.

  * Adverse effect on the fetus and there are no adequate and well-controlled studies in humans, but potential benefits may warrant use of the drug in pregnant women despite potential risks.

approaches that culminate in smoking cessation can consistently affect disease risk. A limited number of randomized trials of e-cigarettes for smoking cessation has been published.[92,93] A study by Hajek and colleagues,[93] using a pragmatic design, showed superior quit rates among smokers using e-cigarettes compared with those using conventional NRT. Findings were compromised by suboptimal use of nicotine replacement in the comparator arm and the high persistence of e-cigarette use in the intervention arm at the end of the trial. Although new trials are ongoing, the current question is whether chronic nicotine delivery is a satisfactory smoking cessation outcome especially in persons at high risk of lung malignancy. One trial of long-term versus standard NRT showed equivalent biochemically verified quit rates at 12 months, establishing questionable therapeutic benefit of long-term regimens.[94] In addition, the likely cumulative morbidity and alarming addictiveness of very high content nicotine delivery systems, such as JUUL, and the substantial prevalence of dual use (combustible tobacco and e-cigarettes) among youth and young adults undermines the practical utility of these products as valid tobacco cessation agents in persons with lung cancer.

High levels of known carcinogens, such as formaldehyde, and DNA damage agents have been detected in e-cigarette solutions.[95,96] Although premarket reviews of currently marketed e-cigarettes were mandated by the FDA under 2016 post-deeming rules, most manufacturers have not submitted applications, thereby delaying the only mechanism that requires listing of all ingredients.[97] Without that information, the spectrum of carcinogen exposure cannot be graded among available products. The long-term health consequences of inhalational exposure to these components are of great concern in persons already at high risk of lung cancer.

One trenchant issue is whether long-term nicotine delivery systems affect lung cancer initiation or progression. Nicotine, the major addictive component of tobacco smoke, is not considered a carcinogen based on animal model data. However, nicotine and selective metabolites possess many tumor-promoting properties both in vitro and in vivo.[98,99] The tumor-promoting functions of nicotine are exerted through the activation of nAChRs. Studies of lung cancer cell lines and tumor xenografts in mouse models show tumor survival and prometastatic effects of nicotine that occur primarily through the $\alpha 7$ subunit of nAChRs.[100] A recent study using lung cancer cell lines showed shared and equivalent induction of tumor-promoting cascades by cigarette smoke and e-cigarette extracts.[101]

Low Nicotine Strategy

The low nicotine strategy for tobacco cessation is anchored on the concept that, by reducing the nicotine content in combustible cigarettes to a nonaddictive level, cessation will be enabled and youth initiation will not result in nicotine addiction or long-term cigarette use.[102,103] The foundational studies employ a cigarette standard with 0.3 mg nicotine per gram; nicotine content of cigarettes from commercially generated American tobacco plants range from 7.5 to 13.4 mg of nicotine per g.[104] Efficacy trials of varying rigor show evidence of either absent or a modest reduction in tobacco product use with this approach but no improved cessation rates compared with conventional approaches.[105–107] Historically, efforts to alter cigarette composition (eg, tar, filters) to create a "healthier product" were undermined by changes in smoking topography that served to maintain adverse levels of toxin exposure. Regarding low nicotine cigarettes, long-term studies are not yet available making concerns about relapse and altered smoking topography unresolved.

SUMMARY

The diagnosis of lung cancer avails not just a teachable moment for the patient but a series of encounters that are fertile contexts for successful tobacco dependence discussions and treatment. The multidisciplinary platform embodied in the tumor board model easily extends to smoking cessation programs provided that caregivers are facile with the critical tenets of pharmacologic and behavioral therapy. Addressing the often-complicating factors of poverty, stigma, shame, and physician discomfort and nihilism can be critical to the management of smoking cessation in the setting of lung cancer. Widespread implementation of guidelines for tobacco dependence treatment on any cancer diagnosis should be a rational and cost-effective goal of care.

CONFLICT OF INTEREST

The authors have no commercial or financial conflicts of interests to disclose.

REFERENCES

1. Centers for Disease Control and Prevention. Available at: https://www.cdc.gov/tobacco/data_statistics/fact_sheets/fast_facts/index.htm#ref. Accessed February 20, 2019.
2. Siegel RL, Miller KD, Jemal A. Cancer statistics, 2019. CA Cancer J Clin 2019;69(1):7–34.
3. Lortet-Tieulent J, Goding Sauer A, Siegel RL, et al. State-level cancer mortality attributable to cigarette smoking in the United States. JAMA Intern Med 2016;176(12):1792–8.
4. Irvin Vidrine J, Reitzel LR, Wetter DW. The role of tobacco in cancer health disparities. Curr Oncol Rep 2009;11(6):475–81.
5. Cokkinides VE, Halpern MT, Barbeau EM, et al. Racial and ethnic disparities in smoking-cessation interventions: analysis of the 2005 National Health Interview Survey. Am J Prev Med 2008;34(5):404–12.
6. Fu SS, Sherman SE, Yano EM, et al. Ethnic disparities in the use of nicotine replacement therapy for smoking cessation in an equal access health care system. Am J Health Promot 2005;20(2):108–16.
7. Alexander LA, Trinidad DR, Sakuma KL, et al. Why we must continue to investigate menthol's role in the African American Smoking Paradox. Nicotine Tob Res 2016;18(Suppl 1):S91–101.
8. Danaei G, Rimm EB, Oza S, et al. The promise of prevention: the effects of four preventable risk factors on national life expectancy and life expectancy disparities by race and county in the United States. PLoS Med 2010;7(3):e1000248.
9. Schütte S, Dietrich D, Montet X, et al. Participation in lung cancer screening programs: are there gender and social differences? A systematic review. Public Health Rev 2018;39:23.
10. Alberg AJ, Shopland DR, Cummings KM. The 2014 Surgeon General's report: commemorating the 50th Anniversary of the 1964 Report of the Advisory Committee to the US Surgeon General and updating the evidence on the health consequences of cigarette smoking. Am J Epidemiol 2014;179(4):403–12.
11. Parsons A, Daley A, Begh R, et al. Influence of smoking cessation after diagnosis of early stage lung cancer on prognosis: systematic review of observational studies with meta-analysis. BMJ 2010;340:b5569.
12. Kawahara M, Ushijima S, Kamimori T, et al. Second primary tumours in more than 2-year disease-free survivors of small-cell lung cancer in Japan: the role of smoking cessation. Br J Cancer 1998;78(3):409–12.
13. Sardari Nia P, Weyler J, Colpaert C, et al. Prognostic value of smoking status in operated non-small cell lung cancer. Lung Cancer 2005;47(3):351–9.
14. Japuntich SJ, Kumar P, Pendergast JF, et al. Smoking status and survival among a national cohort of lung and colorectal cancer patients. Nicotine Tob Res 2019;21(4):497–504.
15. Chen J, Qi Y, Wampfler JA, et al. Effect of cigarette smoking on quality of life in small cell lung cancer patients. Eur J Cancer 2012;48(11):1593–601.
16. Gemine RE, Ghosal R, Collier G, et al. Longitudinal study to assess impact of smoking at diagnosis and quitting on 1-year survival for people with non-small cell lung cancer. Lung Cancer 2019;129:1–7.
17. Shields PG, Herbst RS, Arenberg D, et al. Smoking cessation, Version 1.2016, NCCN clinical practice guidelines in oncology. J Natl Compr Canc Netw 2016;14(11):1430–68.
18. Hanna N, Mulshine J, Wollins DS, et al. Tobacco cessation and control a decade later: American Society of Clinical Oncology policy statement update. J Clin Oncol 2013;31(25):3147–57.
19. Aberle DR, Adams AM, Berg CD, et al. Reduced lung-cancer mortality with low-dose computed

tomographic screening. N Engl J Med 2011;365(5): 395–409.

20. De Koning H, Van Der Aalst C, Ten Haaf K, et al. Effects of volume CT lung cancer screening: mortality results of the NELSON randomised-controlled population based trial. J Thorac Oncol 2018;13(10): S185.

21. Tanner NT, Gebregziabher M, Hughes Halbert C, et al. Racial differences in outcomes within the National Lung Screening Trial. Implications for widespread implementation. Am J Respir Crit Care Med 2015;192(2):200–8.

22. Tanner NT, Kanodra NM, Gebregziabher M, et al. The association between smoking abstinence and mortality in the National Lung Screening Trial. Am J Respir Crit Care Med 2016;193(5):534–41.

23. Centers for Medicare and Medicaid Services. Decision memo for screening for lung cancer with low dose computed tomography (LDCT). Available at: https://www.cms.gov/medicare-coverage-database/details/nca-decision-memo.aspx?NCAId=274. Accessed April 20, 2019.

24. Mazzone P, Powell CA, Arenberg D, et al. Components necessary for high-quality lung cancer screening: American College of Chest Physicians and American Thoracic Society Policy Statement. Chest 2015;147(2):295–303.

25. Ma J, Ward EM, Smith R, et al. Annual number of lung cancer deaths potentially avertable by screening in the United States. Cancer 2013;119(7):1381–5.

26. Wiener RS, Gould MK, Arenberg DA, et al. An official American Thoracic Society/American College of Chest Physicians policy statement: implementation of low-dose computed tomography lung cancer screening programs in clinical practice. Am J Respir Crit Care Med 2015;192(7): 881–91.

27. Fucito LM, Czabafy S, Hendricks PS, et al. Pairing smoking-cessation services with lung cancer screening: a clinical guideline from the Association for the Treatment of Tobacco Use and Dependence and the Society for Research on Nicotine and Tobacco. Cancer 2016;122(8):1150–9.

28. Kathuria H, Detterbeck FC, Fathi JT, et al. Stakeholder research priorities for smoking cessation interventions within lung cancer screening programs. An official American Thoracic Society Research Statement. Am J Respir Crit Care Med 2017;196(9):1202–12.

29. Burris JL, Studts JL, DeRosa AP, et al. Systematic review of tobacco use after lung or head/neck cancer diagnosis: results and recommendations for future research. Cancer Epidemiol Biomarkers Prev 2015;24(10):1450–61.

30. Slatore CG, Baumann C, Pappas M, et al. Smoking behaviors among patients receiving computed tomography for lung cancer screening. Systematic review in support of the U.S. preventive services task force. Ann Am Thorac Soc 2014;11(4):619–27.

31. Ostroff JS, Copeland A, Borderud SP, et al. Readiness of lung cancer screening sites to deliver smoking cessation treatment: current practices, organizational priority, and perceived barriers. Nicotine Tob Res 2016;18(5):1067–75.

32. Chapple A, Ziebland S, McPherson A. Stigma, shame, and blame experienced by patients with lung cancer: qualitative study. BMJ 2004; 328(7454):1470.

33. Hamann HA, Shen MJ, Thomas AJ, et al. Development and preliminary psychometric evaluation of a patient-reported outcome measure for lung cancer stigma: the Lung Cancer Stigma Inventory (LCSI). Stigma Health 2018;3(3):195–203.

34. Ostroff JS, Riley KE, Shen MJ, et al. Lung cancer stigma and depression: validation of the lung cancer stigma inventory. Psychooncology 2019;28(5): 1011–7.

35. Ostroff JS. Innovative approach to reduce lung cancer stigma. ClinicalTrials.gov: a service of the U.S. National Institutes of Health. Available at: https://clinicaltrials.gov/ct2/show/NCT03750 864. Accessed May 5, 2019.

36. Schaap MM, van Agt HM, Kunst AE. Identification of socioeconomic groups at increased risk for smoking in European countries: looking beyond educational level. Nicotine Tob Res 2008;10(2): 359–69.

37. Zhu SH, Anderson CM, Zhuang YL, et al. Smoking prevalence in Medicaid has been declining at a negligible rate. PLoS One 2017;12(5):e0178279.

38. Hovanec J, Siemiatycki J, Conway DI, et al. Lung cancer and socioeconomic status in a pooled analysis of case-control studies. PLoS One 2018;13(2): e0192999.

39. Sanderson M, Aldrich MC, Levine RS, et al. Neighbourhood deprivation and lung cancer risk: a nested case-control study in the USA. BMJ Open 2018;8(9):e021059.

40. Polak M, Genowska A, Szafraniec K, et al. Area-based socio-economic inequalities in mortality from lung cancer and respiratory diseases. Int J Environ Res Public Health 2019;16(10) [pii:E1791].

41. Berry MF, Canchola AJ, Gensheimer MF, et al. Factors associated with treatment of clinical stage I non-small-cell lung cancer: a population-based analysis. Clin Lung Cancer 2018;19(5): e745–58.

42. Rosenstock I. Why people use health services. Millbank Memorial Fund Q 1966;44:94–127.

43. Lasser KE, Kenst KS, Quintiliani LM, et al. Patient navigation to promote smoking cessation among low-income primary care patients: a pilot randomized controlled trial. J Ethn Subst Abuse 2013; 12(4):374–90.

44. Ko NY, Darnell JS, Calhoun E, et al. Can patient navigation improve receipt of recommended breast cancer care? Evidence from the National Patient Navigation Research Program. J Clin Oncol 2014;32(25):2758–64.

45. Brooks DR, Burtner JL, Borrelli B, et al. Twelve-month outcomes of a group-randomized community health advocate-led smoking cessation intervention in public housing. Nicotine Tob Res 2018; 20(12):1434–41.

46. Percac-Lima S, Ashburner JM, Rigotti NA, et al. Patient navigation for lung cancer screening among current smokers in community health centers a randomized controlled trial. Cancer Med 2018;7(3): 894–902.

47. Fraser DL, Fiore MC, Kobinsky K, et al. A randomized trial of incentives for smoking treatment in Medicaid members. Am J Prev Med 2017;53(6):754–63.

48. Lasser KE, Quintiliani LM, Truong V, et al. Effect of patient navigation and financial incentives on smoking cessation among primary care patients at an urban safety-net hospital: a randomized clinical trial. JAMA Intern Med 2017;177(12):1798–807.

49. Available at: https://www.pcori.org/research-results/2018/comparing-smoking-cessation-interventions-among-underserved-patients-referred. Accessed April 21, 2019

50. Wells M, Aitchison P, Harris F, et al. Barriers and facilitators to smoking cessation in a cancer context: a qualitative study of patient, family and professional views. BMC Cancer 2017;17(1):348.

51. Kathuria H, Koppelman E, Borrelli B, et al. Patient-physician discussions on lung cancer screening: a missed teachable moment to promote smoking cessation. Nicotine Tob Res 2018. https://doi.org/10.1093/ntr/nty254.

52. Brain K, Carter B, Lifford KJ, et al. Impact of low-dose CT screening on smoking cessation among high-risk participants in the UK Lung Cancer Screening Trial. Thorax 2017;72(10):912–8.

53. Sitas F, Weber MF, Egger S, et al. Smoking cessation after cancer. J Clin Oncol 2014;32(32):3593–5.

54. Karam-Hage M, Oughli HA, Rabius V, et al. Tobacco cessation treatment pathways for patients with cancer: 10 years in the making. J Natl Compr Canc Netw 2016;14(11):1469–77.

55. Metzl JM, Hansen H. Structural competency: theorizing a new medical engagement with stigma and inequality. Soc Sci Med 2014;103:126–33.

56. Berman M, Crane R, Seiber E, et al. Estimating the cost of a smoking employee. Tob Control 2014; 23(5):428–33.

57. Benowitz NL. Nicotine addiction. N Engl J Med 2010;362(24):2295–303.

58. Benowitz NL, Hukkanen J, Jacob P. Nicotine chemistry, metabolism, kinetics and biomarkers. Handb Exp Pharmacol 2009;(192):29–60.

59. Reid JL, Hammond D, Rynard VL, et al. Tobacco use in Canada: patterns and trends. University of Waterloo, Propel Centre for Population Health Impact; 2014. Available at: https://uwaterloo.ca/tobacco-use-canada/tobacco-use-canada-patterns-and-trends.

60. Fu SS, van Ryn M, Sherman SE, et al. Proactive tobacco treatment and population-level cessation: a pragmatic randomized clinical trial. JAMA Intern Med 2014;174(5):671–7.

61. Nahhas GJ, Wilson D, Talbot V, et al. Feasibility of implementing a hospital-based "Opt-Out" tobacco-cessation service. Nicotine Tob Res 2017;19(8):937–43.

62. Haas JS, Linder JA, Park ER, et al. Proactive tobacco cessation outreach to smokers of low socioeconomic status: a randomized clinical trial. JAMA Intern Med 2015;175(2):218–26.

63. Lewis M. Brain change in addiction as learning, not disease. N Engl J Med 2018;379(16):1551–60.

64. Leone FT, Evers-Casey S. Developing a rational approach to tobacco use treatment in pulmonary practice: a review of the biological basis of nicotine addiction. Clin Pulm Med 2012;19(2):53–61.

65. Stead LF, Koilpillai P, Fanshawe TR, et al. Combined pharmacotherapy and behavioural interventions for smoking cessation. Cochrane Database Syst Rev 2016;(3):CD008286.

66. Gómez-Coronado N, Walker AJ, Berk M, et al. Current and emerging pharmacotherapies for cessation of tobacco smoking. Pharmacotherapy 2018; 38(2):235–58.

67. Schnoll RA, Goelz PM, Veluz-Wilkins A, et al. Long-term nicotine replacement therapy: a randomized clinical trial. JAMA Intern Med 2015; 175(4):504–11.

68. Stahl SM, Pradko JF, Haight BR, et al. A review of the neuropharmacology of bupropion, a dual norepinephrine and dopamine reuptake inhibitor. Prim Care Companion J Clin Psychiatry 2004; 6(4):159–66.

69. Hays JT, Hurt RD, Rigotti NA, et al. Sustained-release bupropion for pharmacologic relapse prevention after smoking cessation. a randomized, controlled trial. Ann Intern Med 2001;135(6): 423–33.

70. Anthenelli RM, Benowitz NL, West R, et al. Neuropsychiatric safety and efficacy of varenicline, bupropion, and nicotine patch in smokers with and without psychiatric disorders (EAGLES): a double-blind, randomised, placebo-controlled clinical trial. Lancet 2016;387(10037):2507–20.

71. de Moura FB, McMahon LR. The contribution of $\alpha 4 \beta 2$ and non-$\alpha 4 \beta 2$ nicotinic acetylcholine receptors to the discriminative stimulus effects of nicotine and varenicline in mice. Psychopharmacology (Berl) 2017;234(5):781–92.

72. Chang PH, Chiang CH, Ho WC, et al. Combination therapy of varenicline with nicotine replacement therapy is better than varenicline alone: a systematic review and meta-analysis of randomized controlled trials. BMC Public Health 2015;15:689.

73. Tonstad S, Tønnesen P, Hajek P, et al. Effect of maintenance therapy with varenicline on smoking cessation: a randomized controlled trial. JAMA 2006;296(1):64–71.

74. Rennard S, Hughes J, Cinciripini PM, et al. A randomized placebo-controlled trial of varenicline for smoking cessation allowing flexible quit dates. Nicotine Tob Res 2012;14(3):343–50.

75. Ebbert JO, Hughes JR, West RJ, et al. Effect of varenicline on smoking cessation through smoking reduction: a randomized clinical trial. JAMA 2015; 313(7):687–94.

76. Lancaster T, Stead LF. Individual behavioural counselling for smoking cessation. Cochrane Database Syst Rev 2017;(3):CD001292.

77. Rigotti NA, Chang Y, Rosenfeld LC, et al. Interactive voice response calls to promote smoking cessation after hospital discharge: pooled analysis of two randomized clinical trials. J Gen Intern Med 2017;32(9):1005–13.

78. Whittaker R, McRobbie H, Bullen C, et al. Mobile phone-based interventions for smoking cessation. Cochrane Database Syst Rev 2016;(4):CD006611.

79. Klesges RC, Krukowski RA, Klosky JL, et al. Efficacy of a tobacco quitline among adult cancer survivors. Prev Med 2015;73:22–7.

80. Anderson CM, Cummins SE, Kohatsu ND, et al. Incentives and patches for Medicaid smokers: an RCT. Am J Prev Med 2018;55(6S2):S138–47.

81. Borrelli B. Advances in smoking cessation, . Motivational interviewing for smoking cessation. London: Future Medicine Ltd; 2013. p. 128–41.

82. Lai DT, Cahill K, Qin Y, et al. Motivational interviewing for smoking cessation. Cochrane Database Syst Rev 2010;(1):CD006936.

83. Klemperer EM, Hughes JR, Solomon LJ, et al. Motivational, reduction and usual care interventions for smokers who are not ready to quit: a randomized controlled trial. Addiction 2017;112(1):146–55.

84. 2008 PHS Guideline Update Panel Liasons, and Staff. Treating tobacco use and dependence: 2008 update U.S. Public Health Service Clinical Practice Guideline executive summary. Respir Care 2008;53(9):1217–22.

85. Carpenter MJ, Hughes JR, Gray KM, et al. Nicotine therapy sampling to induce quit attempts among smokers unmotivated to quit: a randomized clinical trial. Arch Intern Med 2011;171(21):1901–7.

86. Lindson N, Aveyard P, Hughes JR. Reduction versus abrupt cessation in smokers who want to quit. Cochrane Database Syst Rev 2010;(3): CD008033.

87. Hawk L. EVarQuit: extended pre-quit varenicline to assist in quitting smoking (NCT03262662) ClinicalTrials.gov: a service of the U.S. National Institutes of Health. Available at: https://clinicaltrials.gov/ct2/show/NCT03262662. Accessed May 21, 2019.

88. Wu L, Sun S, He Y, et al. Effect of smoking reduction therapy on smoking cessation for smokers without an intention to quit: an updated systematic review and meta-analysis of randomized controlled. Int J Environ Res Public Health 2015; 12(9):10235–53.

89. Hart C, Gruer L, Bauld L. Does smoking reduction in midlife reduce mortality risk? Results of 2 long-term prospective cohort studies of men and women in Scotland. Am J Epidemiol 2013;178(5):770–9.

90. Pisinger C, Godtfredsen NS. Is there a health benefit of reduced tobacco consumption? A systematic review. Nicotine Tob Res 2007;9(6):631–46.

91. Inoue-Choi M, Liao LM, Reyes-Guzman C, et al. Association of long-term, low-intensity smoking with all-cause and cause-specific mortality in the National Institutes of Health-AARP Diet and Health Study. JAMA Intern Med 2017;177(1):87–95.

92. Ghosh S, Drummond MB. Electronic cigarettes as smoking cessation tool: are we there? Curr Opin Pulm Med 2017;23(2):111–6.

93. Hajek P, Phillips-Waller A, Przulj D, et al. A randomized trial of e-cigarettes versus nicotine-replacement therapy. N Engl J Med 2019;380(7):629–37.

94. Ellerbeck EF, Nollen N, Hutcheson TD, et al. Effect of long-term nicotine replacement therapy vs standard smoking cessation for smokers with chronic lung disease: a randomized clinical trial. JAMA Netw Open 2018;1(5):e181843.

95. Korfei M. The underestimated danger of E-cigarettes—also in the absence of nicotine. Respir Res 2018;19(1):159.

96. Lee HW, Park SH, Weng MW, et al. E-cigarette smoke damages DNA and reduces repair activity in mouse lung, heart, and bladder as well as in human lung and bladder cells. Proc Natl Acad Sci U S A 2018;115(7):E1560–9.

97. Gottlieb MA. Regulation of E-cigarettes in the United States and its role in a youth epidemic. Children (Basel) 2019;6(3) [pii:E40].

98. Stepanov I, Carmella SG, Han S, et al. Evidence for endogenous formation of N'-nitrosonornicotine in some long-term nicotine patch users. Nicotine Tob Res 2009;11(1):99–105.

99. Hecht SS, Chen CB, Hirota N, et al. Tobacco-specific nitrosamines: formation from nicotine in vitro and during tobacco curing and carcinogenicity in strain A mice. J Natl Cancer Inst 1978;60(4): 819–24.

100. Schaal C, Chellappan SP. Nicotine-mediated cell proliferation and tumor progression in smoking-related cancers. Mol Cancer Res 2014;12(1):14–23.

101. Schaal CM, Bora-Singhal N, Kumar DM, et al. Regulation of Sox2 and stemness by nicotine and electronic-cigarettes in non-small cell lung cancer. Mol Cancer 2018;17(1):149.

102. Hatsukami DK, Benowitz NL, Donny E, et al. Nicotine reduction: strategic research plan. Nicotine Tob Res 2013;15(6):1003–13.

103. Benowitz NL, Henningfield JE. Reducing the nicotine content to make cigarettes less addictive. Tob Control 2013;22(Suppl 1):i14–7.

104. Kozlowski LT, Mehta NY, Sweeney CT, et al. Filter ventilation and nicotine content of tobacco in cigarettes from Canada, the United Kingdom, and the United States. Tob Control 1998;7(4):369–75.

105. Benowitz NL, Nardone N, Dains KM, et al. Effect of reducing the nicotine content of cigarettes on cigarette smoking behavior and tobacco smoke toxicant exposure: 2-year follow up. Addiction 2015; 110(10):1667–75.

106. Mercincavage M, Lochbuehler K, Wileyto EP, et al. Association of reduced nicotine content cigarettes with smoking behaviors and biomarkers of exposure among slow and fast nicotine metabolizers: a nonrandomized clinical trial. JAMA Netw Open 2018;1(4):e181346.

107. Donny EC, Denlinger RL, Tidey JW, et al. Randomized trial of reduced-nicotine standards for cigarettes. N Engl J Med 2015;373(14):1340–9.

Lung Cancer in Women
A Modern Epidemic

Christina R. MacRosty, DO[a], M. Patricia Rivera, MD[b],*

KEYWORDS

- Lung cancer in women • Lung cancer in nonsmokers • Sex differences in lung cancer
- Hormonal factors • Non-small cell lung cancer in women • Growth factor receptors
- Epidermal growth factor receptor

KEY POINTS

- Although the incidence of lung cancer in women is declining at a slower rate than in men, in many countries the incidence rate is increasing.
- Lung cancer is the leading cause of cancer deaths in women.
- Smoking remains the most important risk factor in women, but nonsmoking women are at higher risk for lung cancer compared with nonsmoking men.
- Sex-based differences in hormonal, environmental, and molecular factors may exist.

INTRODUCTION

Lung cancer remains a significant health problem worldwide for both men and women and is the leading cause of cancer death in many countries. Age-adjusted lung cancer incidence rates have historically been higher in men than in women, but the gap has narrowed, reflecting a decrease in the incidence rate in men and an increase in women. In the last 20 years, lung cancer incidence has been declining in many parts of the world, but the decline has been more notable in men. Smoking remains the most important risk factor, and increasing tobacco use in women in many parts of the world will further exacerbate the incidence and mortality of lung cancer in women. Tobacco exposure alone does not tell the entire story; lung cancer in nonsmokers is more common in women. Data support sex-based differences in the biology of lung cancer, but research has been limited. In this article, the authors summarize sex differences in incidence and mortality; tobacco exposure and risk; biological mechanisms that may affect risk, and differences in histology, prognosis, and treatment of lung cancer in women.

EPIDEMIOLOGY OF LUNG CANCER IN WOMEN
Incidence and Mortality

Although age-adjusted lung cancer incidence rates have historically been higher for men than for women in the United States, the gap has narrowed and incidence rates continue to decline more rapidly in men than in women (2.9 vs 1.5 per 100,000, respectively) (**Fig. 1**), partially explained by historical differences in tobacco cessation and increase in smoking prevalence in women.[1] A population-based study on incidence of lung cancer according to sex, race/ethnic group, and age group (ages 30–54 years) in the United States confirmed the trend of a more rapid decline in incidence among men, but alarmingly, female-to-male incidence rate ratios (IRR) increased from 0.82 (confidence interval [CI] 0.70–0.85) to 1.13 (CI 1.08–1.18) during

[a] Department of Medicine, Division of Pulmonary and Critical Care Medicine, Interventional Pulmonary Program, University of North Carolina at Chapel Hill, 130 Mason Farm Road, Chapel Hill, NC 27599-7020, USA;
[b] Division on Pulmonary and Critical Medicine, University of North Carolina at Chapel Hill, 130 Mason Farm Road, Suite 4125, Chapel Hill, NC 27599-7020, USA
* Corresponding author.
E-mail address: mprivera@med.unc.edu

Clin Chest Med 41 (2020) 53–65
https://doi.org/10.1016/j.ccm.2019.10.005

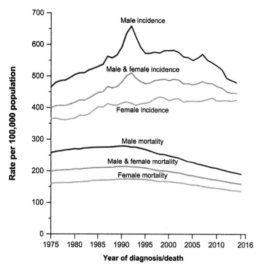

Fig. 1. Trends in cancer incidence (1975–2015) and mortality rates (1975–2016) by sex, United States. (*From* Siegel RL, Miller KD, Jemal A. Cancer Statistics 2019. *CA Cancer J Clin.* 2019 Jan; 69:7-34; with permission.)

health problem well through the first half of this century, particularly in women and in developing countries that continue to observe increasing incidence rates.[3–5] Country-specific data from GLOBOCAN 2012 on temporal trends of lung cancer incidence in 38 countries/regions, stratified by sex, revealed that incidence rates in men had increased in1, decreased in 22, and remained stable in 15 countries, whereas in women, rates had increased in 19, decreased in 1, and remained stable in 18 countries.[3] Highest incidence rates of lung cancer in women are seen in North America, Northern and Western Europe, Australia, and New Zealand, and the epidemic is still in early stages in China, Indonesia, and several African countries (**Fig. 2**).[3]

1995 to 1999 and 2010 to 2014, respectively. Crossover to higher incidence rate of lung cancer in younger women occurred in white women (0.88 [CI 0.84–0.92] to 1.17 [CI 1.11–1.23]) and more notably among Hispanic women (0.79 [CI 0.67–0.92] to 1.22 [CI 01.04–0.1.44]).[2]

Worldwide, lung cancer remains the most common cancer with an estimated 1.2 million new cases in 2018 and is projected to be a major

Lung cancer accounts for about 1.8 million deaths worldwide and is the leading cause of cancer deaths in women in 28 countries (**Fig. 3**).[3,6] In a recent study, age-standardized mortality rates (ASMR) for breast and lung cancer per 100,000 women were calculated from 2008 to 2014 and projected for 2015, 2020, 2025, and 2030 using a Bayesian log-linear Poisson model. Between 2015 and 2030, the median ASMR for lung cancer is projected to increase from 11.2 to 16.0 in 52 countries, whereas declines are expected for breast cancer, from 16.1 to 14.7. In half of the countries analyzed, and in nearly three-quarters of those classified as high-income countries, the ASMR for lung cancer has already surpassed or will surpass the breast cancer ASMR before 2030.[7]

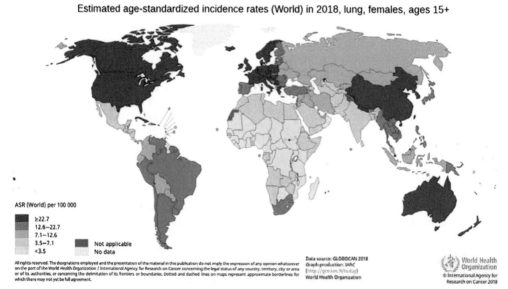

Fig. 2. Estimated lung cancer incidence worldwide 2018. (*From* World Health Organization. International Agency for Research on Cancer. Available at: http://gco.iarc.fr/today/online-analysis-map.)

Estimated age-standardized mortality rates (World) in 2018, lung, females, ages 15+

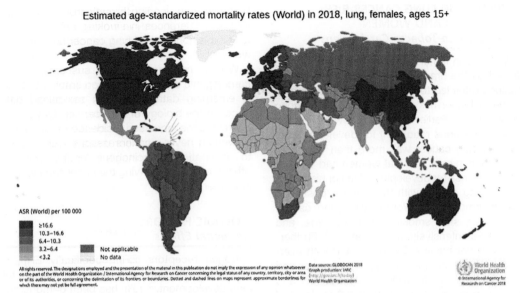

ASR (World) per 100 000

≥16.6
10.3–16.6
6.4–10.3
3.2–6.4   Not applicable
<3.2   No data

Data source: GLOBOCAN 2018
Graph production: IARC
(http://gco.iarc.fr/today)
World Health Organization

World Health Organization
© International Agency for Research on Cancer 2018

Fig. 3. Estimated lung cancer mortality worldwide 2018: women. (*From* World Health Organization. International Agency for Research on Cancer. Available at: http://gco.iarc.fr/today/online-analysis-map.)

Smoking and Lung Cancer Risk

Cigarette smoking is the major cause of lung cancer among female smokers in United States and contributes to about 90% of lung cancer deaths.[8] A study measuring temporal trends in mortality across 3 time periods (1959–1965, 1982–1988, and 2000–2010) among female smokers revealed a large increase (by a factor of 16.8) in deaths from lung cancer over the entire 50-year period, about half of which occurred during the past 20 years.[9] Among women, whites have the highest incidence of tobacco-related lung cancer (54.3%) compared with blacks (49.2%), American Indian/ Alaskan Natives (39%), and Asian/Pacific Islanders (27.9%).[8]

Although the overall prevalence of cigarette smoking in the United States has decreased from 42% in 1964 to 15.5% in 2016 (13.5% in women vs 17.5% in men), smoking rates have remained relatively stable in recent years (2014–2017).[8,10] Using data from the National Health Interview Survey from 1970 through 2016, Jemal and colleagues calculated the prevalence of current smoking and average number of cigarettes smoked daily according to sex, age, and race/ethnic group and found that in younger cohorts, the difference in smoking prevalence between men and women became progressively smaller due to female and male smoking initiation rates converging and decreased smoking cessation rates among women.[2] Although smoking prevalence has been decreasing worldwide, trends in smoking vary dramatically across countries and gender.[11] Women smoke at nearly the same rate as men in high-income countries but they smoke much less than men in many low- and middle-income countries.[12] A major global concern is that projected smoking prevalence rates in women will increase in low- and middle-income countries.[13]

Stabilization of smoking rates in women in some countries and increase in other countries worldwide is alarming considering the 52.7% incidence of new tobacco-related lung cancer cases and indicates a critical need to address factors contributing to female smoking.[8,10]

Lung Cancer in Nonsmokers

Worldwide, an estimated 25% of patients with lung cancer are never smokers, and lung cancer in never-smokers is the seventh most common cause of cancer deaths.[14,15] In the United States, approximately 10% to 15% of non-small cell lung cancer (NSCLC) cases occur annually in non-smokers, more commonly in women than men (17.5% vs 6.9%, respectively; *P*<.001) and more commonly in black than white patients.[16,17] This is in contrast to Asia, where more than 50% of women with lung cancer are never-smokers.[17,18] Although the basis for the high rate of lung cancer in Asian never-smokers is unknown, exposure to fumes from heating cooking oils and burning coal in poorly ventilated areas have been implicated.[19] Adenocarcinoma is the most frequent lung cancer histology in never-smokers, often with specific driver mutations.[14]

DIFFERENCES IN LUNG CANCER RISK BETWEEN MEN AND WOMEN
Susceptibility to Tobacco Carcinogens

The increase in female smoking rates after 1960s followed by the dramatic increase in lung cancer incidence rates led to the hypothesis that women may be at higher risk after exposure to tobacco carcinogens.[20] Earlier studies showed that in smokers, the odds ratio (OR) for development of small cell lung cancer was more than double in women than in men and that women had 1.5 to 2 times higher risk for developing all major histologic types of lung cancer with the same exposure to cigarette smoke.[21–24] Women with lung cancer are younger, start smoking at a later age, and smoke less intensively than men.[24–26] Furthermore, a higher relative risk associated with ever-smoking and level of smoking has been reported in women than men for all lung cancers (12.7 and 9.1 for ever-smoking and 27.9 vs 9.6 for level of smoking, respectively), suggesting that smoking-related morbidity and mortality may have a greater impact on women than men.[27,28]

Increased susceptibility to tobacco carcinogens is controversial, as several studies have found the risk to be similar between men and women. A study evaluating 279,214 men and 184,623 women in the United States showed smoking was associated with similar incidence rates of all histologic subtypes of lung cancer except squamous cell, which had a higher incidence in men.[29] A European study compared 3723 men and women with lung cancer with 4075 controls and found that risk comparing ever-smokers with never-smokers was higher among men than women (OR 16.1 versus 4.2, respectively).[30] A case-control study collected information on lifetime smoking history and evaluated the role of smoking in lung cancer risk combined with environmental and genetic factors. The OR for lung cancer in women was 12.3 compared with 42.2 in men (for all subjects, smokers and nonsmokers), whereas the OR for lung cancer in female ever-smokers was 7.2 compared with 7.1 in male ever-smokers. When evaluated in the context of histologic subtypes, OR for pack-years among adenocarcinoma subtypes was higher in men than in women, with a negative interaction between female sex and smoking ($P = .005$), leading to a conclusion that there is no support for a higher susceptibility to tobacco-related lung cancer in women.[31] A recent study reported that although smoking prevalence was lower in women born after 1965, the incidence rate of lung cancer was significantly higher, especially in white and Hispanic women, who smoke less than young

Hispanic men, leading investigators to conclude that sex differences in smoking behavior do not fully explain increased lung cancer rates in young women.[2]

Women may not be more susceptible to the carcinogenic effects of tobacco smoke, but there is emerging data supporting sex-based differences in the biology of lung cancer. Of particular interest is the increased incidence of lung cancer in women never-smokers despite less exposure to occupational carcinogens lending weight to other mechanisms driving the increased incidence in women (**Box 1**).

BIOLOGIC FACTORS
Hormonal Effects

Estrogen receptors (ER), specifically ERβ, are expressed in the lung and likely play a role in fetal lung development.[32] ERβ has been demonstrated in human NSCLC cell lines; is overexpressed relative to normal lung tissue; is a functional receptor with affinity for the active form of estrogen, β-estradiol; and its activity can be blocked in vitro with the ER inhibitor fulvestrant.[32] Exactly how estrogen is involved in lung carcinogenesis is not well known, but several possible mechanisms have been reported (**Box 2**).[32,33]

Progesterone has been shown to inhibit cell proliferation and induce apoptosis in NSCLC; inhibiting cell migration via progesterone receptors (PR) correlates with longer overall survival.[32] Aromatase plays a role in the conversion of androstenedione to estrone and testosterone to B-estradiol and has been detected in lung tissue.[32] Aromatase-positive NSCLC cells have been shown to produce B-estradiol with decrease in growth of human NSCLC in vitro when treated with aromatase inhibitors indicating potential tumor secretion of estrogens, especially within inflammatory cells responding to cancer cells within the lung.[32] Studies have shown lower incidence of primary lung cancer in patients with breast cancer after treatment with tamoxifen and greater chance of survival in women older than 65 years who expressed lower levels of aromatase in stage I and II NSCLC.[32,34]

A link between hormonal factors and lung cancer risk has been debated. An increased risk of lung cancer in women due to hormone replacement therapy (HRT) and interactions with smoking (OR 1.7 and 32.4 in nonsmokers and smokers, respectively) has been reported.[35] Although a population-based study consisting of 23,244 women undergoing HRT showed an increased risk (relative risk [RR] 1.26) of lung cancer, with most of the cases occurring in women younger

---

Box 1
Plausible biological differences for increased risk of lung cancer in women

Hormonal Factors

- *Estrogen receptors:* overexpressed in human NSCLC cell lines; may play a role in gene regulation, modulation of gene expression in tumor cells, direct carcinogenesis via formation of DNA adducts, growth factor gene activation, stimulating angiogenesis, accelerating metabolism of smoking-related carcinogens.
- *Progesterone:* inhibits cell proliferation and induces apoptosis in NSCLC, inhibits cell migration

Molecular Changes

- *DNA adducts:* formed by activation of polycyclic aromatic hydrocarbons (PAH) that bind to DNA; lead to mutations in tumor growth genes
- *Cytochrome P450 enzymes:*CYP1A1; responsible for activation of PAH
- *Glutathione S-transferases:* detoxify active forms of PAH

Genetic Factors

- *p53 gene:* tumor suppressor gene that, when activated, minimizes damage from DNA, metabolic stressors, or oncogenes; susceptible to mutations that alter its function or cause it to undergo oncogenic activities
- *Kristin rat sarcoma viral oncogene (KRAS) mutation*: oncogenic when overexpressed
- *DNA repair:* essential to repair damage to genome from exogenous and endogenous factors; decreased DNA repair capacity is associated with increased lung cancer risk
- *Growth factors:* involved in signaling pathways related to initiation of the cell cycle, cell proliferation, differentiation, migration, apoptosis; alterations result in unregulated cell growth; gastrin-releasing peptide is X-linked and stimulates growth of bronchial epithelial cells and is involved in mitogenesis of small cell and non-small cell lung cancers; endothelial growth factor receptor has tyrosine kinase activity, and activation triggers a signaling cascade leading to malignant cell proliferation, decreased apoptosis, increased tumor cell motility, and angiogenesis
- *Genetic predisposition*: variations in 3 locations in the genome were associated with lung cancer in Asian female never-smokers

Infections

- *Human papilloma virus (HPV)*: high-risk HPV causes genomic instability that can lead to malignant transformation
- *Nontuberculous mycobacteria*: chronic inflammatory microenvironment may predispose to development of lung cancer

Prior History of Radiation

- *Radiation therapy for breast cancer:* associated with increased risk of second primary lung cancer

---

than 60 years, the higher prevalence of smokers in the cohort compared with the population could have explained the 26% excess of lung cancer.[36] In contrast, 3 cohort studies suggested a protective role of endogenous estrogen with reduction in lung cancer risk with later onset of menopause.[37–39] Schabath and colleagues reported a reduced risk of lung cancer (OR 0.59) in current smokers undergoing HRT, although this protective effect was not seen in former or never smokers.[40] A meta-analysis examining the impact of estrogen therapy, combined estrogen/progestin therapy (EPT), and any HRT on lung cancer risk showed a 27% decrease in women treated with any HRT

regardless of smoking history. Subset analysis of lung adenocarcinoma revealed a significant increased risk (attributable risk of 76%) in women ever treated with HRT and no change in risk among women treated with combined EPT.[41]

Molecular Changes

DNA adducts

Bulky DNA adducts, formed by activation of polycyclic aromatic hydrocarbons (PAHs) to highly reactive compounds that bind to DNA, are higher in women with lung cancer.[42–44] CYP1A1 gene, one of the cytochrome P450 enzymes, activates PAH, whereas the enzyme glutathione

Box 2
Mechanisms by which estrogen may be involved in lung carcinogenesis

- Modulate expression of PH metabolizing enzymes
- Modulate gene expression and regulation
- Act as direct carcinogen via the formation of DNA adducts
- Activate several growth factors genes such a transforming growth factor (TGF) alpha and epidermal growth factor (EGF) that mediate cell division in lung cancer
- Stimulate angiogenesis
- Interact with cigarette smoking by accelerating metabolism of smoking-derived carcinogens

S-transferase (GST) detoxifies active forms of PAH; and individuals with higher inducible CYP1A1 or decreased GSTM1 phenotypes may be at higher risk of lung cancer than those without those phenotypes.[45–47] In vitro studies revealed higher baseline levels of CYP1A1 in cell lines of female origin as well as higher CYP1A1 activity after exposure to cigarette smoke concentrate, indicating increased susceptibility to carcinogens in female cell lines.[43,44] A study of normal lung tissue from 159 patients with lung cancer showed that female and male smokers had higher levels of DNA adducts compared with nonsmokers, although women in the study had lower smoke exposure (22.9 vs 33 pack-years) and were younger (56.2 years vs 62.2 years).[48] Moreover, female smokers had significantly higher levels of DNA adducts compared with male smokers (25.3 vs 12 per 10^8 DNA bases), which correlated with CYP1A1 mRNA expression, indicating sex differences in PAH-DNA adduct formation in the lung.[48] Among nonsmoking women, CYP1A1 polymorphisms are associated with increased risk of lung cancer, thus contributing to the increased overall risk of lung cancer in women, regardless of smoking history.[43]

Genetic mutations

Sporadic cancers occur as a result of spontaneous or DNA-damage associated mutations within somatic cells.[49] The tumor protein 53 gene (p53) is a tumor-suppressor gene that, when activated by certain stressors, causes downstream reactions that counteract or minimize damage from DNA, metabolic stressors, or oncogenes.[49] p53 is susceptible to numerous alterations and oncogenic activities and is a common tumor-associated mutation seen in lung cancer.[49,50] Smoking induces p53 mutations by forming DNA adducts. Kure and colleagues examined 115 surgically resected NSCLCs and demonstrated a higher frequency of p53 mutations and DNA adducts in women than in men despite lower exposure to carcinogens from cigarette smoking in female patients, suggesting that women may be at greater risk for tobacco-related NSCLC regardless of level of smoking exposure.[51] Higher frequency of p53 mutations in female smokers compared with male smokers and female never-smokers has been reported suggesting that lung cancers in female smokers demonstrate more tobacco-related mutations than in male smokers and female nonsmokers.[52]

Kirsten rat sarcoma viral oncogene (K-ras) mutation, within the Ras family of oncogenes, encodes a protein that is oncogenic when overexpressed. K-ras mutations are more common in smokers compared with nonsmokers (35%–43% versus 0%–6%, respectively) and in adenocarcinoma and are associated with DNA adduct formation.[53–55] Among never-smokers, the most common K-ras mutation is a transversion mutation from $G \rightarrow A$ (known as G12D), whereas the most common K-ras mutation in former and current smokers is a $G \rightarrow T$ transversion mutation, known as G12C.[54] The G12C mutation was reported to be more frequent in women than in men with lung cancer although more commonly, women had smoked less and were younger (34 pack-years vs 40 pack-years on average), suggesting that women are more susceptible to smoking-related K-ras mutant lung adenocarcinomas.[54] Nelson and colleagues reported a statistically significant association between female sex and K-ras mutations (OR = 3.3; 95% CI: 1.9–7.9) after adjustment for carcinogen exposures and a strong association between K-ras mutation and decreased survival in stage I lung adenocarcinoma.[55]

DNA repair capacity

DNA repair is critical to repairing damage to the genome from exogenous environmental toxins and endogenous factors.[56] A family of proteins is involved in removing and repairing damaged DNA segments, and a correlation between carcinogenesis and DNA adducts has been reported.[42] Female smokers are reported to have higher levels of DNA adducts than male smokers after adjusting for smoking dose (13.2–17.8 vs 9–9.7 per 10^6, respectively).[51,57,58] A case-control study of 764 patients with lung cancer and 677 controls found significantly lower DNA repair capacity in women than men (7.46% vs 8.15%), and decreased DNA repair capacity was found to be associated with increased lung cancer risk in younger patients, female patients, and those with a family history of lung cancer.[56,58]

Growth factors

Growth factors and their signaling pathways are involved in initiation of the cell cycle, cell proliferation, differentiation, and apoptosis; and genetic aberrations in signaling pathways can lead to unregulated expression of growth and subsequent developmental abnormalities, and chronic diseases.[59] Gastrin-releasing peptide (GRP) is a growth factor within the bombesin-like peptide family that stimulates growth of bronchial epithelial cells and helps regulate human lung development by acting as an autocrine and paracrine growth factor for fetal lung tissue.[60–62] GRP is secreted by pulmonary neuroendocrine cells and is thought to play a role in mitogenesis both in small cell cancers and NSCLCs.[60,62,63] The gene for the GRP receptor (GRPR) is X-linked and located near a cluster of genes that escape X inactivation, thus women can have 2 actively transcribed alleles for the GRPR gene.[64] GRPR mRNA expression was more common in female than in male nonsmokers (55% and 0%, respectively) and in female smokers with less tobacco exposure (1–25 pack-years) compared with men with similar exposure (75% and 20%, respectively).[64] Furthermore, women with GRPR mRNA expression developed lung cancer with significantly less tobacco exposure than men (41 and 59.9 pack-years, respectively).[64] Activation of cells that secrete GRP results in activation of proteins involved in pathways regulating cell proliferation, survival, and migration, suggesting that GRP may play a role in metastasis as well as cell proliferation.[62] Higher levels of GRP are expressed in adenocarcinoma, the most common histology in nonsmokers, and human airway cells exposed to estrogen show increased GRPR expression, suggesting that GRPR gene may be regulated by estrogen.[62,64]

Endothelial growth factor receptor (EGFR/ErbB1) is a member of a family of cell membrane receptors with tyrosine kinase activity that includes HER1, HER2/neu, HER3, and HER4. Activation of EGFR triggers a signaling cascade leading to increased malignant cell proliferation, decreased malignant cell apoptosis, increased tumor cell motility, and angiogenesis.[65] EGFR mutations are found in 10% to 15% of NSCLCs but are more frequent in adenocarcinomas (80.9%), women (69.7%), and never-smokers (66.6%).[66–68] HER-2/Neu is a growth factor receptor that mediates cell proliferation and survival, and overexpression is more common in lung adenocarcinomas in women than in men (20.5% vs 3.2%, respectively).[69–72]

ADDITIONAL RISK FACTORS
Genetic Factors

Although environmental factors such as exhaust from indoor cooking and second-hand tobacco smoke account for some cases of lung cancer in Asian women who have never smoked, they do not account for all cases of lung cancer in this population. Genome-wide association studies (GWAS) compare DNA markers across the genome between people with a disease and people without a disease. One of the largest GWAS studies in female never-smokers, combining data from 14 studies including approximately 14,000 Asian women (6600 with lung cancer and 7500 without lung cancer), found variations at 3 locations in the genome—two on chromosome 6 and one on chromosome 10—that were associated with lung cancer in Asian female never-smokers. The variation at chromosome 10 had never been reported in prior GWAS of lung cancer in Asian or white populations.[73]

Infections

Human papilloma virus (HPV) oncoproteins E6 and E7 disrupt epithelial differentiation and DNA synthesis, causing genomic instability that can lead to malignant transformation.[74] Using polymerase chain reaction (PCR) and in-situ hybridization, HPV DNA was found in tumors of 49% of women with lung cancer who also had a history of high-grade cervical intraepithelial neoplasia.[75] Similarly, in a study of 141 patients with lung cancer and 60 controls, HPV DNA was found in 55% of patients with lung cancer compared with 27% of controls. Stratification by age, gender, and smoking status indicated a higher prevalence of HPV-16 and HPV-18 in nonsmoking women older than 60 years.[76] A meta-analysis including 1094 patients with HPV-positive lung cancer and 484 non-cancer controls found a strong association with HPV-infected lung cancers compared with non-cancer controls (OR 5.67, 95% CI: 3.09–10.4, $P<.001$), an association with HPV-16 and 18 and lung cancer (OR 6.01, 95% CI: 3.32–11.28, $P<.001$), significant association with squamous cell carcinoma (OR 9.78, 95% CI 6.28–15.11, $P<.001$), and a lower prevalence of HPV in normal lung tissue adjacent to HPV-positive lung cancer indicating that HPV likely plays a role in lung carcinogenesis.[74] In contrast, one small study of 32 squamous cell carcinomas and 15 cervical cancers found negative HPVPCR in the lung cancer cases.[77]

Nontuberculous mycobacteria (NTM) are a family of bacteria commonly found in water and soil that cause a variety of infections. Incidence of NTM in the general population is 1.0 to 1.8 per 100,000, with the most common isolate in the United States being *Mycobacterium avium* complex (MAC).[78] Infection occurs more often in patients with compromised immune systems and chronic lung diseases causing structural abnormalities and in women.[78,79] MAC infection and associated chronic inflammatory microenvironment within the lung parenchyma may lead to cellular dysplasia and a predisposition to develop lung cancer; however, factors that make patients susceptible to NTM infection such as derangements in cellular immunity and underlying chronic systemic inflammation may independently increase the risk of lung cancer.[80] A retrospective study evaluating patients with respiratory cultures positive for MAC and newly diagnosed lung cancer showed that 25% of patients diagnosed with lung cancer had MAC in respiratory cultures. When compared with a control group of lung cancer without MAC, female patients with lung cancer who had MAC were more likely to be non-smokers.[81] A retrospective study from Japan reviewed 1382 patients with lung cancer who underwent bronchoscopy with culture evaluation of NTM and found an association between MAC-positive cultures and female sex (OR 0.388; 95% CI, 0.175–0.860; P = .0198) and advanced age.[82] Higher incidence of concomitant lung cancer and NTM diagnoses in women suggests women with NTM infection maybe at increased risk of developing lung cancer.

Breast Cancer and Radiation Therapy

Radiation therapy (RT) for breast cancer has been associated with an increased risk of second primary lung cancer (SPLC). A meta-analysis of patients with breast cancer (N = 631,021) in North America and Europe found that those treated with RT following lumpectomy or mastectomy had a higher risk of SPLC (RR, 1.23; 95% CI, 1.07–1.43), which increased with duration of time following diagnosis.[83] In a study of Asian women with breast cancer, the overall occurrence of SPLC was much higher in the RT group compared with the non-RT group (2.25% vs 0.23%, respectively). After adjusting for age, comorbidities, and location of care, patients with breast cancer treated with RT have a significantly higher risk (hazard ratio [HR] increased 10.078-fold) for lung cancer compared with the non-RT group.[84] A recent meta-analysis estimated the absolute risk of lung cancer following breast cancer with modern RT (average RT doses were 5.7 Gy for whole lung).[85] A lung cancer IRR greater than 10 years after radiotherapy of 2.10 (95% CI, 1.48–2.98; P<.001) was found based on 134 cancers, indicating 0.11 (95% CI, 0.05–0.20) cause-specific mortality and excess IRRs per Gy whole-lung dose. Estimated absolute risk of lung cancer from modern RT for breast cancer was approximately 4% for long-term continuing smokers and 0.3% for nonsmokers, leading the investigators to conclude that the absolute risk of modern RT for breast cancer may outweigh the benefits in women who are long-term smokers.[85]

HISTOLOGIC DISTRIBUTION OF LUNG CANCER IN WOMEN

Adenocarcinoma is the most common histologic subtype of NSCLC. Female smokers are more likely to develop adenocarcinoma, whereas male smokers are more likely to develop squamous cell carcinoma, likely due to differences in tar content of cigarettes as well as mode of inhalation.[22,27,86–88] Rates of small cell lung cancer are similar between men and women (14.8% in women and 13% among men), but case control studies have reported that women smokers have higher OR for development of small cell lung cancer than squamous cell lung cancer.[21,22,27]

TREATMENT RESPONSE, COMPLICATION, AND OUTCOMES

Women are diagnosed with less advanced lung cancer than men, and when adjusted for age, stage, and selected histologic subgroups they have improved outcomes after treatment of lung cancer.[89] Following surgery for stage I NSCLC, mortality rates are reported to be lower among women,[90,91] and 5-year overall survival (OS) rates range from 83% to 91% in women compared with 53% to 74% in men.[92,93] In a National Cancer Database study of lobectomy versus sublobar resection performed between 2003 and 2006 in 11,990 patients with clinical stage IA NSCLC, female sex was associated with long-term survival with a multivariable-adjusted HR in women compared with men of 0.76 (95% CI, 0.72–0.80, P<.0001).[94] In a meta-analysis of randomized trials in advanced NSCLC, women had a higher response to chemotherapy (42% versus 40%, P = .01) and longer survival than men (median OS 9.6 vs 8.6 months, HR 0.86%, P = .002); however, this survival advantage is confined to patients with adenocarcinoma.[95] The increased frequency of EGFR mutations in women with lung adenocarcinoma may explain the improved

OS in women with advanced stage NSCLC.[67] In contrast, a recent meta-analysis including 11,351 patients, 7646 men and 3705 women, with advanced cancer treated with immunotherapy (32% melanoma, 31% had NSCLC) found a pooled overall survival HR of 0.72 (95% CI, 0.65–0.79) in men and 0.86 (95% CI, 0.79–0.93) in women, consistent with a statistically significant decrease in efficacy of immune checkpoint inhibitor in women compared with men (P = .0019).[96]

Women experience higher rates of grade 2 or higher-radiation pneumonitis after stereotactic radiotherapy compared with men (16% vs 13%, respectively; adjusted OR 1.30 [95% CI, 0.53–3.10]).[97]

Combined HRT has been shown to negatively affect lung cancer survival and is associated with a lower age at cancer diagnosis.[32,98] Postmenopausal women in the Women's Health Initiative treated with estrogen monotherapy did not have increased death rate from lung cancer compared with placebo (HR of death 1.07; 95% CI 0.66–1.72, P = .79).[99]

LUNG CANCER SCREENING

The US Preventive Services Task Force (USPSTF) recommends low-dose CT (LDCT) screening in current or former (quit within the last 15 years) smokers aged 55 to 80 years with at least a 30 pack-year smoking.[100] However, use of age and smoking history alone may exclude potentially high-risk patients. In a retrospective study from 2005 to 2011, the proportion of patients with lung cancer who smoked more than 30 pack-years declined and the proportion of former smokers, especially those who had quit smoking more than 15 years before lung cancer diagnosis, increased.[101] The relative proportion of patients meeting USPSTF criteria for LDCT screening was 56.8% from 1984 to 1990 and decreased to 43.3% from 2005 to 2011 (P<.001).[101] When stratified by sex, over time, a more notable decline was found in women meeting lung cancer screening criteria (52.3%–36.6%, P = .005) compared with the decline in men (60%–49.7%, P = .3).[101] The reduced risk of dying from lung cancer following LDCT screening has been shown to be more favorable in women than in men (39%–61% versus 26%, respectively).[102]

IMPACT OF TOBACCO CESSATION

A prospective study assessed the benefits of prolonged smoking cessation at various ages among 1.3 million women and found that women who have smoked cigarettes throughout adult life have 3 times the overall mortality rate of women of the same age who have never smoked or who stopped well before middle age.[103] The excess mortality is mainly due to smoking-related diseases; RR for lung cancer is 21.4 (95% CI 19.7–23.2).[103] Quitting smoking before age 40 years avoids more than 90% of the excess mortality and about 97% if quit before age 30 years. Among smokers who stopped smoking permanently at ages 25 to 34 years or at ages 35 to 44 years, the RRs for lung cancer mortality were significantly reduced at 1.84 (CI 1.45–2.34) and 3.34 (CI 2.76–4.03), respectively, underscoring the critical importance of smoking cessation counseling and treatment in women.[103]

SUMMARY

Lung cancer is a major women's health problem worldwide, with increasing incidence and mortality rates. It is not clear if women are more susceptible to the carcinogenic effects of tobacco; women smokers tend to be younger when diagnosed with lung cancer, and women nonsmokers are more likely to be diagnosed with lung cancer than men nonsmokers. Women may be more susceptible to the influences of hormonal, environmental, and molecular factors. Although research on sex-based differences in the biology, natural history, and response to therapy in lung cancer has been promising, more efforts are needed to better understand the impact of these factors in order to design future trials of therapy and screening in lung cancer. Without doubt, the most effective form of intervention aimed at stopping the lung cancer epidemic in both women and men is to reduce smoking rates to zero. As such, extensive support should be given to campaigns of smoking prevention in all individuals.

DISCLOSURE

The authors have nothing to disclose.

REFERENCES

1. Siegel RL, Miller KD, Jemal A. Cancer statistics 2019. CACancer J Clin 2019;69:7–34.
2. Jemal A, Miller KD, Ma J, et al. Higher lung cancer incidence in young women than young men in the United States. N Engl J Med 2018;378:1999–2009.
3. Bray F, Felay J, Soerjomataram I, et al. Global cancer statistics 2018: GLOBOCAN estimates of incidence and mortality worldwide for 36 cancers in 185 countries. CACancer J Clin 2018;68(6):394–424.
4. Cheng TYD, Cramb SM, Baade PD, et al. The International epidemiology of lung cancer: latest trends,

disparities, and tumor characteristics. J ThoracOncol 2016;11:1653–71.

5. Lortet-Tieulent J, Renteria E, Sharp L, et al. Convergence of decreasing male and increasing female incidence rates in major tobacco-related cancers in Europe in 1988–2010. Eur J Cancer 2015;51: 1144–63.

6. Barta JA, Powell CA, Wisnivesky JP. Global epidemiology of lung cancer. Ann Glob Health 2019; 85(8):1–16.

7. Martin-Sanchez JC, Lunet N, Gonzalez-Marrón A, et al. Projections in breast and lung cancer mortality among women: a Bayesian analysis of 52 countries worldwide. Cancer Res 2018;78:4436–42.

8. Galloway MS, Henley SJ, Steele CB, et al. Surveillance for cancers associated with tobacco use – United States, 2010-2014. MMWRSurveillSumm 2018;67:1–42.

9. Thun MJ, Carter BD, Feskanich D, et al. 50-year trends in smoking-related mortality in the United States. N Engl J Med 2013;368:351–62.

10. Sanford NN, Sher DJ, Xu X, et al. Trends in smoking and e-cigarette use among US patients with cancer, 2014-2017. JAMAOncol 2019;5:426–8.

11. Hitchman SC, Fong GT. Gender empowerment and female smoking prevalence ratios. Bull World Health Organ 2011;89:195–202.

12. WHO report on the global tobacco epidemic, 2008: the MPOWER package. Geneva (Switzerland): World Health Organization; 2008.

13. Warren CW, Jones NR, Eriksen MP, et al. Global Tobacco Surveillance System (GTSS) collaborative group. Patterns of global tobacco use in young people and implications for future chronic disease burden in adults. Lancet 2006;367:749–53.

14. Okazaki I, Ishikawa S, Ando W, et al. Lung adenocarcinoma in never smokers: problems of primary prevention from aspects of susceptible genes and carcinogens. Anticancer Res 2016;36: 6207–24.

15. North CM, Christiani DC. Women and lung cancer: what is new? SeminThoracCardiovasc Surg 2013; 25:87–94.

16. Pelosof L, Ahn C, Gao A, et al. Proportion of never-smoker non-small cell lung cancer patients at three diverse Institutions. J NatlCancerInst 2017;109:1–6.

17. Torok S, Hegedus B, Laszlo V, et al. Lung cancer in never smokers. FutureOncol 2011;7:1195–211.

18. Lee YJ, Kim JH, Kim SK, et al. Lung cancer in never smokers: change of a mindset in the molecular era. Lung Cancer 2011;72:9–15.

19. Sun S, Schiller JH, Gazdar AF. Lung cancer in never smokers–a different disease. Nat Rev Cancer 2007;7:778–90.

20. Ramchandran K, Patel JD. Sex differences in susceptibility to carcinogens. SeminOncol 2009;36: 516–23.

21. Schoenberg JB, Wilcox HB, Mason TJ, et al. Variation in smoking-related lung cancer risk among New Jersey women. Am J Epidemiol 1989;130: 688–95.

22. Osann KE, Anton-Culver H, Kurosaki T, et al. Sex differences in lung cancer risk associated with cigarette smoking. Int J Cancer 1993;54:44–8.

23. Harris RE, Zang EA, Anderson JI, et al. Race and sex differences in lung cancer risk associated with cigarette smoking. Int J Epidemiol 1993;22: 592–9.

24. Zang EA, Wynder EL. Differences in lung cancer risk between men and women: examination of the evidence. J NatlCancerInst 1996;88:183–92.

25. Radzikowska E, Glaz P, Roszkowski K. Lung cancer in women: age, smoking, histology, performance status, stage, initial treatment, and survival: population-based study of 20,561 cases. Ann Oncol 2002;13:1087–93.

26. Mcduffe HH, Klasseen DJ, Dosman JA. Female-male differences in patients with primary lung cancer. Cancer 1987;59:1825–30.

27. Brownson RC, Chang JC, Davis JR. Gender and histologic type variations in smoking-related risk of lung cancer. Epidemiology 1992;3:61–4.

28. Risch HA, Howe GR, Jain M, et al. Are female smokers at higher risk for lung cancer than male smokers? A case-control analysis by histologic type. Am J Epidemiol 1993;138:281–93.

29. Freedman ND, Leitzmann MF, Hollenbeck AR, et al. Cigarette smoking and subsequent risk of lung cancer in men and women: analysis of a prospective cohort study. LancetOncol 2008;9:649–56.

30. Kreuzer M, Boffetta P, Whitley E, et al. Gender differences in lung cancer risk by smoking: a multi-center case-control study in Germany and Italy. Br J Cancer 2000;82:227–33.

31. De Matteis S, Consonni D, Pesatori AD, et al. Are women who smoke at higher risk for lung cancer than men who smoke? Am J Epidemiol 2013;177: 601–12.

32. Siegfried JM, Stabile LP. Estrogenic steroid hormones in lung cancer. SeminOncol 2014;41:5–16.

33. Meireles SI, Gustavo HE, Hirata R, et al. Early changes in gene expression induced by tobacco smoke: evidence for the importance of estrogen within lung tissue. CancerPrev Res (Phila) 2010;3:707–17.

34. Mah V, Marquez D, Alavi M, et al. Expression levels of estrogen receptor beta in conjunction with aromatase predict survival in non-small cell lung cancer. Lung Cancer 2011;74:318–25.

35. Taioli E, Wynder EL. Endocrine factors and adenocarcinoma o the lung in women. J NatlCancerInst 1994;86:869–70.

36. Adami HO, Persson I, Hoover R, et al. Risk of cancer in women receiving hormone replacement therapy. Int J Cancer 1989;44:33–9.

37. Weiss JM, Lacey JV, Shu XO, et al. Menstrual and reproductive factors associated with lung cancer in femal lifetime nonsmokers. Am J Epidemiol 2008;168:1319–25.

38. Baik CS, Strauss GM, Speizer FE, et al. Reproductive factors, hormone use, and risk for lung cancer in postmenopausal women, the Nurses' Health Study. CancerEpidemiolBiomarkers Prev 2010;19:2525–33.

39. Brinton LA, Gierach GL, Andaya A, et al. Reproductive and hormonal factors and lung cancer risk in the NIH-AARP Diet and Health Study Cohort. CancerEpidemiolBiomarkersPrev 2011;20:900–11.

40. Schabath MB, Wu X, Vassilopoulou-Sellin R, et al. Hormone replacement therapy and lung cancer risk: a case-control analysis. ClinCancer Res 2004;10:113–23.

41. Greiser CM, Greiser EM, Doren M. Menopausal hormone therapy and risk of lung cancer – systematic review and meta-analysis. Maturitas 2010;65:198–204.

42. Kriek E, Rojas M, Alexandrov K, et al. Polycystic aromatic hydrocarbons-DNA adducts in humans: relevance as biomarkers for exposure and cancer risk. Mutat Res 1998;400:215–31.

43. Belani CP, Marts S, Schiller J, et al. Women and lung cancer: epidemiology, tumor biology, and emerging trends in clinical research. Lung Cancer 2007;55:15–23.

44. Uppstead H, Osnes GH, Cole KJ, et al. Sex differences in susceptibility to PAHs in an intrinsic property of human lung adenocarcinoma cells. Lung Cancer 2011;71:264–70.

45. Gonzalez FJ, Crespi CL, Gelboin HV. DNA-expressed human cytochrome P450s: a new age of molecular toxicology and human risk assessment. Mutat Res 1991;247:113–7.

46. Hecht SS. Tobacco smoke carcinogens and lung cancer. J NatlCancer Inst 1999;91:1194–210.

47. Seidegard J, Pero RW, Markowitz MM, et al. Isoenzymes of glutathione transferase (class Mu) as a marker for susceptibility to lung cancer: a follow up study. Carcinogenesis 1990;11:33–6.

48. Mollerup S, Ryberg D, Hewer A. Sex differences in lung CYP1a1 expression and DNA adduct levels among lung cancer patients. Cancer Res 1999;59:3317–20.

49. Whibley C, Pharoah PD, Hollstein M. p53 Polymorphisms: cancer implications. Nat Rev Cancer 2009;9:95–107.

50. Takahashi T, Takahashi T, Suzuki H, et al. The p53 gene is very frequently mutated in small-cell lung cancer with a distinct nucleotide substitution pattern. Oncogene 1991;61:775–8.

51. Kure EH, Ryberg D, Hewer A, et al. p53 Mutations in lung tumors: relationship to gender and lung DNA adduct levels. Carcinogenesis 1996;17:2201–5.

52. Tayooka S, Shimizu N, Gazdar A. The TP53 gene, tobacco exposure, and lung cancer. Hum Mutat 2003;21:229–39.

53. Ahrendt SA, Deker PA, Alawi EA, et al. Cigarette smoking is strongly associated with mutation of the K-ras gene in patients with primary adenocarcinoma of the lung. Cancer 2001;92:1525–30.

54. Dogan S, Shen R, Ang DC, et al. Molecular epidemiology of EGFR and KRAS mutations in 3,026 lung adenocarcinomas: higher susceptibility of women to smoking-related KRAS-mutant cancers. ClinCancer Res 2012;18:6169–77.

55. Nelson HH, Christiani DC, Mark EJ, et al. Implications and prognostic value of K-ras mutations for early stage lung cancer in women. J NatlCancerInst 1999;91:2032–7.

56. Spitz MR, Wei Q, Dong Q, et al. Genetic susceptibility to lung cancer: the role of DNA damage and repair. CancerEpidemiolBiomarkersPrev 2003;12:689–98.

57. Ryberg D, Hewer A, Phillips DH, et al. Different susceptibility to smoking-induced DNA damage among male and female lung cancer patients. Cancer Res 1994;54:5801–3.

58. Wei Q, Cheng L, Amos CI, et al. Repair of tobacco carcinogen-induced DNA adducts and lung cancer risk: a molecular epidemiological study. J NatlCancerInst 2000;92:1764–72.

59. Aaronson SA. Growth factors and cancer. Science 1991;254:1146–53.

60. Siegfried JM, DeMichelle MA, Hunt JD, et al. Expression of mRNA for gastrin-releasing peptide receptor by human bronchial epithelial cells; association with prolonged tobacco exposure and responsiveness to bombesin-like peptides. Am J RespirCritCare Med 1997;156:358–66.

61. Ohki-Hamazaki H, Iwabuchi M, Maekawa F. Development and function of bombesin-like peptides and their receptors. Int J DevBiol 2005;49:293–300.

62. Jaeger N, Czepielewski RS, Bagatini M, et al. Neuropeptide gastrin-releasing peptide induces PI3K/reactive oxygen species-dependent migration in lung adenocarcinoma cells. Tumour Biol 2017;39. 1010428317694321.

63. Leyton J, Garcia-Martin LJ, Tapia JA, et al. Bombesin and gastrin releasing peptide increase tyrosine phosphorylation of focal adhesion kinase and paxillin in non-small cell lung cancer cells. CancerLett 2001;162:87–95.

64. Shriver SP, Bordeau HA, Gubish CT, et al. Sex-specific expression of gastrin-releasing peptide receptor: relationship to smoking history and risk of lung cancer. J NatlCancerInst 2000;92:24–33.

65. Scagliotti GV, Selvaggi G, Novello S, et al. The biology of epidermal growth factor receptor in lung cancer. ClinCancer Res 2004;10:4227–32.

66. Paez JG, Janne PA, Lee JC, et al. EGFR mutations in lung cancer: correlation with clinical response to gefitinib therapy. Science 2004;304:1497–500.

67. Rosell R, Moran T, Queralt C, et al. Screening for epidermal growth factor receptor mutations in lung cancer. N Engl J Med 2009;361:958–67.

68. Westover D, Zugazagoitia J, Cho BC, et al. Mechanisms of acquired resistance to first- and second-generation EGFR tyrosine kinase inhibitors. Ann Oncol 2018;29(suppl-1):10–i19.

69. Pellegrini C, Falleni M, Marchetti A, et al. HER-2/Neu alterations in mon-small-cell lung cancer: a comprehensive evaluation by real time RT-PCR, fluorescence in situ hybridization, and immunohistochemistry. ClinCancer Res 2003;9:3645–52.

70. Guinee DG Jr, Travis WD, Trivers GE, et al. Gender comparisons in human lung cancer: analysis of p53 mutations, anti-p53 serum antibodies and C-erbB2 expression. Carcinogenesis 1995;16:993–1002.

71. Hirsch F, Veve R, Varella-Garcia M. Evaluation of Her2/neu expression in lung tumors by immunohistochemistry and fluorescence in situ hybridization [Abstract]. Proc Am SocClinOncol 2000;19:486a.

72. Hseigh CC, Chow KC, Fahn HJ, et al. Prognostic significance of Her-2/neu expression in Stage I adenocarcinoma of lung. Ann ThoracSurg 1998;66:1159–63.

73. Lan Q, Hsiung CA, Matsuo K, et al. Genome-wide association analysis identifies new lung cancer susceptibility loci in never-smoking women in Asia. Nat Genet 2012;44:1330–5.

74. Zhai K, Ding J, Shi HZ. Author's reply to "comments on HPV and lung cancer risk: a meta-analysis". J ClinVirol 2015;63:92–3.

75. Henning EM, Suo Z, Karlsen F, et al. HPV positive bronchopulmonary carcinomas in women with previous high-grade cervical intraepithelial neoplasia (CIN III). ActaOncol 1999;38:639–47.

76. Cheng YW, Hsei LL, Lin PP, et al. Gender differences in DNA adduct levels among non-smoking Taiwanese lung cancer patients. EnvironMolMutagen 2001;37:304–10.

77. Welt A, Hummel M, Niedobitek G, et al. Human papilloma virus infection is not associated with bronchial carcinoma: evaluation by in situ hybridization and the polymerase chain reaction. J Pathol 1997;181:276–80.

78. Griffith DE, Aksamit T, Brown-Elliott BA, et al. An official ATS/IDSA statement: diagnosis, treatment, and prevention of nontuberculous mycobacterial diseases. Am J RespirCritCare Med 2007;175:367–416.

79. Winthrop KL, McNelley E, Kendall B, et al. Pulmonary nontuberculous mycobacterial disease prevalence and clinical features: an emerging public health disease. Am J RespirCritCare Med 2010;182:977–82.

80. Daley CL, Iseman M. Mycobacterium avium complex and lung cancer: chicken or egg? Both? J ThoracOncol 2012;7:1329–30.

81. Lande L, Peterson DD, Gogoi R, et al. Association between pulmonary mycobacterium avium complex infection and lung cancer. J ThoracOncol 2012;7:1345–71351.

82. Tamura A, Hebisawa A, Kusaka K, et al. Relationship between lung cancer and mycobacterium avium complex isolated using bronchoscopy. OpenRespir Med J 2016;10:20–8.

83. Grantzau T, Overgaard J. Risk of second non-breast cancer after radiotherapy for breast cancer: a systematic review and meta-analysis of 762,468 patients. RadiotherOncol 2015;114:56–65.

84. Huang YJ, Huang TW, Lin FH, et al. Radiation therapy for invasive breast cancer increases the risk of second primary lung cancer: a Nationwide population-based cohort analysis. J ThoracOncol 2017;12:782–90.

85. Taylor C, Correa C, Duane FK, et al. Estimating the risks of breast cancer radiotherapy: evidence from modern radiation doses to the lungs and heart and previous randomized trials. J ClinOncol 2017;35:1641–9.

86. Greenberg R, Karson R, Baker J, et al. Incidence of lung cancer by cell type: a population-based study in New Hampshire and Vermont. J NatlCancerInst 1984;72:599–603.

87. Thun MJ, Lally CA, Flannery JT, et al. Cigarette smoking and changes in the histopathology of lung cancer. J NatlCancer Inst 1997;89:1580–6.

88. Stellman SD, Muscat JE, Thompson S, et al. Risk of squamous cell carcinoma and adenocarcinoma to the lung in relation to lifetime filter cigarette smoking. Cancer 1997;80:382–8.

89. Sagerup CMT, Smastuen M, Johannesen TB, et al. Sex-specific trends in lung cancer incidence and survival: a population study of 40118 cases. Thorax 2011;66:301–7.

90. Khullar OV, Liu Y, Gillespi T, et al. Survival after sublobar resection versus lobectomy for clinical stage IA lung cancer: an analysis from the national cancer database. J ThoracOncol 2015;10:1625–101633.

91. Husain ZA, Kim AW, Yu JB, et al. Defining the high-risk population for mortality after resection of early stage NSCLC. ClinLungCancer 2015;16:e183–7.

92. Maeda R, Yoshida J, Ishii G, et al. Influence of cigarette smoking on survival and tumor invasiveness in clinical stage IA lung adenocarcinoma. Ann Thorac Surg 2012;93:1626–32.

93. Chang MY, Mentzer SJ, Colson YL, et al. Factors predicting poor survival after resection of stage IA non-small cell lung cancer. J ThoracCardiovasc Surg 2007;134:850–6.

94. Speicher PJ, Gu L, Gulack BC, et al. Sublobar resection for clinical stage IA non-small-cell lung cancer in the United States. ClinLungCancer 2016;17:47–55.

95. Wheatley-Price P, Blackhall F, Lee SM, et al. The influence of sex and histology on outcomes in non-small cell lung cancer: a pooled analysis of five randomized trials. Ann Oncol 2010;21: 2023–8.

96. Conforti F, Pala L, Bagnardi V, et al. Cancer immunotherapy efficacy and patients' sex: a systematic review and meta-analysis. LancetOncol 2018;19: 737–46.

97. Takeda A, Ohashi T, Kunieda E, et al. Comparison of clinical, tumour-related and dosimetric factors in grade 0–1, grade 2 and grade 3 radiation pneumonitis after stereotactic body radiotherapy for lung tumours. Br J Radiol 2012;85:636–42.

98. Ganti AK, Sahmoun AE, Panwalkar AW, et al. Hormone replacement therapy is associated with decreased survival in women with lung cancer. J ClinOncol 2006;24:59–63.

99. Chlebowski RT, Anderson GL, Manson JAE, et al. Lung cancer among postmenopausal women treated with estrogen alone in the women's health initiative randomized trial. J NatlCancerInst 2010; 102:1413–21.

100. Moyer VA. Screening for lung cancer: U.S. Preventive Services Task Force recommendation statement. Ann Intern Med 2014;160:330–3.

101. Wang Y, Midthun DE, Wampfler JA, et al. Trends in the proportion of patients with lung cancer meeting screening criteria. JAMA 2015;313:853–5.

102. De Koning H, et al. IASLC 19th World Conference on Lung Cancer, Toronto, Canada, September 23–26, 2018.

103. Pirie K, Peto R, Reeves GK, et al. The 21st century hazards of smoking and benefits of stopping: a prospective study of one million women in the UK. Lancet 2013;381:133–41.

Lung Cancer Pathology
Current Concepts

William D. Travis, MD

KEYWORDS

- Lung cancer • Pathology • Adenocarcinoma • Squamous cell carcinoma • Small cell carcinoma
- Large cell neuroendocrine carcinoma • Carcinoid

KEY POINTS

- Small biopsies and cytology specimens now have specific criteria and terminology for diagnosis of lung cancer.
- Immunohistochemistry is recommended to classify most lung cancers, particularly in small biopsies and cytology specimens.
- Precise histologic diagnosis and molecular testing drives personalized therapies for patients.
- Predominant subtyping of resected lung adenocarcinomas has strong correlations with prognosis.
- Although neuroendocrine tumors are grouped together, the carcinoid tumors are very different from the high-grade small cell carcinoma and large cell neuroendocrine carcinoma.

INTRODUCTION

Lung cancer can be diagnosed pathologically based either on histologic biopsy or cytologic specimens.[1,2] In the 2015 World Health Organization (WHO) Classification of Lung Tumors (**Table 1**), the diagnosis of lung cancer was addressed not only in resection specimens but a new approach to small biopsies and cytology specimens was introduced (**Table 2**).[1,2] For these small specimens, diagnostic terms and criteria for all major histologic subtypes of lung cancer were recommended.[1,2] Due to the discovery of driver mutations in many lung cancers, such as *EGFR* mutation and *ALK* rearrangements that represent therapeutic targets, the importance of managing these small specimens for molecular testing is emphasized. Histologically there are 4 major types of lung cancer, including squamous cell carcinoma, adenocarcinoma, small cell carcinoma (SCLC), and large cell carcinoma (see **Table 1**).[2] These major types can be subclassified into more specific subtypes, such as lepidic predominant subtype of adenocarcinoma or the basaloid variant of squamous cell carcinoma.[2]

The 2015 WHO classification introduced multiple new concepts, including (1) widespread requirement of immunohistochemistry for accurate diagnosis for many lung tumors including resected lung cancers; (2) integration of molecular studies, to facilitate personalize treatment strategies for patients with advanced lung cancer; (3) recommendations for diagnosis and tissue management for small biopsies and cytology specimens[1–4]; (4) major changes in the approach to lung adenocarcinoma in resection specimens[1–3]; (5) restricting the diagnosis of large cell carcinoma to resected tumors that lack any clear morphologic or immunohistochemical differentiation or mucin; (6) a new subtyping of squamous cell carcinomas into keratinizing, nonkeratinizing, and basaloid subtypes with the nonkeratinizing tumors requiring immunohistochemical staining of squamous markers; and (7) grouping the neuroendocrine tumors together, although the diagnostic criteria remain the same.[2,3,5]

Thoracic Pathology, Department of Pathology, Memorial Sloan Kettering Cancer Center, Room A525, 1275 York Avenue, New York, NY 10065, USA
E-mail address: travisw@mskcc.org

Clin Chest Med 41 (2020) 67–85
https://doi.org/10.1016/j.ccm.2019.11.001
0272-5231/20/© 2019 Elsevier Inc. All rights reserved.

Table 1
2015 World Health Organization classification of lung tumors

Histologic Type and Subtypes	International Classification of Diseases for Oncology Code
Epithelial tumors	
Adenocarcinoma	8140/3
Lepidic adenocarcinoma	8250/3
Acinar adenocarcinoma	8551/3
Papillary adenocarcinoma	8260/3
Micropapillary adenocarcinoma	8265/3
Solid adenocarcinoma	8230/3
Invasive mucinous adenocarcinoma	8253/3
Mixed invasive mucinous and nonmucinous adenocarcinoma	8254/3
Colloid adenocarcinoma	8480/3
Fetal adenocarcinoma	8333/3
Enteric adenocarcinoma	8144/3
Minimally invasive adenocarcinoma	
Nonmucinous	8256/3
Mucinous	8257/3
Preinvasive lesions	
Atypical adenomatous hyperplasia	8250/0
Adenocarcinoma in situ	
Nonmucinous	8250/2
Mucinous	8253/2
Squamous cell carcinoma	8070/3
Keratinizing squamous cell carcinoma	8071/3
Nonkeratinizing squamous cell carcinoma	8072/3
Basaloid squamous cell carcinoma	8083/3
Preinvasive lesion	
Squamous cell carcinoma in situ	8070/2
Neuroendocrine tumors	
Small cell carcinoma	8041/3
Combined small cell carcinoma	8045/3
Large cell neuroendocrine carcinoma	8013/3
Combined large cell neuroendocrine carcinoma	8013/3
Carcinoid tumors	
Typical carcinoid tumor	8240/3
Atypical carcinoid tumor	8249/3
Preinvasive lesion	
Diffuse idiopathic pulmonary neuroendocrine cell hyperplasia	8040/0
Large cell carcinoma	8012/3
Adenosquamous carcinoma	8560/3
Sarcomatoid carcinomas	
Pleomorphic carcinoma	8022/3
Spindle cell carcinoma	8032/3
Giant cell carcinoma	8031/3

(continued on next page)

Table 1
(continued)

Histologic Type and Subtypes	International Classification of Diseases for Oncology Code
Carcinosarcoma	8980/3
Pulmonary blastoma	8972/3
Other and Unclassified carcinomas	
Lymphoepithelioma-like carcinoma	8082/3
NUT carcinoma	8023/3
Salivary gland-type tumors	
Mucoepidermoid carcinoma	8430/3
Adenoid cystic carcinoma	8200/3
Epithelial-myoepithelial carcinoma	8562/3
Pleomorphic adenoma	8940/0

From Travis WD, Brambilla E, Burke AP, et al. WHO Classification of Tumours of the Lung, Pleura, Thymus and Heart. 4th ed. Lyon: International Agency for Research on Cancer; 2015; with permission.

Table 2
Terminology in small biopsy and cytology versus resection specimens for adenocarcinoma and squamous cell carcinoma

Morphology/Stains	Terminology for Small Biopsies and Cytology Specimens	Terminology for Resection Specimens
Morphologic squamous cell patterns clearly present	Squamous cell carcinoma	Squamous cell carcinoma
Morphologic adenocarcinoma patterns clearly present	Adenocarcinoma (list the patterns in the diagnosis)	Adenocarcinoma Predominant pattern: Lepidic Acinar Papillary Solid Micropapillary
Morphologic squamous cell patterns not present, but supported by stains (ie, p40-positive)	Non–small cell carcinoma, favor squamous cell carcinoma[b]	Squamous cell carcinoma (nonkeratinizing pattern may be a component of the tumor)[b]
Morphologic adenocarcinoma patterns not present, but supported by special stains (ie, TTF1-positive)	Non–small cell carcinoma, favor adenocarcinoma[b]	Adenocarcinoma (solid pattern may be just one component of the tumor)[b]
No clear adenocarcinoma, squamous, or neuroendocrine morphology or staining pattern	Non–small cell carcinoma, not otherwise specified[a,c]	Large cell carcinoma

[a] Metastatic carcinomas should be carefully excluded with clinical and appropriate but judicious immunohistochemical examination.

[b] The categories do not always correspond to solid predominant adenocarcinoma or non-keratinizing squamous cell carcinoma, respectively. Poorly differentiated components in adenocarcinoma or squamous cell carcinoma may be sampled.

[c] The non–small cell carcinoma, not otherwise specified pattern can be seen not only in large cell carcinomas, but also when the solid, poorly differentiated component of adenocarcinomas or squamous cell carcinomas is sampled but does not express immunohistochemical markers or mucin.

Data from Travis WD, Brambilla E, Burke AP, et al. WHO Classification of Tumours of the Lung, Pleura, Thymus and Heart. 4th ed. Lyon: International Agency for Research on Cancer; 2015 and Travis WD, Nicholson AG, Geisinger K, et al. Tumors of the Lower Respiratory Tract. Silver Spring, MD: American Registry of Pathology; 2019.

LUNG CANCER CLASSIFICATION IN SMALL BIOPSIES AND CYTOLOGY

The importance of precise histologic classification of lung cancer in small biopsies and cytology as well as the need for molecular testing in these small tissues has been driven by major progress in therapy for patients with advanced non–small-cell lung carcinoma (NSCLC).[1,2] The first major discovery was the efficacy of tyrosine kinase inhibitors as first-line therapy in patients with advanced lung adenocarcinoma with *EGFR* mutations.[2,3] Subsequently, multiple additional molecular targets have been identified mostly in lung adenocarcinomas, including *ALK* and *ROS1* and *RET* rearrangements, *BRAF* and *MET exon 14* splice site mutations.[2,3] Also, patients with adenocarcinoma or non–small-cell carcinoma (NSCC) not otherwise specified (NOS) have been shown to be more responsive to pemetrexed than those with squamous cell carcinoma.[2,3] In addition, bevacizumab it is contraindicated in patients with lung cancer with squamous cell carcinoma because these patients are at increased risk for life-threatening hemorrhage.[6] Fifth, great promise has been shown with anti-programmed cell death protein 1 (PD-1) and programmed cell death ligand 1 (PD-L1) antibodies, although there is no consistent association with histologic type (adenocarcinoma vs squamous cell carcinoma) and clinical responses are not consistently associated with PD-L1 expression.[7–9]

All of these therapeutic advances made it quite important to develop a new classification of lung cancer in small biopsies and cytology (see **Table 2**). Furthermore, 70% of patients with lung cancer present in advanced stages.[1–3] A fundamental principle of this classification is to manage these small specimens for molecular testing in addition to diagnosis because molecular testing is now routine in lung cancers.

An unequivocal diagnosis of squamous cell carcinoma or adenocarcinoma can be made in small biopsies if the small biopsy or cytology shows tumor cells with keratinizing squamous cell carcinoma or shows a glandular pattern of adenocarcinoma (lepidic, acinar, papillary or micropapillary), respectively. In carcinomas that only show a solid pattern with no clear squamous or glandular features, immunohistochemical stains should be used with one adenocarcinoma marker (such as TTF-1) and one squamous marker (p40), which should allow for classification of most tumors.[1–3,10] Tumors are classified as *NSCC, favor adenocarcinoma* if they lack definite squamous or glandular morphology and show immunohistochemical

staining that favors adenocarcinoma (ie, TTF-1 positive, p40 negative) (**Fig. 1**A, B). Likewise, the tumor is classified as *NSCC, favor squamous cell carcinoma* for tumors lacking any clear morphology that shows a staining pattern that favors squamous cell carcinoma (p40 positive, TTF-1 negative) (**Fig. 1**C, D). In contrast, the term *NSCC-NOS* is used in tumors with no clear differentiation by morphology or special stains or if the stains are conflicting. This term should be used as infrequently as possible, ideally with a frequency of NSCC-NOS in small biopsies or cytology specimens of 5% or less.[1,3,11] Cytology is also very helpful in the diagnosis and classification of poorly differentiated NSCC.[1–3] The use of the term "nonsquamous carcinoma" by pathologists is discouraged, although it is sometimes used for lumping tumors together in some clinical studies.[1–3] The diagnosis of adenocarcinoma or squamous cell carcinomas as well as NSCC-NOS in small biopsies and cytology needs to be made keeping in mind that a variety of other lung cancers, metastatic melanoma, lymphomas, sarcomas, and metastatic tumors can present in the lung.[1–3,10]

Due to the need not only for diagnosis, but also for molecular testing, pathologists should minimize the amount of tissue used for making the diagnosis by performing as few special stains as possible.[1–3] A useful strategy is to cut the block once after review of initial sections to cut as many unstained slides as possible at the time of initial immunohistochemical workup to have enough material to send for molecular testing or to perform additional stains if needed.[1–3] Also, if multiple small pieces of tumor are obtained, it is best to put them in separate blocks. If the tumor shows only a solid pattern by morphology, it may be best to perform one adenocarcinoma (ie, TTF-1) and one squamous (ie, p40) marker to determine if the tumor is adenocarcinoma or squamous cell carcinoma.[1–3] Other more detailed recommendations are found elsewhere.[2,3]

PREINVASIVE LESIONS

Classification of the preinvasive lesions for lung cancer has undergone major changes since the 1967 WHO classification of lung tumors when there were no preinvasive lesions.[2,3,12] Currently it is recognized that there are 3 categories of pre-invasive lesions, including bronchial squamous dysplasia and carcinoma in situ, for squamous cell carcinoma, atypical adenomatous hyperplasia (AAH) and adenocarcinoma in situ (AIS) for adenocarcinoma and diffuse idiopathic pulmonary

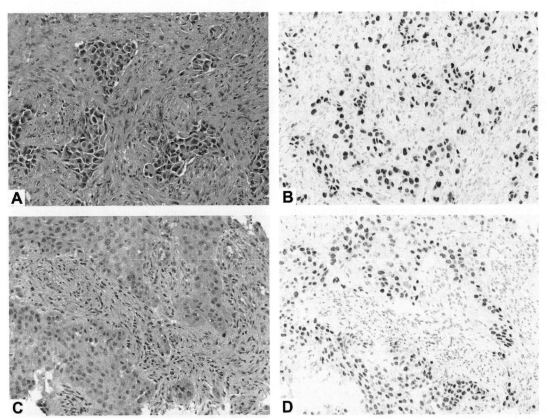

Fig. 1. Non–small cell carcinoma, favor adenocarcinoma. (*A*) This carcinoma shows no clear squamous or glandular differentiation. (hematoxylin-eosin, original magnification ×20). (*B*) The diffuse positive TTF-1 staining, allows for the diagnosis of non–small cell carcinoma, favor adenocarcinoma. Non–small cell carcinoma, favor squamous cell carcinoma. (TTF-1, original magnification ×20). (*C*) This carcinoma shows no clear squamous or glandular differentiation.(hematoxylin-eosin, original magnification ×20). (*D*) The diffuse positive p40 staining and negative TTF-1 staining (not shown) allows for the diagnosis of non–small cell carcinoma, favor squamous cell carcinoma. (TTF-1, original magnification ×20).

neuroendocrine cell hyperplasia (DIPNECH) for carcinoid tumors.[2]

Atypical Adenomatous Hyperplasia

AAH is usually an incidental finding in the lung parenchyma adjacent to resected lung cancers and it consists of a small nodular atypical pneumocyte proliferation that resembles but falls short of

criteria for AIS (**Fig. 2**).[2,3] It occurs in 5.7% to 21.4% of lung adenocarcinoma resection specimens, depending on the extent of lung tissue sampled.[2,3]

Most AAHs are small nodular pneumocyte proliferations usually measuring smaller than 5 mm in diameter. Although there is no absolute size cutoff to separate AAH from AIS, frequently they are

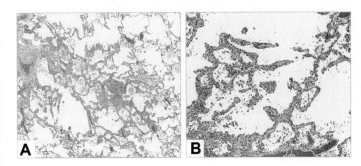

Fig. 2. AAH. (*A*) This millimeter-sized atypical pneumocyte proliferation is ill-defined with mild thickening of the alveolar walls. (hematoxylin-eosin, original magnification ×4). (*B*) The alveolar walls show mild fibrous thickening and the hyperplastic pneumocytes show minimal atypia and there are some gaps between the cells. (hematoxylin-eosin, original magnification ×20).

multicentric.[2,3] AAHs are composed of type II pneumocytes and/or Club (formerly Clara) cells that are cuboidal to low columnar in shape lining alveolar walls and respiratory bronchioles (see **Fig. 2**B).

Adenocarcinoma in Situ

AIS is defined as a small (≤3 cm) proliferation of atypical pneumocytes with pure lepidic pattern without invasion (**Fig. 3**).[1–3] The vast majority are nonmucinous, but rarely they can be mucinous. Nonmucinous tumors consist of a proliferation of type II pneumocytes or Club (formerly Clara) cells. The mucinous AIS cases consist of tall columnar goblet cells having abundant apical mucin. Patients have been reported to have 100% 5-year disease-free survival if these lesions are completely resected.[3,13] By computed tomography (CT), AIS will most often show a pure ground glass nodule if nonmucinous and a solid nodule if mucinous AIS.[1–3]

Squamous Dysplasia and Carcinoma In Situ

Squamous dysplasia and carcinoma in situ represent a continuum of morphologic changes within the bronchial mucosa from normal bronchial mucosa through a series of lesions, including basal cell hyperplasia, squamous metaplasia, dysplasia (mild, moderate, and severe), and carcinoma in situ and ultimately to invasive squamous cell carcinoma.[2,12] As these morphologic changes progress, they occur in parallel with accumulation of genetic changes as well.[2] In squamous carcinoma in situ, the bronchial mucosa shows full-thickness involvement by marked cytologic atypia.

Diffuse Idiopathic Pulmonary Neuroendocrine Cell Hyperplasia (Preinvasive Lesion for Carcinoids)

Carcinoid tumors are rarely found to be associated with the preinvasive lesion called diffuse idiopathic pulmonary neuroendocrine cell hyperplasia (DIPNECH). This is a rare condition characterized by a diffuse proliferation of neuroendocrine cells with multiple tumorlets and neuroendocrine cell hyperplasia in peripheral airways (**Fig. 4**).[14] Clinical presentation can appear as interstitial lung disease or as multiple pulmonary nodules that are frequently incidental findings. The interstitial lung disease presentation is usually associated with small airway obstruction due to bronchiolar fibrosis.[14] Patients who present with clinical manifestations of interstitial lung disease can show a chest CT that is normal or the CT can show mosaic attenuation from air trapping, bronchial wall thickening, and bronchiectasis.[14] The use of the term DIPNECH has recently been proposed to be restricted to patients who present with interstitial lung disease like features including respiratory symptoms, mosaic attenuation on chest CT scans, pulmonary function abnormalities, and constrictive bronchiolitis pathologically.[15]

ADENOCARCINOMA
Adenocarcinoma Classification in Resected Specimens

Invasive adenocarcinoma
Adenocarcinomas account for 50% of all lung cancers in the United States (**Table 3**).[16] They are most often situated in the lung periphery and are often small and subpleural, but they can be large and central (**Fig. 5**). Histologic classification is

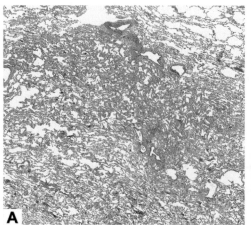
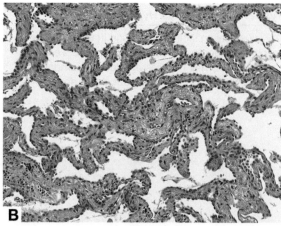

Fig. 3. AIS, nonmucinous. (*A*) This circumscribed nonmucinous tumor grows purely with a lepidic pattern. No foci of invasion or scarring are seen. (hematoxylin-eosin, original magnification ×4). (*B*) High power shows a crowded proliferation of atypical pneumocytes lining the alveolar walls. (hematoxylin-eosin, original magnification ×20).

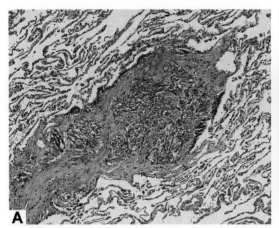 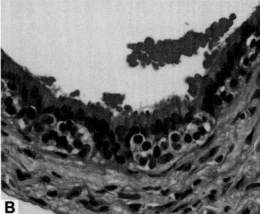

Fig. 4. DIPNECH. (*A*) This carcinoid tumorlet is present in the lung parenchyma adjacent to a carcinoid tumor. (hematoxylin-eosin, original magnification ×4). (*B*) Neuroendocrine cell hyperplasia is seen here as small clusters of neuroendocrine cells at the base of the bronchiolar mucosa. (hematoxylin-eosin, original magnification ×40).

according to the predominant subtype. This is achieved by performing comprehensive histologic subtyping in which each histologic pattern is estimated in a semiquantitative fashion in 5% increments. The term lepidic predominant adenocarcinoma (LPA) is used for tumors that have a predominant lepidic growth pattern consisting of type II pneumocytes and/or Club (formerly Clara) cells where the invasive component is greater than 5 mm (**Fig. 6**A). The other 4 major subtypes consist of acinar (**Fig. 6**B), including the cribriform pattern (**Fig. 6**C), papillary (**Fig. 6**D), and micropapillary patterns (**Fig. 6**E), including the recently described filigree pattern (**Fig. 6**F)[2,3,17] and solid with mucin or TTF-1 expression (**Fig. 6**G, H).[2,3]

Adenocarcinoma variants

There are also 4 lung adenocarcinoma variants, including invasive mucinous adenocarcinoma

(**Fig. 7**), colloid adenocarcinoma, fetal adenocarcinoma, and enteric adenocarcinoma.[1–3]

Invasive mucinous adenocarcinomas differ from nonmucinous invasive adenocarcinomas in several ways including lack of TTF-1 expression in most tumors, frequent multicentric lung lesions, and *KRAS* mutations in most cases. Cytologically the tumor cells have a columnar shape with abundant apical mucin and small basally oriented nuclei. In addition to a lepidic pattern, invasive patterns are also common, including acinar, papillary, or micropapillary patterns (see **Fig. 7**).[1,3] On CT, the tumors frequently show localized or multifocal consolidation with air bronchograms forming nodules and lobar consolidation that can be multilobar and bilateral.[18]

Minimally invasive adenocarcinoma

Minimally invasive adenocarcinoma (MIA) consists of small (≤3 cm) lepidic predominant adenocar

---

Table 3
Percent distribution of lung cancer histologic types from the National Cancer Institute Surveillance, Epidemiology, and End Results Cancer Statistics Review, 2012–2016

Histologic Type	Number	Percentage
Adenocarcinoma	157,488	49.8
Squamous cell carcinoma	71,874	22.7
Small cell carcinoma	39,940	12.6
Other specified carcinomas	17,176	5.4
Non–small cell carcinoma	16,061	5.0
Carcinoma, not otherwise specified	9157	2.9
Large cell carcinoma	4384	1.3
Total	316,080	

From SEER Cancer Statistics Review, 1975-2016. National Cancer Institute, 2018. (Accessed October 30, 2019. (See reference for ICDO codes included for each category)

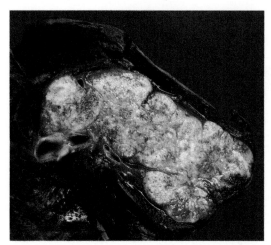

Fig. 5. Adenocarcinoma. Gross features: This adenocarcinoma is large and centrally situated adjacent to a major bronchus.

cinomas with a small area of invasive growth (≤0.5 cm) (**Fig. 8**).[1,2] Although most MIAs are nonmucinous, rare mucinous cases may occur.[1,3] The 5-year disease-free survival is 100% or near 100% if the tumor is completely resected.[2,3,13,19] By CT, nonmucinous tumors should manifest as a ground glass predominant part solid nodule with a small solid component (≤0.5 cm) but mucinous MIA usually shows a solid nodule. If a tumor meets criteria for MIA but is larger than 3.0 cm, it is classified as LPA.[2,3]

Prognosis of adenocarcinoma subtypes in resected specimens

The prognostic significance of the 2011 International Association for the Study of Lung Cancer (IASLC), American Thoracic Society (ATS), and European Respiratory Society (ERS) lung adenocarcinoma classification and 2015 WHO Classification has been validated in multiple clinical studies from independent groups worldwide.[1–3] These studies have consistently shown that lepidic predominant adenocarcinomas have the most favorable prognosis, whereas micropapillary and solid predominant patterns have the worst outcome.[2,3] It has been also shown that even small amounts of the micropapillary pattern are associated with poor outcome, particularly in patients who undergo limited resection.[20] Recently a new filigree pattern has been recognized in addition to the traditional floret and stromal patterns because it shows a similar poor outcome.[17] An intermediate prognosis is seen with the acinar and papillary predominant patterns. The cribriform pattern is included as a high-grade acinar pattern associated with poor

prognosis.[21] For invasive mucinous adenocarcinoma and colloid adenocarcinoma, the reported prognosis is variable, with some showing intermediate and others poor prognosis.[19,22]

Potential impact of classification on TNM staging

There are 2 ways this classification of lung adenocarcinoma impacts on TNM staging.[1–3] First, it helps in the setting of multiple adenocarcinomas to compare the histologic features using comprehensive histologic subtyping. When 2 tumors have similar percentages of histologic subtypes, this tends to support the tumors are related, whereas if they are different, it supports separate primaries. In addition to distribution of histologic subtypes, cytologic and stromal characteristics also can be helpful. In addition to morphologic features, the ultimate decision on whether tumors are related or separate primaries requires a multidisciplinary approach, including clinical, radiologic, and molecular findings.[23–25]

For nonmucinous adenocarcinomas with a lepidic component, it was recommended to use invasive size rather than total size for the size T-factor, in the eighth edition TNM Classification.[26] The reason is that invasive size has been shown to be a better predictor of clinical outcome than the total size formerly recommended in the seventh edition TNM.[27] In tumors in which the invasive size cannot be measured on a single slide, it is recommended to estimate the invasive tumor size by multiplying the total tumor size times the percentage of the invasive components, which results in subtraction of the lepidic component.[26] In one large study of p-Stage I-IIA patients, it was shown that 22% of patients were downstaged using invasive size compared with total size and invasive size also gave a better separation of the survival curves than total size.[27]

Spread through air spaces

Spread through air spaces (STAS) is a pattern of tumor invasion into the lung parenchyma beyond the edge of the tumor (**Fig. 9**).[2,28] Although first described in lung adenocarcinoma,[28] it has now been shown to be of prognostic importance in all major histologic types of lung cancer studies, including squamous cell carcinoma,[29] atypical carcinoid,[30] large cell neuroendocrine carcinoma,[30] small cell carcinoma,[30] and pleomorphic carcinoma.[31] It is required to have more than 1 cluster of tumor cells at least 1 airspace beyond the tumor edge. The criteria for STAS includes exclusion of artifacts, including (1) mechanically induced tumor floaters that are randomly situated, often at the edge of the tissue section or out of the

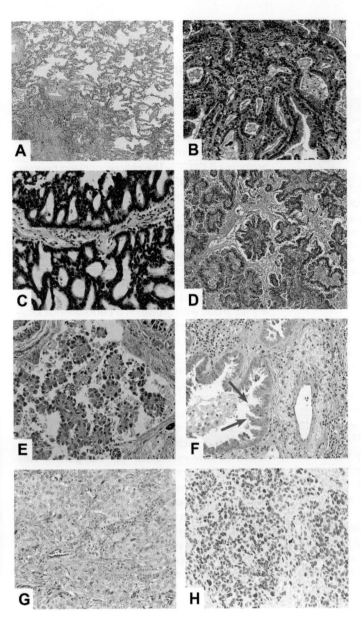

Fig. 6. Major histologic patterns of invasive adenocarcinoma. (*A*) Lepidic predominant pattern with mostly lepidic growth (*left*) and an area of invasive acinar adenocarcinoma (*right*). (hematoxylin-eosin, original magnification ×4). (*B*) Acinar pattern consists of infiltrative glands with tumor cells surrounding a space in the center of the malignant glands. (hematoxylin-eosin, original magnification ×20). (*C*) Cribriform pattern is included within the acinar pattern. Area of invasive acinar adenocarcinoma. (hematoxylin-eosin, original magnification ×20). (*D*) Papillary adenocarcinoma consists of malignant cuboidal to columnar tumor cells growing on the surface of fibrovascular cores. (hematoxylin-eosin, original magnification ×10). (*E*) Micropapillary adenocarcinoma, classical floret type, consists of small papillary clusters of glandular cells growing within this airspace, most of which do not show fibrovascular cores. (hematoxylin-eosin, original magnification ×40). (*F*) Micropapillary adenocarcinoma, filigree type, demonstrates narrow stacks of tumor cells at least 3 tumor cells high protruding into the air space. *Red arrows* highlight areas of filigree pattern. (hematoxylin-eosin, original magnification ×20). (*G*) Solid adenocarcinoma consists of sheets of tumor cells with no glandular formation. (hematoxylin-eosin, original magnification ×20). (*H*) The same tumor cells from part G stain positively with TTF-1, confirming adenocarcinoma differentiation. (TTF-1, original magnification ×20).

plane of section; (2) tumor cell clusters with jagged edges that suggest tumor fragmentation or edges of a knife cut during specimen processing; (3) the presence of isolated tumor clusters at a distance from the tumor rather than in a continuous manner from the tumor edge; and (4) linear strips of tumor cells that are lifted off alveolar walls favors an artifact.

A rapidly accumulating number of studies have demonstrated the poor prognostic significance of STAS. Data suggest that the survival implication of STAS is particularly important in patients who have undergone limited resection more than lobectomy.[32–35] It remains to be seen how this will be implemented into clinical practice, but it is possible this could impact intraoperative and postoperative setting management for both pathologists and surgeons.[32]

SQUAMOUS CELL CARCINOMA

Squamous cell carcinoma represents 23% of all lung cancers in the United States (see **Table 3**).[16] There has been a shift in the location of squamous cell carcinomas from a central (**Fig. 10**) to a predominantly peripheral location.[3] There are 3 subtypes of squamous carcinomas, including keratinizing, nonkeratinizing, and basaloid.[2]

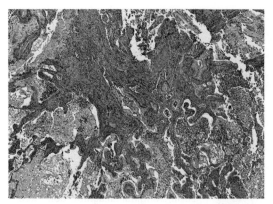

Fig. 7. Invasive mucinous adenocarcinoma. This area of invasive mucinous adenocarcinoma demonstrates an acinar pattern. The tumor consists of columnar cells filled with abundant mucin in the apical cytoplasm and shows small basal oriented nuclei. (hematoxylin-eosin, original magnification ×4).

Keratinizing squamous carcinoma shows intercellular bridging, squamous pearl formation, and keratinization (**Fig. 11**A). Nonkeratinizing squamous cell carcinomas show solid sheets of tumor cells that lack keratinization or glandular morphology (**Fig. 11**B). The diagnosis can be made only if immunohistochemistry shows expression of squamous markers, such as p40 (**Fig. 11**C) with negative TTF-1.[2,3,10] Basaloid squamous cell carcinomas are mostly nonkeratinizing with frequent peripheral palisading, organoid nesting (**Fig. 11**D), small tumor cells with scant cytoplasm. Abrupt keratinization and bands of hyaline stroma can be seen.

The histologic subtypes have not been shown to have prognostic significance. The suggestion by some studies that basaloid squamous carcinomas had a poor survival has not been validated.[2,3] Tumor budding and small nest size are the only histologic features consistently shown to be associated with poor prognosis.[36,37]

NEUROENDOCRINE LUNG TUMORS

Neuroendocrine lung tumors embrace a spectrum of low-grade and intermediate-grade typical and atypical carcinoid, respectively (see **Box 1**). These tumors must be separated from the high-grade small cell carcinoma and large cell neuroendocrine carcinoma (LCNEC). The only recognized preinvasive lesion is DIPNECH, and this is associated only with carcinoid tumors.

SMALL CELL CARCINOMA

SCLC accounts for 13% of all lung cancers (see **Table 3**) with the diagnosis of more than 29,600 new cases anticipated in the United States in 2019.[16,38] In most cases, it presents as a central perihilar mass with growth in a peribronchial location with infiltration of the bronchial submucosa and peribronchial tissue. Lymph node metastases are common and often extensive. The cut surface is usually white-tan with frequent extensive necrosis and hemorrhage. The tumor can present as a solitary coin lesion in 5% of cases.[3]

There are 2 major histologic types of SCLC: SCLC in which the entire tumor shows only SCLC, and combined SCLC in which there is a mixture of any non–small cell component (see **Box 1**).[2] SCLC consists of small tumor cells with a round to spindled shape, scant cytoplasm, nuclear chromatin that is finely granular, and nucleoli are inconspicuous or absent (**Fig. 12**).[2] Necrosis is frequent and often extensive. Mitotic counts are characteristically very high, averaging 80 mitoses per 2 mm² area or more.[2,39] Because most patients present in advanced stages, in the vast majority of cases the diagnosis is usually established

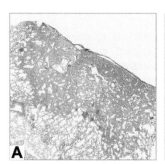
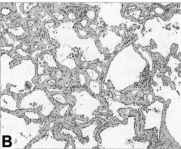
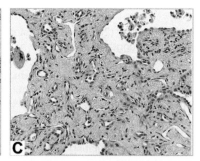

Fig. 8. MIA. (*A*) This MIA is lepidic predominant with a small focus of invasion. (hematoxylin-eosin, original magnification ×2). (*B*) The lepidic component consists of a proliferation of type II pneumocytes and Club (formerly Clara) cells along intact alveolar walls. (hematoxylin-eosin, original magnification ×10). (*C*) The invasive component consists of an acinar pattern with glands infiltrating fibrous stroma. (hematoxylin-eosin, original magnification ×20).

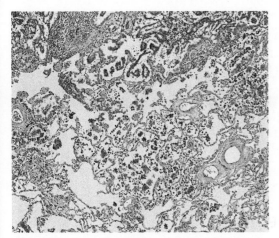

Fig. 9. STAS. Extending within air spaces beyond the edge of this lung adenocarcinoma there are nests and clusters of tumor cells within airspaces. (hematoxylin-eosin, original magnification ×10).

on transbronchial biopsy and/or cytology. The diagnosis is quite reliable in these small specimens. It is unusual to encounter surgically resected SCLC.

Although immunohistochemistry is helpful in the diagnosis, the most important stain is a good quality hematoxylin-eosin stain. Pancytokeratin is positive in virtually all cases, as well as at least 1 neuroendocrine marker such as chromogranin, synaptophysin, CD56, or INSM1 (see **Fig. 12B**) in more than 90% of cases.[10] Keratin expression helps to exclude lymphocytes in chronic inflammation or lymphoma. TTF-1 expression is seen in 70% to 80% of cases, but it can be positive in extrapulmonary SCLC, so it cannot be used as a lung-specific marker.[2,10] SCLC typically shows a high Ki-67 proliferation rate of 70% to 90% (see **Fig. 12C**).[40,41]

SCLC can be diagnosed well in small biopsies and cytology specimens. However, in these small specimens, immunohistochemistry is particularly important in the differential diagnosis with other tumors, especially crushed carcinoid tumors or lymphoid lesions. Ki-67 is particularly useful in these settings because SCLC should show a high proliferation rate of usually more than 50%, but often closer to 80% to 100%.[2,40,41] In addition, keratin versus lymphoid markers can help separate SCLC from lymphoid lesions such as chronic inflammation or lymphoma.[10]

Neuroendocrine markers are useful in a panel consisting of chromogranin, synaptophysin, CD56, and INSM1. However, if the workup includes CD56 and INSM1, all neuroendocrine markers can be negative in up to 10% of cases.[10] So it is possible in the minority of cases to diagnose SCLC if all neuroendocrine markers are negative.[2,3] In such cases, if TTF-1 is also negative, it is important to exclude basaloid squamous cell carcinomas by performing p40 staining.[10]

COMBINED SMALL CELL LUNG CANCER

Combined SCLC can be found in 10% to 28% of cases depending on the extent of histologic sampling. The highest percentage was reported in a series of 100 resected SCLC, in which combined SCLC and large cell carcinoma was most the most common encountered in 16% of cases followed by adenocarcinoma in 9% (see **Fig. 12D**) and squamous cell carcinoma in 3% of cases.[39] At least 10% large cells are required for the diagnosis of combined SCLC and large cell carcinoma.[2,39] However, for combined SCLC and adenocarcinoma or squamous cell carcinoma there is no requirement for a minimum percentage of adenocarcinoma or squamous cell carcinoma.

LARGE CELL NEUROENDOCRINE CARCINOMA

LCNEC comprises 3% of resected lung cancers.[3,42] In the spectrum of neuroendocrine lung tumors, it is a high-grade non–small cell

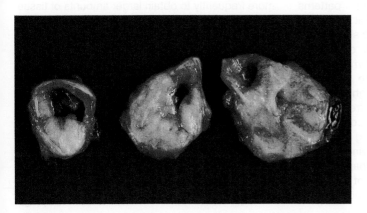

Fig. 10. Squamous cell carcinoma. Gross features: This central tumor surrounds the bronchus and was cut in multiple serial sections.

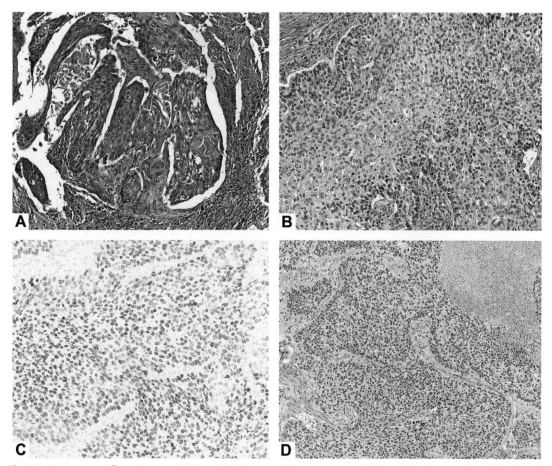

Fig. 11. Squamous cell carcinoma. (*A*) Keratinizing type. These tumor cells have abundant eosinophilic keratinized cytoplasm and form nests and keratin pearls characteristic of squamous differentiation. (hematoxylin-eosin, original magnification ×20). (*B*) Nonkeratinizing type. Sheets of tumor cells have moderate amounts of eosinophilic cytoplasm with uniform nuclei showing vesicular chromatin. (hematoxylin-eosin, original magnification ×20). (*C*) The tumor cells of the tumor in part B stain diffusely with p40 confirming squamous differentiation. (p40, original magnification ×20). (*D*) Basaloid type. The tumor shows prominent peripheral palisading with some organoid nesting. Many tumor cells have scant cytoplasm. The tumor stained diffusely for p40. (hematoxylin-eosin, original magnification ×20).

neuroendocrine carcinoma (see **Box 1**). Diagnostic criteria include the following: (1) neuroendocrine morphology, including organoid, palisading, trabecular, or rosettelike growth patterns (**Fig. 13**A); (2) cytologic features that fit for a non–small cell carcinoma: large tumor cell size, polygonal shape, moderate to abundant cytoplasm, coarse or vesicular nuclear chromatin, and frequent nucleoli; (3) the mitotic rate should be high (11 or more per 2 mm^2), although the mean is usually 60 mitoses per 2 mm^2; (4) frequent necrosis; and (5) immunohistochemical confirmation of neuroendocrine differentiation using a panel of markers where at least 1 of the following are positive: chromogranin (**Fig. 13**B), synaptophysin, CD56, or INSM1.[2,3,43] The diagnosis of LCNEC in small biopsy specimens is difficult because it is usually very difficult to identify the neuroendocrine morphology in such small tissues. However, in recent years now that core biopsies are performed more frequently to obtain larger amounts of tissue for molecular testing, the diagnosis of LCNEC is being made more frequently.

The term combined LCNEC is used if the tumor shows other non–small cell carcinoma components, such as adenocarcinoma or squamous cell carcinoma (see **Table 3**).[2,3] If SCLC is present, the diagnosis becomes combined SCLC.

TYPICAL AND ATYPICAL CARCINOID TUMORS

Carcinoid tumors account for 1% to 2% of all lung cancers.[3,44] The average age at presentation is 45 to 55 years, but carcinoids can occur at any age

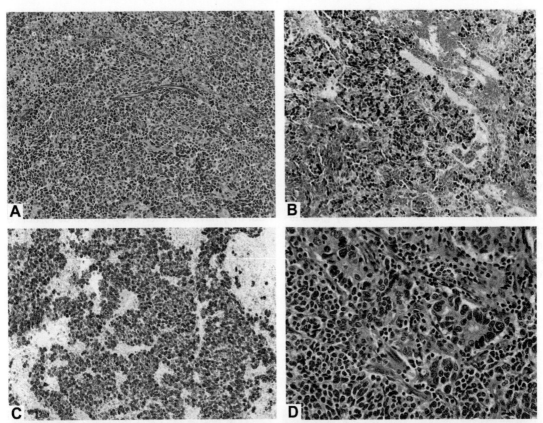

Fig. 12. Small cell carcinoma. (*A*) This tumor is composed of small cells with scant cytoplasm, finely granular chromatin and frequent mitoses. Nucleoli are absent. (hematoxylin-eosin, original magnification ×10). (*B*) Tumor cells nuclei stain strongly with immunohistochemistry for INSM1. (INSM1, original magnification ×20). (*C*) The Ki-67 proliferation rate is more than 90%. (Ki-67, original magnification ×20). (*D*) This combined SCLC and adenocarcinoma shows a mixture of small cell carcinoma and acinar adenocarcinoma. (hematoxylin-eosin, original magnification ×40).

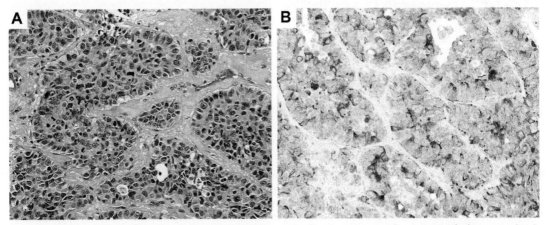

Fig. 13. LCNEC. (*A*) This tumor shows necrosis and tumor cells showing neuroendocrine morphology growing in nests with peripheral palisading and prominent rosettelike structures. Numerous mitoses are present and elsewhere the tumor showed necrosis. (hematoxylin-eosin, original magnification ×20). (*B*) The tumor cells show strong staining with chromogranin. (Chromogranin, original magnification ×20).

and there is no sex predilection. Patients present with hemoptysis, postobstructive pneumonitis, and dyspnea, but half of patients are asymptomatic.[3] Paraneoplastic syndromes, such as the carcinoid and Cushing syndrome, are uncommon.[42,45]

Carcinoid tumors may be situated peripherally, in the mid portion or centrally in the lung (Fig. 14). Central tumors are often associated with postobstructive manifestations and can have a polypoid endobronchial component. Carcinoids can show a variety of histologic patterns, most often an organoid nesting pattern. The cytologic features are uniform, consisting of moderate eosinophilic, finely granular cytoplasm. Nuclei have a finely granular chromatin pattern (Box 1, see Fig. 14B–D, Table 4). In addition tumors can show palisading, trabecular, spindle cell, rosettelike, papillary, glandular, sclerosing, and follicular patterns.[3,43]

Lung carcinoids are classified as either typical (TC) (see Fig. 14A, B) or atypical (AC) (see Fig. 14C, D). ACs are diagnosed in carcinoid tumors that show (1) mitoses between 2 and 10 per 2 mm^2 in areas of viable tumor (see Fig. 14D), or (2) the presence of necrosis that is usually punctate (see Fig. 14C).[2,3,46] TCs lack necrosis and mitotic figures are less than 2 per 2 mm^2 (see Table 4).[2,3,46]

Carcinoids stain for neuroendocrine immunohistochemical markers, such as chromogranin, synaptophysin, CD56, and INSM1 and the staining is usually diffuse and strong except for some ACs. Ki-67 proliferation rates tend to be higher in AC but they have not been shown to be as reliable a way compared with mitoses to distinguish TC from AC and it is not part of the diagnostic criteria.[40] TCs usually show a low proliferation rate (≤5%). In contrast, AC Ki-67 proliferation

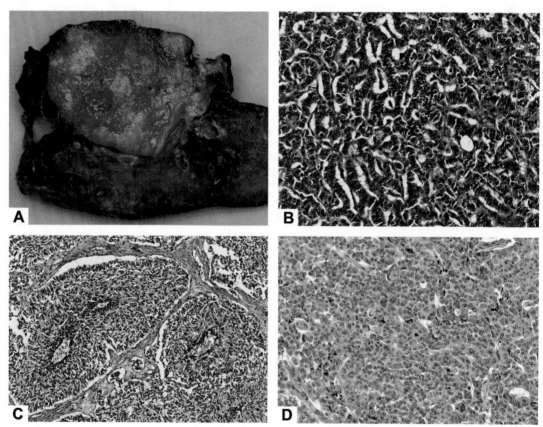

Fig. 14. Carcinoid tumor. (A) Gross features: This 5.2 cm left upper lobe typical carcinoid tumor shows a smooth tan-yellow cut surface with no necrosis or hemorrhage. (B) Typical carcinoid shows organoid nesting and trabecular arrangement. Tumor cells are uniform with moderate eosinophilic cytoplasm. Nuclei have salt and pepper chromatin. No necrosis or mitoses are seen. (hematoxylin-eosin, original magnification ×20). (C) Atypical carcinoid shows organoid nesting with prominent rosettelike structures. Punctate necrosis is present. (hematoxylin-eosin, original magnification ×20). (D) This atypical carcinoid shows a single mitotic figure (center). The surrounding tumor cells have moderate eosinophilic cytoplasm and nuclei with salt and pepper chromatin. (hematoxylin-eosin, original magnification ×40).

<table>
<tr><td>

Box 1
The spectrum of neuroendocrine tumors of the lung

Small cell carcinoma

  Combined small cell carcinoma

Large cell neuroendocrine carcinoma

  Combined large cell neuroendocrine carcinoma

Typical carcinoid (size 0.5 cm or larger)

Atypical carcinoid

Preinvasive lesion for carcinoid tumors

  Diffuse idiopathic pulmonary neuroendocrine cell hyperplasia

</td></tr>
</table>

a criterion for distinguishing TC from AC.[47] Rarely, lung carcinoids present with metastatic disease and in biopsies of metastatic tumor from these patients it is recommended to diagnose metastatic carcinoid tumor rather than to use the terms TC and AC. However, it is recommended to record the mitotic rate per 2 mm^2, the presence of necrosis, and the Ki-67 proliferation rate.[48] In the progression of lung carcinoid tumors as they metastasize, sometimes the mitotic rate and Ki-67 proliferation rate increase, but they are still distinguished from the high-grade LCNECs and SCLCs.[48]

Survival is worse for patients with AC (30%, ranging from 27% to 47%) compared with TC (more than 90%).[3,45,46] Furthermore, ACs have a higher rate of lymph node and other distant metastases.[3,45,46]

rates are usually between 5% and 10% but may be up to 20%.[2,41] In the diagnosis of lung neuroendocrine tumors, the most useful role for Ki-67 staining is in the separation of carcinoids from the high-grade LCNECs or SCLCs, which have very high proliferation rates.[40,41] This is particularly useful in small crushed biopsies.[40,41]

The primary therapeutic approach for lung carcinoids is surgical resection, because the vast majority present in early stages.[47] An excellent prognosis is seen in most patients with TC who only rarely die of tumor.[42,45] Because 5% to 20% of TCs have regional lymph node metastases, the finding of metastases should not be used as

LARGE CELL CARCINOMA

Large cell carcinoma is defined as a poorly differentiated non–small cell carcinoma that does not meet criteria for any other non–small cell carcinoma or small cell carcinoma. It lacks glandular or squamous differentiation by morphology or immunohistochemistry.[2,3] The diagnosis cannot be made on small biopsies or cytology and it requires a resection specimen.[49] According to a recent report of the US National Cancer Institute, Surveillance, Epidemiology, and End Results (SEER) data, it comprises 1.5% of all lung

Table 4
Typical and atypical carcinoid: distinguishing features

Histologic or Clinical Feature	Typical Carcinoid	Atypical Carcinoid
Histologic Patterns: Organoid, Trabecular, Palisading and Spindle cell	Characteristic	Characteristic
Mitoses	Absent or <2 per 2 mm^2 area of viable tumor	2–10 per 2 mm^2 or area of viable tumor
Necrosis	Absent	Characteristic, usually focal or punctate
Nuclear pleomorphism, hyperchromatism	Usually absent, not sufficient by itself for diagnosis of atypical carcinoid	Often present
Regional lymph node metastases at presentation	5%–15%	40%–48%
Distant metastases at presentation	Rare	20%
Survival at 5 y	90%–95%	50%–60%
Disease-free survival at 10 y	90%–95%	35%

From Travis WD. Pathology of lung cancer. Clin Chest Med 2002; 23:65-81; with permission.

carcinomas.[16] This marks a major decrease from 9% reported in the SEER monograph for 1983 to 1987.[44,49] It should be kept in mind though that the SEER data include unresectable tumors that would have been diagnosed on small biopsies or cytology as well as resected tumors, realizing that the diagnosis of large cell carcinoma cannot be made in such specimens. Other surgical series also report a frequency for large cell carcinoma of approximately 3%.[50,51] In the 2015 WHO Classification, tumors formerly classified as large cell carcinoma that express TTF-1 or p40 are now classified as solid adenocarcinoma or nonkeratinizing squamous cell carcinoma, respectively.[2]

Large cell carcinoma is a diagnosis of exclusion, in which the presence of squamous cell or glandular differentiation (**Fig. 15**) needs to be excluded by light microscopy, immunohistochemistry, and/or mucin stains.[52–54] The tumor cells grow in sheets and nests with a round to polygonal shape, vesicular nuclear chromatin, and prominent nucleoli (see **Fig. 15**),[2] so these tumors should be negative for TTF-1 and p40 to exclude glandular or squamous differentiation, respectively. The presence of 5 or more mucin-positive cells in at least 2 high-power fields would favor solid adenocarcinomas with mucin rather than large cell carcinoma.[2]

ADENOSQUAMOUS CARCINOMA

Adenosquamous carcinoma comprises 0.6% to 2.3% of all lung cancers and is diagnosed in non–small cell carcinomas that show at least 10% components of both squamous cell carcinoma and adenocarcinoma (**Fig. 16**).[2,3] The diagnosis can be made only on a resection specimen, so on small biopsies or cytology this diagnosis can only be suggested. Morphologic features on hematoxylin-eosin–stained slides that reflect clear differentiation, such as glandular patterns or keratinization, may be present in either one or both components. Similarly, these components may be defined by a solid pattern that shows expression of TTF-1/mucin or p40, respectively.

SARCOMATOID CARCINOMAS

Sarcomatoid carcinomas account for 0.3% of all invasive lung malignancies.[2,44] This category includes 3 different tumors: (1) pleomorphic carcinoma, (2) carcinosarcoma, and (3) pulmonary blastoma.[2,3] Pleomorphic carcinomas are defined as non–small cell carcinomas that contain mixtures of different components, such as adenocarcinoma and squamous cell carcinoma in addition to least 10% spindle cell and/or giant cell carcinoma (**Fig. 17**).[2] The typical presentation is as a large, peripheral tumor with frequent chest wall invasion.[2] These tumors need to be sampled generously, with at least 1 section per centimeter of the tumor diameter to demonstrate the different histologic components. The diagnosis requires a resection specimen and cannot be made on small biopsies or cytology. Tumors consisting of pure giant cell or spindle cell patterns are classified as giant cell or spindle cell carcinoma, respectively. Giant cell carcinomas are composed of tumor cells

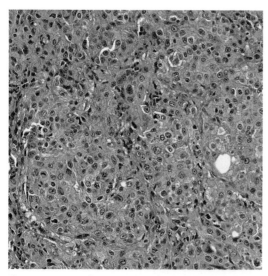

Fig. 15. Large cell carcinoma. This resected lung cancer consists of diffuse sheets of tumor cells with abundant cytoplasm, vesicular chromatin, and prominent nucleoli. No glandular or squamous morphology are seen and stains for TTF-1, p40, and mucin were negative. (hematoxylin-eosin, original magnification ×40).

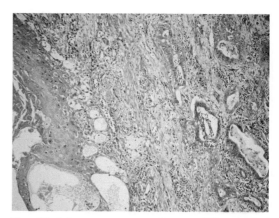

Fig. 16. Adenosquamous carcinoma. This resected lung cancer shows adenocarcinoma with a lepidic pattern (*left*) and squamous cell carcinoma (*right*). Both components were present in at least 10% of the tumor. (hematoxylin-eosin, original magnification ×10).

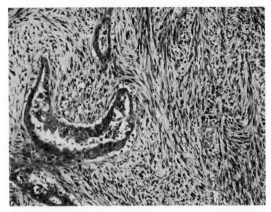

Fig. 17. Pleomorphic carcinoma. This resected lung cancer was composed of a mixture of acinar adenocarcinoma and malignant spindle cells. (hematoxylin-eosin, original magnification ×40).

with large cell size and nuclei and frequent multinucleated tumor giant cells.[2,3]

CARCINOSARCOMA AND PULMONARY BLASTOMA

Carcinosarcoma is composed of a mixture of carcinoma and sarcoma. Heterologous elements are required to recognize the sarcomatous component including chondrosarcoma, osteosarcoma, or rhabdomyosarcoma.[2,3] Pulmonary blastomas are biphasic tumors consisting of primitive sarcomatous elements as well as a glandular component that resembles well-differentiated fetal adenocarcinoma.[2,3] In cases in which the carcinoma or sarcoma components are poorly differentiated, immunohistochemistry can be helpful. In such cases, epithelial markers, such as keratin, may demonstrate epithelial differentiation, or stains such as TTF-1 or p40 may support adenocarcinoma or squamous differentiation. For the sarcomatous component, desmin and myogenin may help confirm the presence of rhabdomyosarcoma.[2,3]

DISCLOSURE

Nothing to disclose.

REFERENCES

1. Travis WD, Brambilla E, Noguchi M, et al. The new IASLC/ATS/ERS international multidisciplinary lung adenocarcinoma classification. J Thorac Oncol 2011;6:244–85.
2. Travis WD, Brambilla E, Burke AP, et al. WHO classification of tumours of the lung, pleura, thymus and heart. 4th edition. Lyon (France): International Agency for Research on Cancer; 2015.
3. Travis WD, Nicholson AG, Geisinger K, et al. Tumors of the lower respiratory tract. Silver Spring (MD): American Registry of Pathology; 2019.
4. Lindeman NI, Cagle PT, Aisner DL, et al. Updated molecular testing guideline for the selection of lung cancer patients for treatment with targeted tyrosine kinase inhibitors: guideline from the College of American Pathologists, the International Association for the Study of Lung Cancer, and the Association for Molecular Pathology. J Thorac Oncol 2018;13: 323–58.
5. Travis WD, Brambilla E, Nicholson AG, et al. The 2015 World Health Organization classification of lung tumors: impact of genetic, clinical and radiologic advances since the 2004 classification. J Thorac Oncol 2015;10:1243–60.
6. Johnson DH, Fehrenbacher L, Novotny WF, et al. Randomized phase II trial comparing bevacizumab plus carboplatin and paclitaxel with carboplatin and paclitaxel alone in previously untreated locally advanced or metastatic non-small-cell lung cancer. J Clin Oncol 2004;22:2184–91.
7. Kerr KM, Hirsch FR. Programmed death ligand-1 immunohistochemistry: friend or foe? Arch Pathol Lab Med 2016;140:326–31.
8. Hirsch FR, McElhinny A, Stanforth D, et al. PD-L1 immunohistochemistry assays for lung cancer: results from phase 1 of the blueprint PD-L1 IHC assay comparison project. J Thorac Oncol 2017;12: 208–22.
9. Rimm DL, Han G, Taube JM, et al. A prospective, multi-institutional, pathologist-based assessment of 4 immunohistochemistry assays for PD-L1 expression in non-small cell lung cancer. JAMA Oncol 2017;3:1051–8.
10. Yatabe Y, Dacic S, Borczuk AC, et al. Best practices recommendations for diagnostic immunohistochemistry in lung cancer. J Thorac Oncol 2019;14: 377–407.
11. Rekhtman N, Brandt SM, Sigel CS, et al. Suitability of thoracic cytology for new therapeutic paradigms in non-small cell lung carcinoma: high accuracy of tumor subtyping and feasibility of EGFR and KRAS molecular testing. J Thorac Oncol 2011;6:451–8.
12. Travis WD. Lung. In: Henson DE, Albores-Saavedra J, editors. Pathology of incipient neoplasia. New York: Oxford University Press, Inc.; 2001. p. 295–318.
13. Kadota K, Villena-Vargas J, Yoshizawa A, et al. Prognostic significance of adenocarcinoma in situ, minimally invasive adenocarcinoma, and nonmucinous lepidic predominant invasive adenocarcinoma of the lung in patients with stage I disease. Am J Surg Pathol 2014;38:448–60.
14. Rossi G, Cavazza A, Spagnolo P, et al. Diffuse idiopathic pulmonary neuroendocrine cell hyperplasia syndrome. Eur Respir J 2016;47:1829–41.

15. Mengoli MC, Rossi G, Cavazza A, et al. Diffuse idiopathic pulmonary neuroendocrine cell hyperplasia (DIPNECH) syndrome and carcinoid tumors with/without NECH: a clinicopathologic, radiologic, and immunomolecular comparison study. Am J Surg Pathol 2018;42:646–55.

16. Howlader N, Noone AM, Krapcho M, et al. SEER Cancer Statistics Review, 1975-2016. Bethesda (MD): National Cancer Institute; 2018.

17. Emoto K, Eguchi T, Tan KS, et al. Expansion of the concept of micropapillary adenocarcinoma to include a newly recognized filigree pattern as well as the classical pattern based on 1468 Stage I lung adenocarcinomas. J Thorac Oncol 2019; 14(11):1948–61.

18. Koo HJ, Kim MY, Koo JH, et al. Computerized margin and texture analyses for differentiating bacterial pneumonia and invasive mucinous adenocarcinoma presenting as consolidation. PLoS One 2017;12:e0177379.

19. Yoshizawa A, Motoi N, Riely GJ, et al. Impact of proposed IASLC/ATS/ERS classification of lung adenocarcinoma: prognostic subgroups and implications for further revision of staging based on analysis of 514 stage I cases. Mod Pathol 2011;24:653–64.

20. Nitadori J, Bograd AJ, Kadota K, et al. Impact of micropapillary histologic subtype in selecting limited resection vs lobectomy for lung adenocarcinoma of 2cm or smaller. J Natl Cancer Inst 2013;105: 1212–20.

21. Kadota K, Kushida Y, Kagawa S, et al. Cribriform subtype is an independent predictor of recurrence and survival after adjustment for the eighth edition of TNM staging system in patients with resected lung adenocarcinoma. J Thorac Oncol 2019;14: 245–54.

22. Boland JM, Maleszewski JJ, Wampfler JA, et al. Pulmonary invasive mucinous adenocarcinoma and mixed invasive mucinous/nonmucinous adenocarcinoma-a clinicopathological and molecular genetic study with survival analysis. Hum Pathol 2018;71:8–19.

23. Detterbeck FC, Nicholson AG, Franklin WA, et al. The IASLC lung cancer staging project: summary of proposals for revisions of the classification of lung cancers with multiple pulmonary sites of involvement in the forthcoming eighth edition of the TNM classification. J Thorac Oncol 2016;11:639–50.

24. Nicholson AG, Viola P, Torkko K, et al. Interobserver variation among pathologists and refinement of criteria in distinguishing separate primary tumors from intrapulmonary metastases in lung. J Thoracic Oncol 2018;13:205–17.

25. Chang JC, Alex D, Bott M, et al. Comprehensive next-generation sequencing unambiguously distinguishes separate primary lung carcinomas from intra-pulmonary metastases: comparison with standard histopathologic approach. Clin Cancer Res 2019;25(23):7113–25.

26. Travis WD, Asamura H, Bankier AA, et al. The IASLC lung cancer staging project: proposals for coding T categories for subsolid nodules and assessment of tumor size in part-solid tumors in the forthcoming eighth edition of the TNM classification of lung cancer. J Thorac Oncol 2016;11:1204–23.

27. Kameda K, Eguchi T, Lu S, et al. Implications of the eighth edition of the TNM proposal: invasive versus total tumor size for the T descriptor in pathologic stage I-IIA lung adenocarcinoma. J Thorac Oncol 2018;13:1919–29.

28. Kadota K, Nitadori J, Sima CS, et al. Tumor spread through air spaces is an important pattern of invasion and impacts the frequency and location of recurrences after limited resection for small stage I lung adenocarcinomas. J Thorac Oncol 2015;10: 806–14.

29. Kadota K, Kushida Y, Katsuki N, et al. Tumor spread through air spaces is an independent predictor of recurrence-free survival in patients with resected lung squamous cell carcinoma. Am J Surg Pathol 2017;41:1077–86.

30. Aly R, Eguchi T, Kadota K, et al. Impact of tumor spread through air spaces (STAS) in lung neuroendocrine tumors (NETs). J Thorac Oncol 2018;13: S434–5.

31. Yokoyama S, Murakami T, Tao H, et al. Tumor spread through air spaces identifies a distinct subgroup with poor prognosis in surgically resected lung pleomorphic carcinoma. Chest 2018;154:838–47.

32. Eguchi T, Kameda K, Lu S, et al. Lobectomy is associated with better outcomes than sublobar resection in Spread through air spaces (STAS)-Positive T1 lung adenocarcinoma: a propensity score-matched analysis. J Thorac Oncol 2019;14:87–98.

33. Kadota K, Kushida Y, Kagawa S, et al. Limited resection is associated with a higher risk of locoregional recurrence than lobectomy in stage I lung adenocarcinoma with tumor Spread through air spaces. Am J Surg Pathol 2019;43:1033–41.

34. Liu H, Yin Q, Yang G, et al. Prognostic impact of tumor spread through air spaces in non-small cell lung cancers: a meta-analysis including 3564 patients. Pathol Oncol Res 2019;25(4):1303–10.

35. Bains S, Eguchi T, Warth A, et al. Procedure-specific risk prediction for recurrence in patients undergoing lobectomy or sublobar resection for small (≤2 cm) lung adenocarcinoma: an international cohort analysis. J Thorac Oncol 2019;14:72–86.

36. Kadota K, Miyai Y, Katsuki N, et al. A grading system combining tumor budding and nuclear diameter predicts prognosis in resected lung squamous cell carcinoma. Am J Surg Pathol 2017;41:750–60.

37. Kadota K, Nitadori J, Woo KM, et al. Comprehensive pathological analyses in lung squamous cell

carcinoma: single cell invasion, nuclear diameter, and tumor budding are independent prognostic factors for worse outcomes. J Thorac Oncol 2014;9: 1126–39.

38. Siegel RL, Miller KD, Jemal A. Cancer statistics, 2019. CA Cancer J Clin 2019;69:7–34.

39. Nicholson SA, Beasley MB, Brambilla E, et al. Small cell lung carcinoma (SCLC): a clinicopathologic study of 100 cases with surgical specimens. Am J Surg Pathol 2002;26:1184–97.

40. Rindi G, Klimstra DS, Abedi-Ardekani B, et al. A common classification framework for neuroendocrine neoplasms: an International Agency for Research on Cancer (IARC) and World Health Organization (WHO) expert consensus proposal. Mod Pathol 2018;31:1770–86.

41. Pelosi G, Rindi G, Travis WD, et al. Ki-67 antigen in lung neuroendocrine tumors: unraveling a role in clinical practice. J Thorac Oncol 2014;9:273–84.

42. Travis WD. Advances in neuroendocrine lung tumors. Ann Oncol 2010;21(Suppl 7):vii65–71.

43. Travis WD, Linnoila RI, Tsokos MG, et al. Neuroendocrine tumors of the lung with proposed criteria for large-cell neuroendocrine carcinoma. An ultrastructural, immunohistochemical, and flow cytometric study of 35 cases. Am J Surg Pathol 1991;15: 529–53.

44. Travis WD, Travis LB, Devesa SS. Lung cancer [published erratum appears in Cancer 1995 Jun 15; 75(12):2979]. Cancer 1995;75:191–202.

45. Pietanza MC, Krug L, Wu AJ, et al. Small cell and neuroendocrine tumors of the lung. In: DeVita VT, Lawrence TS, Rosenberg SA, editors. Devita, Hellman, and Rosenberg's cancer: principles and practice of oncology. 10th edition. Philadelphia: Wolters Kluwer; 2015. p. 536–59.

46. Travis WD, Rush W, Flieder DB, et al. Survival analysis of 200 pulmonary neuroendocrine tumors with clarification of criteria for atypical carcinoid and its separation from typical carcinoid. Am J Surg Pathol 1998;22:934–44.

47. Chi Y, Gao S, Du F, et al. Diagnosis, treatment, and prognosis of bronchopulmonary carcinoid: an analysis of 74 patients. Anticancer Drugs 2016;27:54–9.

48. Rekhtman N, Desmeules P, Litvak AM, et al. Stage IV lung carcinoids: spectrum and evolution of proliferation rate, focusing on variants with elevated proliferation indices. Mod Pathol 2019;32:1106–22.

49. Rekhtman N, Travis WD. Large no more: the journey of pulmonary large cell carcinoma from common to rare entity. J Thorac Oncol 2019;14:1125–7.

50. Sun Z, Aubry MC, Deschamps C, et al. Histologic grade is an independent prognostic factor for survival in non-small cell lung cancer: an analysis of 5018 hospital- and 712 population-based cases. J Thorac Cardiovasc Surg 2006;131:1014–20.

51. Sawabata N, Asamura H, Goya T, et al. Japanese Lung Cancer Registry Study: first prospective enrollment of a large number of surgical and nonsurgical cases in 2002. J Thorac Oncol 2010;5:1369–75.

52. Carvalho L. Reclassifying bronchial-pulmonary carcinoma: differentiating histological type in biopsies by immunohistochemistry. Rev Port Pneumol (2006) 2009;15:1101–19.

53. Hwang DH, Szeto DP, Perry AS, et al. Pulmonary large cell carcinoma lacking squamous differentiation is clinicopathologically indistinguishable from solid-subtype Adenocarcinoma. Arch Pathol Lab Med 2013;138:626–35.

54. Rekhtman N, Tafe LJ, Chaft JE, et al. Distinct profile of driver mutations and clinical features in immunomarker-defined subsets of pulmonary large-cell carcinoma. Mod Pathol 2013;26:511–22.

Lung Cancer Screening
Patient Selection and Implementation

Nina A. Thomas, MD[a], Nichole T. Tanner, MD, MSCR[a,b],*

KEYWORDS

- Lung cancer • Screening • Patient selection • Risk prediction • Shared decision making
- Implementation science

KEY POINTS

- The goal of lung cancer (LC) screening is to detect early-stage LC in patients at high risk for LC who are healthy enough to undergo evaluation and successful treatment, while minimizing adverse effects of screening.
- Several randomized controlled trials have demonstrated lung-cancer mortality benefit of screening for LC with low-dose computed tomography in select patients.
- Professional societies and the US Preventive Services Task Force recommend LC screening in individuals based on age, smoking history, and ability to undergo curative treatment of a screen-detected LC.
- Patient selection for LC screening may be improved with the use of validated risk prediction calculators, which incorporate additional risk factors for LC.
- Implementation of LC screening requires multidisciplinary input to ensure that the essential components of a LC screening program are incorporated.

INTRODUCTION

The combined 5-year survival for lung cancer (LC) remains low, at 18%, because most patients present with advanced disease at the time of diagnosis.[1] In those with early-stage disease, however, the 5-year survival is as high as 80%, making early detection ideal.[2] The results of the National Lung Screening Trial (NLST) provided the evidence for screening, with annual low-dose computed tomography (LDCT) demonstrating a 20% reduction in LC mortality.[3] Due to these results, the US Preventive Services Task Force (USPSTF) provided a grade B recommendation in favor of screening, and the Centers for Medicare and Medicaid Services (CMS) approved LC screening in their eligible beneficiaries.[4] Both the USPSTF and CMS highlight the importance of proper patient selection and, in conjunction with

professional societies, outlined components necessary for an effective LC screening program.[5] This article focuses on patient selection for and implementation of LC screening.

EVIDENCE FOR LUNG CANCER SCREENING

The Prostate, Lung, Colorectal and Ovarian (PLCO) Cancer Screening Trial was the first large randomized trial to examine LC screening with the use of chest radiography versus usual care. Screening with chest x-ray did not result in a significant decrease in LC incidence or mortality. There were also similar rates of stage and histology between the 2 groups.[6] This study provided definitive evidence that screening with chest x-ray is not effective.

Following the PLCO, there have been several cohort studies evaluating outcomes from

[a] Division of Pulmonary, Critical Care, Allergy and Sleep Medicine, Medical University of South Carolina, 96 Jonathan Lucas Street, CSB Suite 816, MSC 630, Charleston, SC 29425, USA; [b] Health Equity and Rural Outreach Innovation Center (HEROIC), Ralph H. Johnson Veterans Affairs Hospital, 109 Bee Street, Charleston, SC 29401, USA
* Corresponding author.
E-mail address: tripici@musc.edu

Clin Chest Med 41 (2020) 87–97
https://doi.org/10.1016/j.ccm.2019.10.006
0272-5231/20/© 2019 Elsevier Inc. All rights reserved.

screening with computed tomography (CT) that suggested a benefit to LDCT screening but were inconclusive in the absence of a comparator arm.[7–9] In addition, there were several randomized controlled trials (RCTs) of LDCT that failed to demonstrate mortality benefit due to their lack of power and low enrollment.[10–13] The largest and most often cited RCTs are highlighted.

The NLST randomized 53,454 patients at high risk for developing LC to chest x-ray versus LDCT annually for 3 years. Inclusion criteria to define individuals at high risk of developing LC included (1) ages 55 years to 74 years, (2) history of cigarette smoking of at least 30 pack-years, and (3) if former smokers, whether they had quit within the last 15 years. There was no usual care group in this study. The trial met its predetermined endpoint of a 20% reduction in LC-related mortality in the LDCT arm with a number needed to screen of 320 to prevent 1 LC death.[3,14] These findings provided the impetus for broad-based implementation of LC screening programs in the United States.

Simultaneous to the NLST, the Dutch-Belgian Randomized Lung Screening Trial (NELSON) was another large randomized trial in the Netherlands and Belgium that aimed to show that screening with LDCT would decrease 10-year mortality. Patient eligibility included analysis. The NELSON trial randomized 15,822 participants to LDCT or usual care and found a mortality benefit with a 26% reduction in LC mortality.[15] This study was unique compared with the NLST and many other previous trials in that all pulmonary nodules were monitored with 3-dimensional volumetric analysis. Nodules were characterized by nodule size and volume doubling time, which was found to be more accurate than the 2-dimensional monitoring of nodules. The participants were also followed at longer intervals, at 1 year, 3 years, and 5.5 years from enrollment. This method of risk stratification for LC screening was novel in that it included patients' CT findings as a part of their risk assessment for LC.[16]

The Detection and Screening of Early Lung Cancer by Novel Imaging Technology and Molecular Essays trial was an RCT comparing usual care with LDCT annually for 5 years. This Italian study, which was not powered to detect a difference between the 2 groups, randomized 2472 men to LDCT or usual care. Eligible participants ages 60 years to 74 years with at least a 20 pack-year smoking history were followed for a median of 8 years. Although more early-stage and advanced-stage LCs were discovered in the LDCT arm, there was no significant stage shift compared with the usual care arm and there was no difference in LC or all-cause mortality.[13]

Finally, the Multicentric Italian Lung Detection trial was a single-center trial that included 4099 smokers, ages 49 years and older, with a greater than 20 pack-year smoking history, and randomized them to annual CT, biennial CT, or usual care.[17] The relative risk (RR) for dying of LC was lower in the biennial CT and annual CT groups compared with the usual care group, but all-cause mortality did not significantly differ when comparing the combined screening groups with the usual care group.

PATIENT SELECTION FOR LUNG CANCER SCREENING
Current Lung Cancer Screening Recommendations

Several professional societies have endorsed LC screening in the United States, each having slightly different age criteria for patient selection and some including other risk factors. **Table 1** summarizes the current recommendations for patient selection for LC screening based on different professional societies.

US Preventive Screening Task Force

In 2013, largely based on the results of the NLST, the USPSTF recommended screening for LC with LDCT in a high-risk population. The criteria recommended for screening remained mostly true to inclusion criteria for the NLST. As a result of the Cancer Intervention and Surveillance Modeling Network for health care research, however, the age criterion for inclusion was increased from 55 years to 74 years to 55 years to 80 years to balance the benefits of screening with the risk of false-positive results.[4]

National Comprehensive Cancer Network

The National Comprehensive Cancer Network (NCCN) was the first major organization to recommend and develop official guidelines for LC screening. The NCCN recommends screening with LDCT for 2 separate groups of individuals felt to be at high risk for developing LC. The first group are those meeting the age and smoking history criteria for NLST inclusion. The second group, given a category 2A recommendation, includes younger individuals (ages 50 years and older) with lighter smoking histories (minimum 20 pack years) and an additional risk factor for LC. Additional risk factors include a personal history of cancer or lung disease, family history of LC, radon exposure, or occupational exposure to carcinogens. The inclusion of these additional risk factors

Table 1
Recommendations for lung cancer screening

Guideline	Inclusion Criteria	Exclusion Criteria	When to Stop Screening
NLST	• Age 55–74 y • ≥30 pack-year smoking history • Quit smoking <15 y ago	• History of LC • Chest imaging within 18 mo • Hemoptysis, weight loss >7 kg	
USPSTF	• Age 55–80 y • ≥30 pack-year smoking history • Quit smoking <15 y ago	• Condition limits life expectancy • Unable or unwilling to undergo screening/treatment	• Stopped smoking for 15 y • Age 80 • Unable to undergo evaluation/treatment
CMS	• Age 55–77 y • ≥30 pack-year smoking history • Quit smoking <15 y ago	• Condition limiting life expectancy • Unable or unwilling to undergo screening/treatment	• Stopped smoking for 15 y • Age 80 • Unable to undergo evaluation/treatment
NCCN	Group 1 • Age 55–74 y • ≥30 pack-year smoking history • Quit smoking <15 y ago Group 2 • Age ≥50 • ≥20 pack-year smoking history • One additional risk factor (personal cancer history, family history, exposure, chronic lung disease)		
CHEST	• Age 55–77 y • ≥30 pack-year smoking history • Quit smoking <15 y ago	• History of LC • Chest imaging within 18 mo • Hemoptysis weight loss >7 kg	
AATS	Group 1 • Age 55–79 y • ≥30 pack-year smoking history • Quit smoking <15 y ago Group 2 • LC survivors without recurrence after 4 y of surveillance Group 3 • Age 50–79 y • ≥20 pack-year smoking history • Additional comorbidities that produce a 5% risk of developing LC within 5 y		

was based on previous studies, which showed association with higher risk for LC.[18]

Occupational carcinogens, such as arsenic, chromium, asbestos, nickel, cadmium, beryllium, silica, diesel fumes, coal smoke, and soot, have a calculated mean RR of 1.59 for development of LC.[19–21] Among these patients with occupational exposures, smokers have an even higher risk for developing LC. A 2005 meta-analysis showed that the amount of radon exposure had a linear relationship with the risk of development of LC, which again was even higher in smokers.[22] Patients with a personal history of cancer, whether lung primary, head and neck, lymphoma, or other smoking-related cancers, also have increased risk of developing LC due to both genetic susceptibility and treatment, including radiation and alkylating chemotherapy agents.[23] Although there is no specific genetic syndrome associated with LC, a family history of a first-degree relative with LC portends an RR of 1.8 (95% CI, 1.6–2.0) of developing LC.[24] Finally, underlying lung disease, specifically COPD and pulmonary fibrosis, have been associated with higher risk for developing LC.[21]

American College of s Physicians (CHEST)

American College of Chest Physicians (CHEST) guidelines for patient selection for LC are in line with the NLST entry criteria, including patients ages 55 years to 77 years, patients who have smoked at least 30 pack-years or more, and patients who are current smokers or have quit within the past 15 years. This differs from the age cutoff of 80 years recommended by the USPSTF but is reflective of what is covered by the CMS. The guidelines do remark on the improved efficiency of identifying high-risk patients using risk prediction calculators; however, they do not currently recommend using these calculators to qualify high-risk patients who do not meet the NLST criteria for LC screening. This is attributed to the idea that the risk factors included in many of these calculators also portend a higher risk of death from competing comorbidities or morbidity from evaluation of the nodules, mitigating the benefit and increasing the harm of LC screening in this population. Additionally, for patients who meet these criteria, but have comorbidities that disallow them to tolerate evaluation or treatment of early-stage cancer, or substantially decrease life expectancy, the guidelines recommend against screening.[25]

American Association for Thoracic Surgery

The American Association for Thoracic Surgery (AATS) recommendations for inclusion in LC screening also reflect the inclusion criteria for the NLST, with the main difference of age cutoff from ages 55 years to 79 years. Although the NLST screened patients with LDCT annually for 3 years, the risk of developing LC after 3 years does not decrease. By the end of follow-up in the trial, 5 years after the third annual screen, the percentage of stage I LCs detected had decreased from 63% to 50% whereas the rate of diagnosis of stage IIIB/IV LC had increased from 21% to 33%.[26] This suggests that continued surveillance with annual LDCT after the third scan may lead to greater mortality reduction if said cancers had been diagnosed at earlier stages. Thus, the AATS recommends the higher age cutoff of 79 years old, because risk of LC increases linearly with the age and the average life expectancy in the United States is 78.6 years, with an additional 9 years for Americans who reach age 79 years. The AATS also specifically recommends annual screening with LDCT for LC survivors starting 5 years after treatment, because these patients maintain a high risk for recurrence or secondary LC and were excluded from most trials. Additionally, they recommend screening for patients ages 50 years to 79 years with a 20 pack-year smoking history and an additional risk factor that produces at least a 5% risk of developing LC over the next 5 years. They do recommend the use of clinical risk calculators to assist in determining patient risk.[26]

Risk Prediction Models for Patient Selection

Following the publication of the NLST, there have been several investigations into developing and validating risk prediction calculators to be more efficient (eg, find more cancers while screening less people) than the selection criteria of age and smoking history. By enriching the pool of patients screened for LC, there is the potential to both reduce the number of false positives and the number needed to screen. Furthermore, providing a person with an individual risk of developing LC can be beneficial in facilitating informed decision making around LC screening.

In the United States, the number of screen-eligible patients from 2010 to 2015 decreased by 1.5 million. The decrease in number of patients with a 5-year LC risk of at least 2%, however, was only 0.8 million, suggesting there are patients at high risk of developing LC who are not being screened.[27] Beyond age and smoking history, other risk factors identified to increase risk of LC include family history, ethnicity, level of education, socioeconomic status, body mass index (BMI), chronic obstructive pulmonary disease (COPD), personal history of cancer, and smoking intensity. Although many models have been developed, external validation and comparison of these models to each other are somewhat limited. A study from Ten Haaf and colleagues,[28] published in 2017, compared the performance of 9 of the more prevalent risk models on the NLST and PLCO trial populations.

Table 2 identifies the 9 different risk models, their inclusion risk factors, and the prediction

Table 2
Comparison of seven risk prediction models

Model	Predicted Outcome	Prediction Time Frame	Risk Factors Included
Bach model	LC incidence	1 y	Age, gender, smoking duration, years since cessation, asbestos exposure
Liverpool Lung Project	LC incidence	5 y	Age, gender, smoking duration, personal history of LC, personal history of pneumonia, asbestos exposure
PLCO$_{m2012}$	LC incidence	6 y	Age, race, education, BMI, COPD, personal history of cancer, family history of LC, smoking status, smoking duration, smoking intensity, years since cessation
TSCE lung incidence model	LC incidence	1 y (iterative)	Age, gender, smoking status, smoking duration, smoking intensity, years since cessation
Knoke model	LC death	1 y (iterative)	Age, gender, smoking status, smoking duration, smoking intensity, years since cessation
TSCE lung cancer death model	LC death	1 y (iterative)	Age, gender, smoking status, smoking duration, smoking intensity, years since cessation
TSCE Nurses' Health Study/Health Professionals Follow-Up Study lung cancer death model	LC death	1 y (iterative)	Age, gender, smoking status, smoking duration, smoking intensity, years since cessation

Adapted from Ten Haaf K, Jeon J, Tammemagi MC, et al. Risk prediction models for selection of lung cancer screening candidates: A retrospective validation study. *PLoS Med.* 2017;14(4):e1002277; with permission.

time frame. All these models outperformed the NLST eligibility criteria with higher sensitivity for all models and higher specificity for some models. **Fig. 1** compares the sensitivity and specificity of the different models to the NLST criteria. The PLCO$_{m2012}$, Bach, and two-stage clonal expansion (TSCE) incidence models had the best overall performance in that order with highest sensitivity and specificity for prediction 6-year LC incidence. These 3 models had the best discriminative performance (based on areas under the curve >0.68–0.77) when coupled with specific risk thresholds. For example, the PLCOm2012 risk threshold for

screening is at least a 1.5% 6-year risk. The study concluded that LC risk prediction models, when considering their specific riskh thresholds, outperform current recommended LC screening criteria.[28]

Although these risk models performed best, they can be somewhat time consuming and complex to use. The Pittsburgh Predictor model is a 4-factor risk model that is less complicated to use. The factors included are duration of smoking, smoking status, smoking intensity, and age. In a study from Wilson and Weissfeld[29] in 2016, the Pittsburgh Predictor represented risk equally to

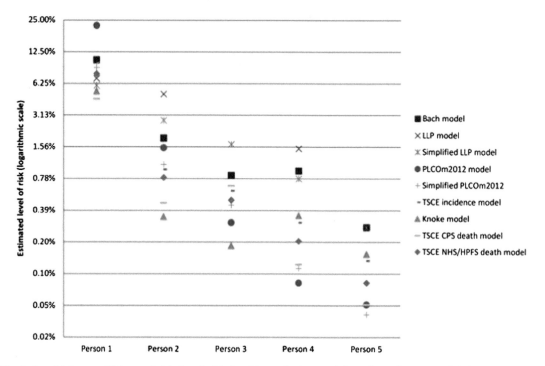

Fig. 1. Sensitivity, specificity, and risk thresholds for risk prediction models. Risk prediction models for selection of LC screening candidates: a retrospective validation study. CPS, american cancer society cancer prevention studies; LLP, liverpool lung project; NHS/HPFS- nurses health study/health professionals' follow-up study; SCE, two-stage clonal expansion. (*From* Ten Haaf K, Jeon J, Tammemagi MC, et al. Risk prediction models for selection of lung cancer screening candidates: A retrospective validation study. PLoS Med. 2017;14(4):e1002277.)

the Bach and $PLCO_{m2012}$ models but with a small reduction in prediction accuracy. The investigators suggested that this simpler model may facilitate implementation of prediction models as part of standard procedures without hindering use.

Most risk models do not incorporate the actual findings on LDCT into the risk calculation. As referenced previously, the NELSON trial demonstrated that radiologic features, such as volume-doubling time and 3-dimensional volumetric analysis, was associated with increased incidence of LC over 5 years.[16] Subsequently, the COSMOS trial demonstrated that certain nodule features on an initial LDCT screen predicted LC risk on subsequent screens. The predictive radiologic features included the presence of emphysema, nodule type (solid, partial solid, nonsolid, and noncalcified), and nodule size greater than 8 mm.[30]

In 2019, Tammemägi and colleagues[31] demonstrated that patients with increased risk calculated by $PLCO_{m2012}$ of at least 2.6% with an initial negative CT scan warrant continued annual screening because their risk of developing LC did not fall below 1.5% despite 3 negative CT scans. They also showed that using a $PLCO_{m2012}$ adjusted model that includes the initial LDCT screening

result, as outlined by the American College of Radiology structured reporting Lung-RADS criteria, can improve risk prediction over the next 3 years to 6 years and reduce cost and radiation exposure. An easy-to-use, spreadsheet risk calculator that incorporates the $PLCO_{m2012}$ risk calculator and recent LC screening results is available online, called the Brock model (https://brocku.ca/lung-cancer-risk-calculator).[31,32]

Who Is Currently Being Screened for Lung Cancer Screening?

The United States is the only country that has implemented LC screening nationally. Although Canada recommends screening high-risk individuals, an organized program has not yet been established and European countries do not yet recommend organized LC screening. This wide variability derives from the complexity of patient selection for LC screening. The goal of LC screening is to identify patients at high risk for LC who are healthy enough to undergo evaluation and successful treatment of early-stage cancer, while minimizing adverse effects of screening. Despite growing implementation efforts, the uptake for LC screening in the United States has been low, with estimates ranging from 1.9% to 4% of eligible persons undergoing screening.[27,33,34] Although it may be that LC screening is novel and adoption efforts are early, there are several other potential barriers to uptake, including the patient population. This is the first time selection for a cancer screening test has been linked to a health behavior. When compared with never smokers and former smokers, current smokers are less educated, less likely to identify a primary health care provider, and less likely to want to be screened for LC or undergo surgery for a screen-detected cancer.[35] Smokers experience stigma and self-blame related to LC diagnosis and this may have an impact on screening uptake.[36]

IMPLEMENTATION OF LUNG CANCER SCREENING

Since the 2013 USPSTF recommendation for LC screening, implementation of organized, formal LC screening programs has been met with significant challenges. In a study evaluating implementation of LC screening in the US veteran population, Kinsinger and colleagues[37] found that only 57.7% of patients offered LC screening agreed and only 86% completed their first LDCT. Reasons patients did not pursue screening included concerns about the need for screening, exposure to radiation, psychological distress, and the effort required to attend screening examinations. A qualitative comparison study of 3 Veterans Affairs hospital sites helped identify certain barriers to implementation. One barrier identified was the management and distribution of workload. Solutions included hiring a dedicated LC screening coordinator and additional staff with protected time for screening work, utilizing registries to monitor results, and facilitating communication of results using multidisciplinary committees. Primary care physician (PCP) buy-in was another barrier identified, which showcases the need for education involving current research and guidelines, regular feedback addressing PCP concerns, and plans for follow-up of screening results. Education about LC screening should be multifaceted, with the goal of encouraging PCP buy-in while discouraging unwarranted screening of low-risk patients, where harm outweighs benefit at an increased cost to the health care system.[38]

The American Thoracic Society (ATS) and CHEST published a policy statement to assist in the implementation of new LC screening programs in clinical practice. It focuses on 3 necessary stages: planning, implementation, and maintenance.[5]

Planning

Given the immense reallocation of resources and changes in workload that will be involved in starting a new LC screening program, planning is paramount to success. The ATS/CHEST recommends creation of a multidisciplinary steering committee to help facilitate working relationships and proper communication channels among the necessary members of different clinical expertise. The committee should include representation from pulmonary, radiology, thoracic surgery, interventional radiology, and medical and radiation oncology as well as primary care. The committee should engage PCPs to help educate and solicit feedback or concerns prior to implementing a system. They also should engage local leadership and program marketing to discuss possible costs and requirements from each department as well as careful marketing strategies, especially if direct-to-consumer marketing is planned.

Implementation

ATS/CHEST emphasizes 9 core components necessary for proper implementation of an LC screening program[39]:

1. Who is offered LC screening?
   - Lung cancer screening should be offered in general to those meeting USPSTF criteria. This includes current and former smokers having quit within the past 15 years ages 55 to 80 years with a minimum 30 pack year history. Consideration should be given based on possible payers. For example, CMS offers reimbursement up to age 77 while some private insurers offer reimbursement up to 80 years of age.
   - Screening should only be offered to those healthy enough to derive benefit. In the NLST, all participants were asymptomatic and medically fit to undergo curative surgery for a screen-detected cancer. One study has suggested that those who cannot undergo surgery will have worse outcomes.[40] Many patients eligible for LCS are at high risk for other disease due to their smoking histories, including coronary artery disease, respiratory disease, and other cancers. The very habit that makes them eligible for LC screening puts them at risk from dying from other disease. How to incorporate competing causes of death and comorbid conditions into patient selection is an area of active research.[41]
   - Programs should collect data regarding enrolled patients' risk of developing cancer.
2. How often and for how long to screen?

- Screening should be offered until patients reach the upper age limit of screening (age 80 years, per USPSTF), until they are greater than 15 years out from quitting smoking or until they are no longer healthy enough to undergo screening.
- Electronic medical record tools can be utilized to identify eligibility and set reminders for follow-up.
- Human review by midlevel providers is useful to determine eligibility, counsel low-risk patients, and follow-up results.

3. How is the CT performed?
- American College of Radiology technical specifications: noncontrast, helical CT with radiation dose less than or equal to 3 mGy, less than or equal to 2.5-mm slice thickness (1 mm preferred)

4. Lung nodule identification
- Each program should have a policy on size and characteristics of a nodule used to label it positive.
- Data should be collected regarding size, characteristics, and number of positive nodules.

5. Structured reporting
- A structured and standardized reporting system should be used, for example Lung-RADS.
- Data should be collected on reporting.

6. Lung nodule management algorithms
- Identify which providers are responsible for results and further management (PCP vs pulmonologist).
  ○ Can dichotomize low-risk small nodules less than or equal to 8 mm to PCP or screening coordinators and higher-risk nodules greater than or equal to 8 mm or growing nodules to specialists
- Develop lung nodule care pathways.
- ACCP and British Thoracic Society have algorithms for nodule management.
- Available multidisciplinary specialties to review nodules and establish further evaluation or management plans (many have a tumor board conference)
- Tracking nodule follow-up with registries and a designated coordinator
- Resources should be available to further characterize or diagnose nodules, like positron emission tomography, nonsurgical or minimally invasive procedures, and surgical evaluation.
- A system of communication of results and follow-up plans with the patient that is timely and sensitive with delivery (this includes lung nodule results as well as incidental findings)

- Collect data on use, outcomes, surveillance, further imaging, and procedures.

7. Shared decision making (SDM)
- Discuss benefits and harms of screening prior to enrollment in person.
- Should include information regarding the frequency of finding a nodule (25%–50% of screens) and likelihood of benign findings (90% of nodules)
- Should include information about the detection of nodules and subsequent evaluation that may be needed, including possible harms for evaluation or treatment and possible patient distress
- An SDM visit currently is required by CMS for reimbursement. Providers should be adequately educated to identify appropriate patients for screening, discuss the benefits and harms of screening, and counsel patients who do not qualify for screening, that is, low-risk patients.
- Providers should be prepared to counsel patients on the importance of adherence to annual LDCT screening and the risks, benefits, and the patient's willingness to undergo appropriate diagnostic or therapeutic procedures.
- Discussions regarding who should perform the SDM visit should occur during the planning stage. Some programs rely on PCPs to facilitate the discussion. The benefit is that they may already have an established relationship with the patient. They have less expertise, however, regarding the nuances of evaluation and treatment and are time limited in their visit. Another option is using midlevel providers, such as screening coordinators dedicated to SDM with adequate expertise, but this could result in an additional visit for the patient.
- Supplemental materials available for providers/patients, including paper and Web-based decision aids (see http://shouldIscreen.com)

8. Smoking cessation corollary
- LC screening is a potential teachable moment for current smokers and tobacco dependence is a predictor of higher LC incidence and mortality.[42]
- The benefit of LCS is enhanced with tobacco cessation.[43]
- Integrated smoking cessation programs either on-site or established referral
  ○ Best strategy is not known but can include written or phone counseling, medication treatment, and/or motivational interviewing by trained providers.

- Collect data on smoking cessation interventions offered and success.
- The SDM visit also should include sufficient counseling on tobacco cessation. Providers should be trained in motivational interviewing skills and should be knowledgeable about resources available as well as pharmacologic and nonpharmacologic treatment.

Maintenance

9. Data collection and maintenance
   - Data should be collected, including elements from previous 8 components, and outcomes, including details of cancer diagnoses and complications.
   - Annual review of data and quality improvement
   - Annual summary of data should be submitted to an oversight body with authority to credential.
   - Must meet following metrics:
     1. Appropriateness of screening greater than or equal to 90%
     2. Adherence to structured reporting greater than or equal to 90%
     3. Appropriateness of nodule evaluation
     4. Adherence with smoking cessation interventions

FUTURE

Patient selection for LC screening will continue to evolve with further research. Changes in identification of the high-risk patient population require further research on the performance of risk prediction models and data collection regarding outcomes of LC screening. Inclusion of volumetric analysis may be more widely incorporated into risk stratification and further evaluation. Additionally, further study into cost-effectiveness, resource allocation, and adherence may influence changes in screening. A recent study from Caverly and colleagues in 2018[44] identified circumstances in which LDCT screening is more patient preference–sensitive. Patient preference influenced outcomes for patients with an annual risk less than 0.3% for LC or life expectancy less than 10.5 years. For higher-risk patients with longer life expectancy, the benefits of LDCT outweighed any negative impact of patient preference. A unique component to this study is that outcomes were measured by lifetime quality-adjusted life-year gains, which is perhaps a more patient-centered outcome than mortality. Furthermore, development and research of new biologic markers that can be incorporated into screening may drastically change the environment of patient selection.

SUMMARY

There is strong evidence for LC screening with LDCT; however, proper patient selection is necessary to ensure optimal benefit with minimal harm. Although age and smoking criteria are the most common metrics used to identify those eligible for screening, ensuring that an individual is also well enough to undergo curative treatment and is willing to participate in repeat annual screening is important. There are several risk prediction calculators that have been shown more efficient in selecting patients for LC screening that also can be utilized to convey personal risk to individuals for LC screening during SDM. Although these are promising, risk-based patient selection currently is not recommended routinely. As hospital systems and practices consider implementing LC screening, careful multidisciplinary planning is warranted up-front to achieve all components necessary for an effective LC screening program.

DISCLOSURES

The authors have nothing to disclose.

REFERENCES

1. Siegel RL, Miller KD, Jemal A. Cancer statistics, 2018. CA Cancer J Clin 2018;68(1):7–30.
2. Cancer facts & figures 2017. 2017. Available at: https://www.cancer.org/content/dam/cancer-org/research/cancer-facts-and-statistics/annual-cancer-facts-and-figures/2017/cancer-facts-and-figures-2017.pdf. Accessed July 22, 2019.
3. National Lung Screening Trial Research Team, Aberle DR, Adams AM, Berg CD, et al. Reduced lung-cancer mortality with low-dose computed tomographic screening. N Engl J Med 2011; 365(5):395–409.
4. Moyer VA, U.S. Preventive Services Task Force. Screening for lung cancer: U.S. Preventive Services Task Force recommendation statement. Ann Intern Med 2014;160(5):330–8.
5. Wiener RS, Gould MK, Arenberg DA, et al. An official American Thoracic Society/American College of Chest Physicians policy statement: implementation of low-dose computed tomography lung cancer screening programs in clinical practice. Am J Respir Crit Care Med 2015;192(7):881–91.
6. Oken MM, Hocking WG, Kvale PA, et al. Screening by chest radiograph and lung cancer mortality: the Prostate, Lung, Colorectal, and Ovarian (PLCO) randomized trial. JAMA 2011;306(17):1865–73.
7. Gohagan JK, Marcus PM, Fagerstrom RM, et al. Final results of the lung screening study, a randomized feasibility study of spiral CT versus chest X-ray

screening for lung cancer. Lung Cancer 2005;47(1): 9–15.

8. Lopes Pegna A, Picozzi G, Mascalchi M, et al. Design, recruitment and baseline results of the ITA-LUNG trial for lung cancer screening with low-dose CT. Lung Cancer 2009;64(1):34–40.

9. Veronesi G, Bellomi M, Mulshine JL, et al. Lung cancer screening with low-dose computed tomography: a non-invasive diagnostic protocol for baseline lung nodules. Lung Cancer 2008;61(3):340–9.

10. Paci E, Puliti D, Lopes Pegna A, et al. Mortality, survival and incidence rates in the ITALUNG randomised lung cancer screening trial. Thorax 2017; 72(9):825–31.

11. Pedersen JH, Ashraf H, Dirksen A, et al. The Danish randomized lung cancer CT screening trial–overall design and results of the prevalence round. J Thorac Oncol 2009;4(5):608–14.

12. Pastorino U, Sverzellati N. Lung cancer: CT screening for lung cancer–do we have an answer? Nat Rev Clin Oncol 2013;10(12):672–3.

13. Infante M, Cavuto S, Lutman FR, et al. Long-term follow-up results of the DANTE Trial, a randomized study of lung cancer screening with spiral computed tomography. Am J Respir Crit Care Med 2015; 191(10):1166–75.

14. Aberle DR, DeMello S, Berg CD, et al. Results of the two incidence screenings in the national lung screening trial. N Engl J Med 2013;369(10): 920–31.

15. de Koning DB, Van Der Aalst C, Ten Haaf K, et al. Effects of volume CT lung cancer screening: Mortality results of the NELSON randomized-controlled population based trial. Paper presented at: World Conference on Lung Cancer. Toronto, Canada, September 25, 2018.

16. Yousaf-Khan U, van der Aalst C, de Jong PA, et al. Risk stratification based on screening history: the NELSON lung cancer screening study. Thorax 2017;72(9):819–24.

17. Pastorino U, Rossi M, Rosato V, et al. Annual or biennial CT screening versus observation in heavy smokers: 5-year results of the MILD trial. Eur J Cancer Prev 2012;21(3):308–15.

18. Wood DE. National Comprehensive Cancer Network (NCCN) clinical practice guidelines for lung cancer screening. Thorac Surg Clin 2015;25(2):185–97.

19. Straif K, Benbrahim-Tallaa L, Baan R, et al. A review of human carcinogens–part C: metals, arsenic, dusts, and fibres. Lancet Oncol 2009;10(5):453–4.

20. Steenland K, Loomis D, Shy C, et al. Review of occupational lung carcinogens. Am J Ind Med 1996; 29(5):474–90.

21. Wood DE, Kazerooni EA, Baum SL, et al. Lung cancer screening, version 3.2018, NCCN clinical practice guidelines in oncology. J Natl Compr Canc Netw 2018;16(4):412–41.

22. Darby S, Hill D, Auvinen A, et al. Radon in homes and risk of lung cancer: collaborative analysis of individual data from 13 European case-control studies. BMJ 2005;330(7485):223.

23. Wu GX, Nelson RA, Kim JY, et al. Non-small cell lung cancer as a second primary among patients with previous malignancy: who is at risk? Clin Lung Cancer 2017;18(5):543–50.e3.

24. Matakidou A, Eisen T, Houlston RS. Systematic review of the relationship between family history and lung cancer risk. Br J Cancer 2005;93(7):825–33.

25. Mazzone PJ, Silvestri GA, Patel S, et al. Screening for lung cancer: CHEST guideline and expert panel report. Chest 2018;153(4):954–85.

26. Jacobson FL, Austin JH, Field JK, et al. Development of the American Association for Thoracic Surgery guidelines for low-dose computed tomography scans to screen for lung cancer in North America: recommendations of the American Association for Thoracic Surgery Task Force for lung cancer screening and surveillance. J Thorac Cardiovasc Surg 2012;144(1):25–32.

27. Jemal A, Fedewa SA. Lung cancer screening with low-dose computed tomography in the United States-2010 to 2015. JAMA Oncol 2017;3(9): 1278–81.

28. Ten Haaf K, Jeon J, Tammemagi MC, et al. Risk prediction models for selection of lung cancer screening candidates: a retrospective validation study. PLoS Med 2017;14(4):e1002277.

29. Wilson DO, Weissfeld J. A simple model for predicting lung cancer occurrence in a lung cancer screening program: the Pittsburgh Predictor. Lung Cancer 2015;89(1):31–7.

30. Maisonneuve P, Bagnardi V, Bellomi M, et al. Lung cancer risk prediction to select smokers for screening CT–a model based on the Italian COSMOS trial. Cancer Prev Res (Phila) 2011;4(11): 1778–89.

31. Tammemägi MC, Ten Haaf K, Toumazis I, et al. Development and validation of a multivariable lung cancer risk prediction model that includes low-dose computed tomography screening results: a secondary analysis of data from the national lung screening trial. JAMA Netw Open 2019;2(3): e190204.

32. ACR: lung cancer screening resources. 2019. Available at: http://www.acr.org/Quality-Safety/ Resources/Lung-Imaging-Resources. Accessed Juy 19 2019.

33. Huo J, Shen C, Volk RJ, et al. Use of CT and chest radiography for lung cancer screening before and after publication of screening guidelines: intended and unintended uptake. JAMA Intern Med 2017; 177(3):439–41.

34. Pham D, Bhandari S, Oechsli M, et al. Lung cancer screening rates: Data from the lung cancer

screening registry. Paper presented at: Journal of Clinical Oncology 2018.

35. Silvestri GA, Nietert PJ, Zoller J, et al. Attitudes towards screening for lung cancer among smokers and their non-smoking counterparts. Thorax 2007; 62(2):126–30.

36. Scott N, Crane M, Lafontaine M, et al. Stigma as a barrier to diagnosis of lung cancer: patient and general practitioner perspectives. Prim Health Care Res Dev 2015;16(6):618–22.

37. Kinsinger LS, Anderson C, Kim J, et al. Implementation of lung cancer screening in the veterans health administration. JAMA Intern Med 2017;177(3): 399–406.

38. Gesthalter YB, Koppelman E, Bolton R, et al. Evaluations of implementation at early-adopting lung cancer screening programs: lessons learned. Chest 2017;152(1):70–80.

39. Mazzone P, Powell CA, Arenberg D, et al. Components necessary for high-quality lung cancer screening: American College of Chest Physicians and American Thoracic Society Policy Statement. Chest 2015;147(2):295–303.

40. Tanner NT, Dai L, Bade BC, et al. Assessing the generalizability of the National Lung Screening trial: comparison of patients with stage 1 disease. Am J Respir Crit Care Med 2017;196(5):602–8.

41. Rivera MP, Tanner NT, Silvestri GA, et al. Incorporating coexisting chronic illness into decisions about patient selection for lung cancer screening. an official American Thoracic Society Research statement. Am J Respir Crit Care Med 2018; 198(2):e3–13.

42. Rojewski AM, Tanner NT, Dai L, et al. Tobacco dependence predicts higher lung cancer and mortality rates and lower rates of smoking cessation in the National Lung Screening Trial. Chest 2018; 154(1):110–8.

43. Tanner NT, Kanodra NM, Gebregziabher M, et al. The association between smoking abstinence and mortality in the national lung screening trial. Am J Respir Crit Care Med 2016;193(5):534–41.

44. Caverly TJ, Cao P, Hayward RA, et al. Identifying patients for whom lung cancer screening is preference-sensitive: a microsimulation study. Ann Intern Med 2018;169(1):1–9.

Approach to the Subsolid Nodule

Vincent J. Mase Jr, MD, Frank C. Detterbeck, MD*

KEYWORDS

- Ground glass nodule • Atypical adenomatous hyperplasia • Adenocarcinoma in situ
- Minimally invasive adenocarcinoma • Lepidic adenocarcinoma

KEY POINTS

- Most ground glass nodules (GGNs) do not progress.
- Traditional (ie, solid, spiculated) lung cancers, GGNs that progress, and GGNs that do not progress seem to be different disease entities.
- Observation of GGNs that are predominantly ground glass to identify those that gradually progress is safe.
- Lung cancers that have a GGN component have distinctly better long-term outcomes than completely solid lung cancers.
- The incidence of recurrence is minimal for completely resected GGNs that have a consolidated portion size of less than 10 mm (on lung windows) or a solid portion size of less than 5 mm (on mediastinal windows).

INTRODUCTION

There has been growing awareness that ground glass nodules (GGNs) are a clinically distinct group of pulmonary nodules. Increased use of chest computed tomography (CT) has led to an increase in nodule detection, which will likely continue with broader adoption of lung cancer screening. Management of GGNs is increasingly relevant in clinical care. The lung cancer community have learned much about how GGNs behave. This chapter reviews relevant evidence that informs the clinical management of patients with a GGN.

This chapter focuses on persistent, focal GGNs with distinct borders in middle-aged to older adults. Such GGNs are strongly correlated with the adenocarcinoma spectrum of non-small cell lung cancer (NSCLC). GGNs due to inflammatory processes (which generally are transient and appear as an infiltrate with indistinct borders) and regional, patchy, or extensive ground glass opacities that indicate focal or diffuse pneumonitis or interstitial lung disease are not included.

THE NATURE OF GROUND GLASS NODULES
Imaging Features

A GGN, as defined by the Fleischner Society, is a hazy increased opacity of lung, with preservation of bronchial and vascular margins.[1] This radiographic appearance can be caused by any condition that decreases air in the lung parenchyma without total obstruction of the alveoli, such as interstitial thickening (due to fluid, cells, and/or fibrosis), partial collapse of alveoli, increased capillary blood volume, or a combination thereof.[1]

Assessment of GGNs requires attention to technical details of the CT scan (eg, slice thickness). One study found that more than 50% of lesions considered pure GGNs (without a solid component) on 5 mm slices actually had a solid component on 1 mm slices.[2] Recent guidelines recommend a thin-slice CT (1–1.25 mm) for lung imaging because of such discrepancies.[3] Likewise, small differences cannot be reliably identified when comparing CT scans using different techniques (eg, a 5-mm and a 1-mm thickness

Department of Surgery, Division of Thoracic Surgery, Yale University School of Medicine, PO Box 208062, New Haven, CT 06520-8062, USA
* Corresponding author.
E-mail address: frank.detterbeck@yale.edu

Clin Chest Med 41 (2020) 99–113
https://doi.org/10.1016/j.ccm.2019.11.004
0272-5231/20/© 2019 Elsevier Inc. All rights reserved.

scan or a diagnostic CT and the CT done with positron emission tomography [PET] for attenuation correction). Furthermore, there is interobserver variability; one representative study noted 36% discordance for size or presence of a solid area (160 nodules, median diameter 12 mm [5–33] ranging from pure GGN to solid).[4]

Different methods of categorizing GGNs have been used. One approach is to classify GGNs as pure (only ground glass on lung windows), heterogeneous (having both a ground glass and a denser area of consolidation on lung windows), and part-solid (having a solid area that is visible on mediastinal windows, all using thin-slice [1 mm] CT).[5] Another method divides GGNs into quartiles by the percentage of the lesion that is consolidated (on lung windows): 0% to 24% (pure ground glass), 25% to 49%, 50% to 74%, and greater than or equal to 75%.[6] Another strategy estimates the ratio of the size of the ground glass component on lung windows to the solid component on mediastinal windows, called the tumor disappearance ratio (TDR),[7,8] or the proportion of consolidation (on lung windows) to ground glass, called a consolidation/tumor ratio (CTR).[9] An older classification distinguishes 6 categories based on the density, morphology, and proportion of a solid component.[10]

In this review, mixed GGN refers to lesions that are neither pure ground glass nor completely solid, that is, containing both a ground glass component and either a consolidated (lung windows) or a solid (mediastinal windows) component. To avoid confusion, the authors specify whether size in cited studies refers to the overall lesion, the consolidated, or the solid component. Finally, unless otherwise noted, the current definition of T-stage categories (based on consolidated or invasive component only) is used instead of the older definition based on overall size.[11]

Pathology of Ground Glass Nodules

The lung adenocarcinoma spectrum begins with premalignant lesions including atypical adenomatous hyperplasia (AAH) and adenocarcinoma in situ (AIS).[12] AAH is a localized, small ($\leq$5 mm) proliferation of mildly to moderately atypical type II pneumocytes. AIS has a predominantly lepidic pattern of neoplastic cells growing along alveolar walls without stromal, vascular, or pleural invasion and less than or equal to 3 cm overall. Minimally invasive adenocarcinoma (MIA) has less than or equal to 5 mm of invasion ($\leq$3 cm overall) in a lepidic background. The diagnosis of AIS or MIA cannot be established from a small biopsy; the entire tumor must be available for histologic

examination.[13] Invasive lung adenocarcinomas are typically mixed, and although lepidic predominant adenocarcinoma is most common in GGNs, any subtype can be present and even predominant (lepidic, acinar, papillary, micropapillary, and solid).[13]

The degree of correlation between the radiographic and histologic appearance is not reliable. Resected pure GGNs harbor invasive cancer in 10% to 40% of cases, and 20% to 60% of mixed GGNs are not invasive cancer (**Fig. 1**).[14–25] The inclusion of other imaging characteristics (eg, solid size, margin, mass, density) have not identified a reliable way to predict histologic subtype.[14,15] Another large study found no correlation between the amount of ground glass on imaging and the lepidic proportion among 465 pIA mixed GGNs (average CTR 0.68).[26]

CT-guided biopsy of GGNs provides reasonable results in several studies, involving either pure or mixed GGNs with a CTR less than or equal to 0.5 and an average overall lesion size of ~15 mm.[27–29] In general, about 10% of attempts were nondiagnostic; excluding these, the reported sensitivity is 67% to 95%, and the false-negative rate for a diagnosis of malignancy is 20% to 40%. Sensitivity was only slightly better in larger or more consolidated lesions. Identification of adenocarcinoma subtype or invasiveness was lower, but it is inappropriate to attempt to make such diagnoses on a limited biopsy.

However, a persistent, focal GGN can be predicted to be a form of adenocarcinoma with a high degree of reliability. Adenocarcinoma (of some subtype along the spectrum) is found in ~95% of mixed GGNs (CTR <0.5) and ~85% of pure GGNs in multiple studies; these often included cases that underwent immediate biopsy/resection, so the rate of adenocarcinoma in GGNs that have been demonstrated to be persistent is likely even higher.[14]

Natural History of Ground Glass Nodules

Multiple clinical observational studies have found that the majority (60%–90%) of pure or mixed GGNs do not progress during periods of observation for 5 to 10 years.[5,16,17,30–33] A long-term prospective study found progression in 19% of 243 GGNs (accrued 2000–2005, followed until 2015; progression was defined as increased consolidation on lung windows or growth, usually $\geq$2 mm).[31] A multicenter prospective study of 1253 GGNs (median 7.8 mm overall size, 85% pure, 7% heterogeneous, 8% part-solid) reported that at 5 years, development of a new solid component ($\geq$2 mm on mediastinal windows)

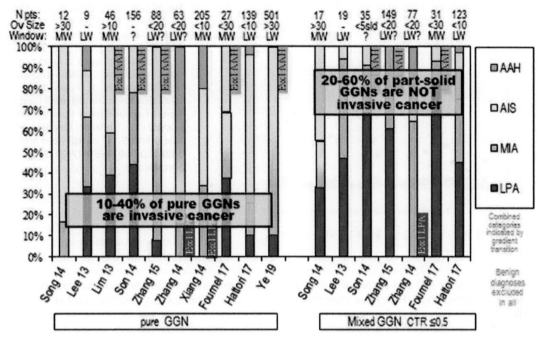

Fig. 1. Comparison of imaging and histologic categories of GGNs. Histologic diagnoses in resected GGNs. Inclusion criteria: studies of GGNs correlating the imaging characteristics with histologic subtypes using the current adenocarcinoma classification. Excl, excluding; LPA, lepidic predominant adenocarcinoma; LW, lung windows; MW, mediastinal windows; pts, patients; Ov size, overall size (mm); sld, solid. (*Data from* Refs.[16–25])

occurred in 6% and 14% of pure and heterogenous GGNs, and growth of a solid component (≥2 mm) was seen in 1%, 5%, and 22% of pure, heterogenous, and part-solid GGNs, respectively.[5] The overall lesion size grew (≥2 mm) in 14% of pure GGNs, 24% of heterogenous, and 48% of part-solid GGNs.[5] A retrospective study of 109 GGNs found that 37% progressed (median observation 4.2 years, **Fig. 2**).[30,34] Similar results have been reported by others.[17,32]

These clinical observations confirm multiple basic science observations. GGNs that did or did not progress reveal markedly different genetic patterns (90% harboring epidermal growth factor receptor [EGFR] mutations vs 20%, respectively)[35]; others have corroborated genetic differences.[36] Mouse models demonstrate similar findings: Kirsten rat sarcoma gene (Kras)-mutated mice develop AAH that does not progress, whereas EGFR-mutated mice develop AAH that progresses to lung adenocarcinoma.[37–40] These data, together with other studies, suggest varied behavior among premalignant lesions and lung cancers, corresponding to different genetic underpinnings (**Fig. 3**).[35,41]

Among GGNs that progress, the rate of progression is characteristically very slow. The median time to detection of growth (typically 2–3 mm) was 2 years in one long-term prospective study

(range <1–9 years).[31] Similar results were noted in another prospective study: median time to development of a solid component (≥2 mm on mediastinal windows) was 3.8 and 2.1 years for pure and heterogenous GGNs, respectively.[5] Expressed differently, the time until development or growth of a solid component (on mediastinal windows) to greater than or equal to 3.3 mm (a proposed trigger for intervention) was 4.2, 4.2, and 2.5 years for pure, heterogeneous, and part-solid GGNs, respectively; the minimum time to this endpoint was 1.8 and 2.5 years for pure and heterogeneous GGNs and 6 months for part-solid GGNs.[5]

The rate of growth is reported to be ~2 mm/y among GGNs that grew.[17] In one study 2% were observed to exhibit more rapid growth (>5 mm/y) at least once.[17] Among GGNs that grow, the volume doubling times (VDT) are long (mean 800–1800 days).[5,16,17] Similar indolent growth rates of GGNs have also been noted in CT screening studies.[42–45] However, the specific VDT of the solid component (on mediastinal windows) of mixed lesions is reported to be similar to traditional solid lung cancers (100–300 days).[5]

Several studies have investigated predictors of growth by multivariate analysis.[17,32,46] The most consistent predictors are initial overall lesion size and a history of lung cancer; less consistent

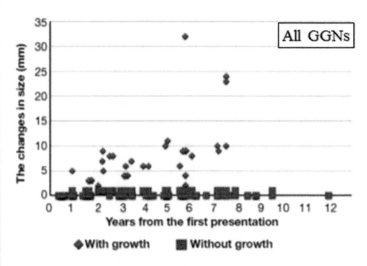

Fig. 2. Outcomes of GGNs over time. Changes in the sizes of 108 evaluated lesions from the time of the first presentation to the last CT scan in patients with a lung cancer and additional GGNs. (*Adapted from* Kobayashi Y, Fukui T, Ito S, et al. How long should small lung lesions of ground-glass opacity be followed? J Thorac Oncol. 2013 Mar;8(3):309-14. https://doi.org/10.1097/JTO.0b013e31827e2435; with permission.)

predictors are older age and a consolidated/heterogeneous appearance. Few have investigated predictors of progression (increased density, growth of or development of a consolidated or solid component)[5]; it must be concluded that predictors of progression are insufficiently defined.

In summary, most of the GGNs do not progress, likely reflecting underlying genetic characteristics. The rate of growth among those that grow is slow, with rare exceptions. Predictors of growth include initial overall GGN size and a history of lung cancer.

HOW SHOULD WE MANAGE PATIENTS?
Can Histologic Features Be Used?

Histology is of limited use in patient management for multiple reasons. Persistent focal GGNs are almost always lesions along the adenocarcinoma spectrum. Bronchoscopic or CT-guided biopsy of small opaque lesions can be difficult, and there is a substantial false-negative rate. The histologic

subtype cannot be determined until after resection (ie, after a therapeutic decision has been made). Most importantly, most GGNs do not progress, and a biopsy does not define how a lesion will behave.

The argument that identification of invasive cancer or the histologic subtype is critical is flawed. Evidence of a prognostic impact comes from studies that have included both GGNs and completely solid cancers.[47–50] Applying these data to predominantly ground glass tumors is inappropriate. Those studies that have examined the behavior of predominantly ground glass tumors have demonstrated no difference in outcomes for invasive cancer versus AIS or MIA (**Fig. 4**A).[19,51]

Can Baseline Imaging Characteristics Be Used?

Completely solid cIA lung cancers clearly pose a threat and thus warrant prompt treatment, even for tumors less than 1 cm. Node involvement is

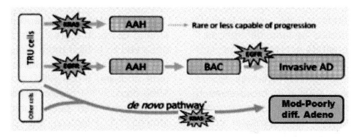

Fig. 3. Model for development of lung adenocarcinoma. Evidence suggest there are several different pathways for development of tumors on the lung adenocarcinoma spectrum: AAH that does not progress (associated with *Kras* mutations), AAH that progresses to adenocarcinoma (associated with *EGFR* mutations), and yet another pathway(s) for the traditional moderately or poorly differentiated lung adenocarcinoma (also *Kras* associated). AD, adenocarcinoma; BAC, bronchioloalveolar carcinoma; Mod-poorly diff Adeno, moderately or poorly differentiated adenocarcinoma; TRU, terminal respiratory unit. (*From* Yatabe Y, Borczuk AC, Powell CA. Do all lung adenocarcinomas follow a stepwise progression? *Lung Cancer.* 2011;74(1):7-11; with permission.)

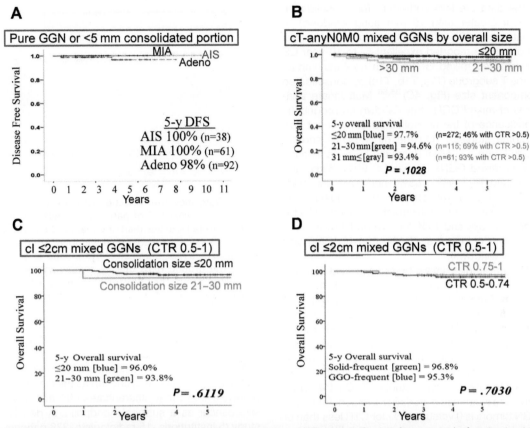

Fig. 4. Outcomes after resection of GGNs with consolidation. (*A*) Ten-year disease-free survival of patients with pure GGNs or small consolidated component (<5 mm) by histologic category. (*B*) Five-year overall survival among patients with mixed GGNs by overall size. Number of patients and percent with CTR >0.5 shown in parentheses. (*C*) Five-year overall survival among patients with a GGN, by ratio of ground glass to consolidated component (lung windows, 2 mm slices, n = 177). (*D*) Five-year overall survival among patients with a GGN, CTR 0.5 to 1, by size of consolidation (lung windows). Adeno, adenocarcinoma; DFS, disease-free survival. (*From* Refs.[19,55,66])

found in ~10%, 20%, and 30% of solid cl T1a, T1b, and T1c tumors, respectively.[52,53] Despite resection, 5-year overall survival (OS) is approximately 85%, 70%, and 60% for cl T1a, T1b, and T1c tumors, respectively.[52,54,55]

However, most GGNs do not pose an imminent threat. Multiple studies demonstrate that a ground glass component correlates with excellent outcomes after resection, much better size-for-size or by T subgroup when compared with solid tumors (either overall or consolidated size).[25,26,52,53,55–57] Several studies[25,52,53,55] have reported such excellent outcomes for resected GGNs—with little impact of the consolidated component size or proportion thereof—that it is unclear where an inflection point lies at which survival diminishes.

Pure GGNs consistently have excellent survival without recurrence, regardless of overall lesion size (but only rare cases are >3 cm).[14,55,58–63] In a prospective study of lobectomy (Japan Cooperative

Oncology Group [JCOG] 0201), 5-year recurrence-free survival (RFS) did not vary significantly by overall lesion size if the CTR was less than or equal to 0.25 (97% for cl ≤ 2 cm, 94% for >2–3 cm).[64] Others have noted that overall tumor size has no impact, even with inclusion of some with higher CTR ratios (**Fig. 4**B).[55]

Several studies suggest that clA1 mixed GGNs remain highly curable even with consolidated components of 6 to 10 mm. For cl T1a mixed GGNs a 5-year OS of 97.5% was reported (n = 123, 45% invasive carcinoma, 39% lobectomy, 40% segmentectomy).[53] This was confirmed in another study of mixed clA1 GGNs (n = 102, mean consolidated size 8.3 mm on lung windows [2 mm slices], 71% invasive carcinoma, 55% lobectomy).[65] No node involvement was noted for mixed cl T1a GGN tumors.[53,65] Recurrence has been noted in 1.6% of clA1 mixed GGNs (on lung windows, 2 mm slices) and a 5-year RFS of 94% to 95%.[53,65]

The data are less consistent for consolidation size of greater than 10 mm (lung windows) or greater than 50% of the total lesion size. Several studies have reported excellent 5- to 10-year OS for resected mixed GGNs, with no clear impact of the T subgroup (T1a, T1b, T1c) by consolidated component size (**Fig. 4**C).[55,66] Multivariate analyses of mixed GGNs have shown no prognostic significance of the consolidated component size in some studies.[25] On the other hand, another study found a survival decrease by consolidation size in mixed GGNs (5-year OS 99%, 89%, and 89% and RFS 95%, 85%, and 72% for cIA1, cIA2, and cIA3, respectively).[53] In addition, the incidence of node involvement for mixed GGN tumors was 3% and 14% for T1b and T1c tumors, respectively, in one study (by consolidation size on lung windows).[53]

Several studies have reported excellent 5- to 10-year OS for resected mixed GGNs with no clear impact of the consolidated proportion (CTR $\leq$0.5 vs >0.5 (**Fig. 4**D).[25,55,66] A small trend toward slightly inferior RFS was noted for CTR greater than 0.5 and larger consolidation size (20–30 mm).[25,66] Multivariate analyses of mixed GGNs have shown no prognostic significance of the CTR ratio in some studies.[25] On the other hand, the incidence of node involvement for mixed GGN tumors is 0 versus ~5% for CTR less than or equal to 0.5 versus greater than 0.5.[10,67] Others have noted decreasing survival for cIA mixed GGNs according to the CTR (5-year RFS of 99% and 91% for CTR $\leq$0.5 vs > 0.5).[67] Furthermore, a study of large, mostly consolidated cN0 GGNs (average consolidated size 23 mm, CTR >0.75) found that although node involvement occurred in only 3% and outcomes were much better than completely solid similar-sized lung cancers, the 5-year OS was 87%.[56] Taken together, it seems that a consolidated portion of greater than or equal to 10 mm or a CTR of greater than 0.5 in a mixed GGN warrants consideration of intervention.

Less data are available regarding the impact of a solid portion on mediastinal windows. Specific survival after resection by solid portion size has not been reported. One study noted little impact of the TDR on RFS after resection (mostly lobectomy) in mixed GGNs with an overall size less than or equal to 1 cm (specifically TDR of 0 to <0.4 vs 0.4–0.8, **Fig. 5**).[48] This implies a 5- to 10-year RFS of ~90% for small ($\leq$1 cm overall) resected GGNs with a solid portion of ~2 to 6 mm (on mediastinal windows). Larger mixed GGNs exhibited clearly worse survival, although there was still no clear difference between TDR categories.[48] Taken together, a solid component on mediastinal windows that is less than ~5 mm

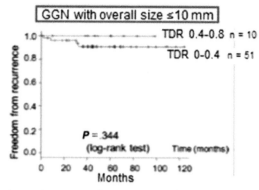

Fig. 5. Outcomes after resection of GGNs with solid portion. A 10-year RFS of patients with mixed GGNs with an overall size less than or equal to 10 mm (solid portion assessed on mediastinal windows, "thin-slice CT", n=61). (*From* Murakawa T, Konoeda C, Ito T, et al. The ground glass opacity component can be eliminated from the T-factor assessment of lung adenocarcinoma. *Eur J Cardiothorac Surg.* 2013;43(5):925-932; with permission.)

appears to result in excellent survival, but this may not be true with a larger solid component.

Another approach is using the 5 mm threshold that has (arbitrarily) been chosen as the dimension of invasiveness that differentiates MIA from invasive cancer as a surrogate endpoint. A detailed study (5 institutions, 15 radiologists, 378 patients, multiple blinded assessments) found that a size of 8 mm on lung windows and 6 mm on mediastinal windows correlated best with 5 mm on histologic examination (with ~80% sensitivity and ~80% specificity for each).[68] These dimensions are roughly in alignment with the thresholds discussed in the preceding paragraphs. GGNs below these thresholds seem to pose little risk.

Can Assessment of How a Ground Glass Nodule Behaves Be Used?

The observation that most GGNs do not progress and the good outcomes after resection of GGNs suggest a surveillance strategy may be best to identify those GGNs that progress. This section addresses questions raised by such an approach.

An initial period of observation is usually indicated, because about 30% of GGNs resolve, typically within a few months.[14,69] However, the evidence considered in this chapter pertains to persistent GGNs (ie, that did not resolve).

In considering a surveillance approach, it is helpful to consider that the clinical and pathologic T stage category, respectively, is defined by the size of the solid (by imaging, CT parameters not specified) or invasive component, based on multiple studies demonstrating that this determines prognosis).[11] This means that pure GGNs are classified as T0 and many mixed GGNs as Tis or Tmi. However, further analysis suggests that classification by solid/invasive tumor size does not bring GGNs and solid lung cancers prognostically into alignment—the presence of a ground glass component consistently results in better survival for each stage subgroup.[25,26,53,66] This effect is noted even with only a minor ground glass component (ie, CTR >0.5).[25,66] Furthermore, good OS and RFS is reported whenever a ground glass component is present, with the consolidated component size having relatively little impact.[66]

Is a surveillance approach safe?
The safety of observation to assess for progression is a critical question if we adopt a surveillance strategy. The evidence presented earlier that most of the GGNs do not change, even over many years, and that change is gradual in those that do supports this approach. Most studies reporting rates of growth report only indolent growth,[5,16,17] but some report rare cases (~2%) with growth of ~5 mm/y—although it seems this was not necessarily sustained and the subsequent outcomes of these patients is unknown.[17,70] It seems that a change from a pure GGN to a mixed GGN is a predictor of more rapid growth.[17] This is consistent with a recent study that suggests that the VDT of the solid component in mixed GGNs is similar to that of traditional NSCLC (~6 months).[5]

Two prospective studies provide strong evidence that observation is safe (**Fig. 6**).[5,31] These studies involved predominantly pure GGNs, with few having a CTR greater than 0.5 or a solid portion on mediastinal windows. Of the small subset of patients in these studies that eventually underwent resection, all were stage pIA, with less than 2% being T2aN0M0 due to visceral pleural invasion (which has unclear prognostic impact in small lesions). The average size of the solid component in one prospective study at the time of resection was 3.7 mm (mediastinal windows), and the average total size was 16 mm[5]; this was not reported in the other study.[31] Subsequent follow-up of the resected patients found that all were cured in one study[5] and 98.4% in the other.[31] (Two patients [1.6%] in the latter study[31] developed recurrence and died about 2.5 and 4 years postresection. Both exhibited increasing CTR over ~3 years, beginning from a total size of 5 mm and a CTR of 0.75 in one patient and a 27 mm pure GGN in the other. Imaging characteristics of the tumors at the time of resection was not provided, leaving it unclear if earlier intervention could have altered the outcome.) Thus, prospective studies suggest that surveillance, with intervention when there is a change, does not result in stage progression or affect curability, with a rate of exceptions that is similar to the rate of major morbidity/mortality from anatomic pulmonary resection.

How well can we assess change?
Thin-slice (~1 mm) CT scans are needed to assess GGNs. In addition, small differences cannot be reliably assessed when comparing CT scans done with different thicknesses (eg, a 5 mm and a 1 mm scan, or a diagnostic CT and the CT of a PET scan). Differences of less than 2 mm cannot be reliably assessed even for solid nodules and thin-slice scans.[3,71,72] Small differences are harder to assess with GGNs[44,73];

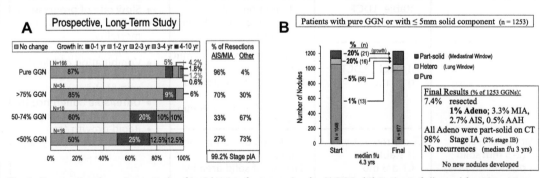

Fig. 6. Prospective, long-term study of incidence of progression by %GGO. (*A*) Patients followed for 10 to 15 years (accrued 2000–2005); pure or mixed GGNs less than or equal to 3 cm. Progression defined as either growth or increased consolidation (usually ~2–3 mm ↑); proportion of consolidation assessed on lung windows. (*B*) Multicenter prospective study of patients with pure GGN or with less than or equal to 5 mm solid component. Adeno, adenocarcinoma; f/u, follow-up; yrs, years. (*Data from* Sawada S, Yamashita N, Sugimoto R, et al. Long-term outcomes of patients with ground-glass opacities detected using computed tomography. *Chest.* 2017;151(2):308-315. *Data from* Kakinuma R, Noguchi M, Ashizawa K, et al. Natural History of Pulmonary Subsolid Nodules: A Prospective Multicenter Study. J Thorac Oncol. 2016;11(7):1012-1028.)

intra-/interobserver variability of 15% to 30% has been noted with respect to overall volume[16,74] and a 36% rate of discordance for the size and/or presence of solid component.[4] Two studies of GGNs have suggested that an increase in mass is associated with less variability than growth overall or development of a solid component, but this has not been adopted.[16,44]

Observation interval and duration

A schedule of serial imaging is proposed in **Table 1**. The interval between scans is based on the observed rates of growth or progression in GGNs. The initial interval represents a safe interval for the short end of the range of observed rates— that is, detection of a change but before this alters prognosis. An interval of 1 year is proposed for pure GGNs, 6 months for heterogeneous GGNs, and 3 months for part-solid GGNs (on mediastinal windows). If no change occurs, subsequent intervals can be doubled, especially for pure GGNs.[16] Often a few time points are needed to establish stability or gradual change, given the inter/intraobserver variability of subtle changes.

Whether surveillance can be discontinued at some point is unclear. NCCN and Fleischner guidelines do not recommend continuation if a GGN has been stable for 5 years.[75,76] A long-term prospective study found that all mixed GGNs that grew demonstrated growth within 3 years,[31] and this seems to be corroborated by others.[30] However, 2 studies of late growth of initially stable GGNs suggest further follow-up is needed.[46,70] One study noted late growth in 7% of 218 patients with GGNs that were stable for 3 years (mostly mixed GGNs).[46] The other study involved 208 predominantly pure GGNs that were stable for 5 years; growth (>2 mm) was seen in 13% (median of 3.2 mm over a median of 8.2 years) and development of a solid component (presumably on mediastinal windows) in 16%.[70] Note that in both studies few patients underwent resection (1.5% and 1.4% of all), suggesting that the late changes were less clinically concerning.[46,70] At this point, it seems reasonable to continue surveillance in healthy individuals beyond 5 years, albeit perhaps at protracted intervals.

TREATMENT OF GROUND GLASS NODULES
Triggers for Intervention

What are appropriate triggers for intervention? There is a growing consensus for surveillance rather than intervention for pure GGNs.[75–77] The Fleischner society recommends surveillance of mixed GGNs with a consolidated component up to 6 mm (presumably assessed on lung windows although not explicitly stated).[75] The proposed schema in **Table 1** focuses on the development or growth of a solid component on thin-cut mediastinal windows, and to a lesser extent a rate of growth and consolidation.[78]

Table 1
Surveillance schema for GGNs

GGN Type	Follow-up Schedule	Triggers for Intervention[a]	Relative Considerations
Pure GGN[b]	LDCT q 12 mo if stable, LDCT q 24 mo	New consolidation ≥6–10 mm on LW New solid area ≥2-5 mm on MW	Favoring no intervention: • Slow rate of progression • Competing causes of mortality Favoring intervention: • Combination of triggers (↑size, ↑ CTR/TDR, ↑ rate of change) • Unreliable adherence to surveillance imaging • Rapid growth (eg, ≥25% growth per year)[c]
Heterogeneous GGN	CT q 6 mo × 2 y; if stable, LDCT q 12 mo	Consolidation of ≥10 mm on LW Growth of consolidated area by ≥2 mm New solid area ≥2–6 mm on MW	
Part-solid GGN (2–5 mm solid portion on MW)	CT q 3 mo × 1 y; if stable, CT q 6 mo	Solid area of ≥5 mm on MW Growth of solid area by ≥2 mm on MW	

Note: CT should be done with 1 to 1.25 mm slice thickness.
Abbreviations: CT, computed tomography; CTR, consolidation/tumor ratio (all on lung windows); GGN, ground glass nodule; LDCT, low dose CT; LW, lung windows; MW, mediastinal windows; TDR, tumor disappearance ratio (size on MW/LW).
[a] Assuming no doubt about measurement (generally requires ≥2 interval scans)
[b] there appears to be limited value of surveillance of pure GGNs of <5 mm overall size
[c] speculative recommendation, based on limited data

Arguments for the solid component as the main trigger include the following: (1) multiple studies[48,49,79–82] demonstrate that outcomes correlate with the solid/invasive component size; (2) several studies suggest development of a solid component signals less indolent growth[5,17,46]; (3) studies focused on an area of consolidation have found that the size or proportion of consolidation has little prognostic impact[19,26,66]; and (4) prospective studies with similar criteria for intervention have demonstrated excellent outcomes.[5,31] (However, these prospective studies were designed to evaluate the incidence of progression of GGNs rather than the utility of a strict management algorithm.) Because of unreliability of subtle changes (<2 mm), when there is doubt, additional serial imaging is generally best to differentiate a consistent trend from measurement noise.

Management of an individual patient must consider multiple aspects specific to that patient. With indolent lung cancers, the risk to health posed by the lung cancer must be weighed against the person's estimated lifespan (ie, competing threats to health). The risk of an intervention is important, as is the risk that the patient will not adhere to serial imaging. The patient may have preferences to avoid surgery or to minimize uncertainty. However, a high degree of patient anxiety should be managed by reassurance rather than resection. Reassurance is really what such patients are seeking, and the accumulated knowledge of GGN behavior and the excellent outcomes with observation provides this. Establishing an appropriate mindset regarding a GGN is very effective; undertaking resection of GGNs that raise little concern to a knowledgeable clinician generally promotes ongoing patient fear of having had "lung cancer" that is not apropos for the situation.

PET has no role in management of GGNs. The small consolidated/solid size, low cellularity of the ground glass component, and indolent behavior result in low avidity on PET imaging.[83] The performance characteristics for PET in determining malignancy in GGNs are poor (sensitivity 10%, specificity 20%, false-negative rate 90%, false-positive rate 80%).[84] Using faint uptake to make subjective judgments is unfounded and capricious in the face of the extensive evidence regarding CT characteristics of GGNs.

What Intervention Is Appropriate?

Many retrospective reports have consistently documented excellent outcomes after surgical resection of predominantly ground glass lung cancers (5-year survival >95% with no recurrences).[14] These reports have often involved a mixture of lobectomy, segmentectomy, and wedge resection. One cannot determine the impact of one resection type versus another because of multiple sources of confounding (eg, limited resection may be selected in compromised patients or for tumors thought to be biologically less active). Although the excellent results support the concept that lobectomy may not be needed, we need clinical trials in specific patient cohorts to define what type of resection is appropriate.

For small (cl, ≤2 cm total lesion size) pure or predominantly GGNs (CTR ≤0.25), 2 prospective studies have demonstrated similar results: 5-year RFS was 97% after lobectomy in one (JCOG 0201, subset analysis)[64] and 99.7% after sublobar resection (82% wedge) in the other (JCOG 0804, **Fig. 7**).[85] Although this seems to justify sublobar resection for such lesions, this should be considered carefully. In JCOG 0804 very careful attention was given to the margins (median 15 mm). Long-term results of another prospective trial, involving similar tumors (≤2 cm, pure or predominantly ground glass) and careful exploration of sublobar resection (that satisfied stringent margin and invasiveness criteria), demonstrated

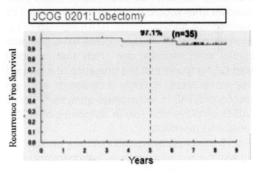

Fig. 7. Outcomes by type of resection; patients with less than or equal to 2 cm cIA GGN, CTR less than or equal to 0.25. RFS after lobectomy in a prospective trial (JCOG 0201); subset of 35 patients with less than or equal to 2 cm cIA pure GGN or CTR less than or equal to 0.25. (*Adapted from* Asamura H, Hishida T, Suzuki K, et al. Radiographically determined noninvasive adenocarcinoma of the lung: survival outcomes of Japan Clinical Oncology Group 0201. J Thorac Cardiovasc Surg. 2013;146(1):24-30; with permission. *From* Suzuki K, Watanabe S, Wakabayashi M, et al. A nonrandomized confirmatory phase III study of sublobar surgical resection for peripheral ground glass opacity dominant lung cancer defined with thoracic thin-section computed tomography. Paper presented at: ASCO2017; Chicago, IL; with permission.)

that late recurrences occurred between 5 and 10 years in 19% of R0 sublobar resections (88% wedge, 12% segment).[86,87] A randomized controlled trial (RCT) (JCOG 0802) designed to answer this question (lobectomy vs segmentectomy for cl, ≤2 cm total lesion size pure or predominantly GGNs [CTR of ≤0.25]) has completed accrual (n = 1106); outcome results are expected in 2021.

Well-defined outcomes for patients with larger or more consolidated tumors are not available. JCOG 1211 is a prospective trial of segmentectomy for mixed GGNs (CTR 0.25–0.5 for ≤2 cm and CTR ≤0.25 for 2–3 cm total lesion size). Accrual is complete (n = 390); results should become mature in 2021. Until then, the less well-defined data discussed earlier regarding the impact of consolidation or solid component size and increasing CTR (>0.50) must be used. This demonstrates a ∼5% incidence of nodal involvement and recurrences at least in some studies in such patients, suggesting caution in applying sublobar resection liberally to such tumors at this time. In addition, lobectomy for cl tumors with a CTR of greater than 0.25 to 1 in a prospective trial (JCOG 0201) resulted in 5-year RFS of 88% and 76% for less than or equal to 2 cm and greater than 2- to 3-cm tumors, respectively; however, it is unclear how many completely solid tumors were included.[64]

Recently, concern has been raised about poor outcomes after sublobar resection in the event of a microscopic finding termed STAS (spread of tumor in airspaces).[88] These studies have primarily included solid cancers; one study that included mixed GGNs found that the presence of a ground glass component strongly correlated with an absence of STAS in multivariate analysis.[89] Thus, STAS likely plays little role in outcomes of GGNs after limited resection.

Both limited resection and lobectomy are associated with the same low rates of perioperative mortality and morbidity in good-risk patients. Two RCTs of lobectomy versus sublobar resection have reported no differences: 90-day mortality of 0 versus 0 and complications in 26% versus 27% (≥grade 2) in one study[90] and 1.7% versus 1.2% and 15% versus 14% (≥grade 3) in the other.[91] These results do not apply to patients with limited pulmonary reserve. A decrease in FEV1 at 6 months of 2% versus 9% was observed for sublobar resection versus lobectomy in an earlier RCT.[92]

Taken together, although it seems reasonable to perform a sublobar resection for pure or nearly pure GGNs, careful attention must be paid to the margin given the suggestion of late local recurrences. Achieving an adequate margin can be difficult because these lesions are usually not palpable and thus require use of intraoperative localization techniques. The CHEST lung cancer guideline makes a weak recommendation for sublobar resection for pure or nearly pure GGNs with a margin of greater than 2 cm or greater than the tumor diameter for GGNs less than 2 cm.[93] The appropriate type of resection is unclear when a minor consolidated or solid component is present (ie, CTR ∼0.25 or ∼2 mm solid portion). It may turn out that segmentectomy is adequate, but this is not yet established. Particularly, if the anatomic location is unfavorable or there is concern about achieving a wide margin, there should be a low threshold to choosing lobectomy.

There is no clear data regarding stereotactic body radiotherapy (SBRT) for GGNs, although it is used selectively, especially in patients with limited pulmonary reserve or multifocal ground glass/lepidic adenocarcinoma. In patients with severe COPD, it is questionable whether treatment of a GGN is beneficial due to competing health risks. Multiple intermediate-term studies of SBRT have shown excellent local control rates, and multiple studies suggest that GGN cancers have a low propensity for nodal and distant metastases, leading to a rationale for using SBRT. However, the late local recurrences noted in the previous paragraphs signal a degree of caution. In addition, it is often difficult to differentiate a residual or slowly progressing ground glass lung cancer from SBRT treatment artifact on subsequent CT scans.

MULTIFOCAL GROUND GLASS NODULES

Patients with GGNs often have several lesions. These are classified as multifocal ground glass/lepidic adenocarcinomas and are viewed as separate primary cancers, although their multiplicity suggests an as yet unclear relationship (field cancerization?).[94–96] A review demonstrates a markedly diminished incidence of spread to nodes or distant sites and excellent long-term survival.[95,96] Each lesion should be managed separately, with intervention or observation depending on the amount of change over time as described in preceding sections; lesions that remain pure GGNs generally do not warrant intervention.[14,97] Chemotherapy has no role in this setting; this would imply a chemopreventative effect for indolent, preinvasive cancers that are probably biologically different than traditional aggressive lung cancers.[15]

SUMMARY

Multiple sources of evidence demonstrate that lung cancers with a ground glass appearance are a fundamentally different disease than traditional solid lung cancers. There is likely a different cause (lack of association with smoking, different demographics), a different genetic pattern, and different clinical behavior (indolent or lack of progression, low propensity for node or distant metastases, markedly better survival than solid lung cancers when matched by invasive size). In fact, even among GGNs it seems there are different types, which either do or (more commonly) do not progress. This indicates that the threat posed by a GGN is fundamentally different than that of a solid lung cancer. This shift in mindset is crucial to appropriately approach GGNs, both for the treating physician as well as for the patient.

The fact that most GGNs do not progress, and those that do behave in an indolent manner calls for restraint regarding therapeutic intervention. The management is not binary (malignant vs benign); it is nuanced. The potential threat posed by the GGN must be balanced against other potential health hazards. In contrast to solid lung cancers, biopsy is of limited use. Persistent, focal GGNs are invariably tumors along the adenocarcinoma spectrum; a biopsy provides little guidance regarding how it will behave. The language we use is important to foster the right mindset: most GGNs are "inconsequential" types of lung cancer, at worst they are "well-behaved" lung cancers. Conveying this is crucial to allaying a patient's fear, which is a key component of effective management.

Although the detection of a completely solid lung cancer justifies prompt intervention, it is less clear what characteristics of mixed GGNs warrant intervention on initial detection. It seems that outcomes are potentially slightly diminished if there is a solid component greater than 5 mm (mediastinal windows), an area of consolidation (lung windows) of greater than 10 mm, or a CTR greater than 0.5, especially when in combination with larger size. Intervention is reasonable for such lesions, but it should be noted that not all studies show worse outcomes above these thresholds, and the effect is minor even in those that do.

Observation of mixed GGNs, with intervention on progression, has been demonstrated to be safe in several prospective studies (involving predominantly pure GGNs with a minority having a CTR >0.5 or a solid portion on mediastinal windows). Appropriate triggers for intervention seem to be development of or growth of a solid portion or a substantial area of consolidation. Differences of less than 2 mm are unreliable and warrant additional interval imaging to distinguish a consistent trajectory from measurement noise. One must be careful to compare scans that have been done

with similar parameters (eg, thin slices). With this approach, no intervention is needed in most patients, and there is no evidence of stage progression or loss of curability in those that are eventually resected. The rate of progression should be considered, balanced against the patient's estimated life expectancy.

A wide resection may be considered for pure or mostly pure GGNs, but it seems that generally no resection is needed for these lesions. Although some evidence supports a wedge or segmentectomy for mixed predominantly ground glass lesions, evidence of late local recurrences signals caution in adopting this too aggressively. For lesions with a more substantial area of consolidation or solid component, segmentectomy is reasonable, but there should be a low threshold to perform lobectomy given the current evidence (eg, if not anatomically well localized to a segment, more rapid growth, larger size, CTR, or TDR).

DISCLOSURE

There are no financial or commercial conflicts of interest for either author or funding sources to report.

REFERENCES

1. Hansell DM, Bankier AA, MacMahon H, et al. Fleischner Society: glossary of terms for thoracic imaging. Radiol 2008;246(3):697–722.
2. Lee HY, Goo JM, Lee HJ, et al. Usefulness of concurrent reading using thin-section and thick-section CT images in subcentimetre solitary pulmonary nodules. Clin Radiol 2009;64(2):127–32.
3. Bankier AA, MacMahon H, Goo JM, et al. Recommendations for measuring pulmonary nodules at CT: a statement from the Fleischner Society. Radiology 2017;285(2):584–600.
4. van Riel S, Sanchez C, Bankier A, et al. Observer variability for classification of pulmonary nodules on low-dose Ct images and its effect on nodule management. Radiol 2015;277(3):863–71.
5. Kakinuma R, Noguchi M, Ashizawa K, et al. Natural history of pulmonary subsolid nodules: a prospective multicenter study. J Thorac Oncol 2016;11(7):1012–28.
6. Suzuki K, Teruaki K, Takashi A, et al. A prospective radiological study of thin-section computed tomography to predict pathological noninvasiveness in peripheral clinical IA lung cancer (Japan Clinical Oncology Group 0201). J Thorac Oncol 2011;6(4):751–6.
7. Takamochi K, Nagai K, Yoshida J, et al. Pathologic N0 status in pulmonary adenocarcinoma is

predictable by combining serum carcinoem-bryonic antigen level and computed tomographic findings. J Thorac Cardiovasc Surg 2001;122(2): 325–30.

8. Okada M, Nishio W, Sakamoto T, et al. Discrepancy of computed tomographic image between lung and mediastinal windows as a prognostic implication in small lung adenocarcinoma. Ann Thorac Surg 2003;76(6):1828–32 [discussion: 1832].

9. Kodama K, Higashiyama M, Yokouchi H, et al. Prognostic value of ground-glass opacity found in small lung adenocarcinoma on high-resolution CT scanning. Lung Cancer 2001;33(1):17–25.

10. Suzuki K, Kusumoto M, Watanabe S-i, et al. Radiologic classification of small adenocarcinoma of the lung: radiologic-pathologic correlation and its prognostic impact. Ann Thorac Surg 2006;81(2): 413–9.

11. Travis D, Asamura H, Bankier AA, et al. The IASLC lung cancer staging project: proposals for coding T categories for subsolid nodules and assessment of tumor size in part solid tumors in the forthcoming eighth edition of the TNM Classification of Lung Cancer. J Thorac Oncol 2016;11(8):1204–23.

12. Travis WD, Brambilla E, Noguchi M, et al. International Association for the Study of Lung Cancer/American Thoracic Society/European Respiratory Society International Multidisciplinary Classification of Lung Adenocarcinoma. J Thorac Oncol 2011; 6(2):244–85.

13. Travis W, Brambilla E, Burke A, et al. WHO classification of tumours of the lung, pleura, thymus and heart. 4th edition. Lyon (France): International Agency for Research on Cancer (IARC); 2015.

14. Detterbeck FC, Homer RJ. Approach to the ground-glass nodule. Clin Chest Med 2011;32(4):799–810.

15. Chiang A, Detterbeck F, Stewart T, et al. Non-small cell lung cancer. In: Devita V Jr, Lawrence T, Rosenberg S, editors. Cancer: principles & practice of oncology. 11th edition. Baltimore (MD): Lippincott, Williams & Wilkins; 2019. p. 618–70.

16. Song YS, Park CM, Park SJ, et al. Volume and mass doubling times of persistent pulmonary subsolid nodules detected in patients without known malignancy. Radiology 2014;273(1):276–84.

17. Lee SW, Leem CS, Kim TJ, et al. The long-term course of ground-glass opacities detected on thin-section computed tomography. Respir Med 2013; 107(6):904–10.

18. Lim H-j, Ahn S, Lee KS, et al. Persistent pure ground-glass opacity lung nodules ≥ 10 mm in diameter at ct scan: Histopathologic comparisons and prognostic implications. Chest 2013;144(4): 1291–9.

19. Son JY, Lee HY, Lee KS, et al. Quantitative CT analysis of pulmonary ground-glass opacity nodules for the distinction of invasive adenocarcinoma from pre-invasive or minimally invasive adenocarcinoma. PLoS One 2014;9(8):e104066.

20. Zhang Y, Shen Y, Qiang J, et al. HRCT features distinguishing pre-invasive from invasive pulmonary adenocarcinomas appearing as ground-glass nodules. Eur Radiol 2016;26(9):2921–8.

21. Zhang Y, Qiang JW, Ye JD, et al. High resolution CT in differentiating minimally invasive component in early lung adenocarcinoma. Lung Cancer 2014; 84(3):236–41.

22. Xiang W, Xing Y, Jiang S, et al. Morphological factors differentiating between early lung adenocarcinomas appearing as pure ground-glass nodules measuring ≤10 mm on thin-section computed tomography. Cancer Imaging 2014;14:33.

23. Fournel L, Etienne H, Mansuet Lupo A, et al. Correlation between radiological and pathological features of operated ground glass nodules. Eur J Cardiothorac Surg 2017;51(2):248–54.

24. Hattori A, Matsunaga T, Takamochi K, et al. Surgical management of multifocal ground-glass opacities of the lung: correlation of clinicopathologic and radiologic findings. Thorac Cardiovasc Surg 2017;65(2): 142–9.

25. Ye T, Deng L, Wang S, et al. Lung adenocarcinomas manifesting as radiological part-solid nodules define a special clinical subtype. J Thorac Oncol 2019; 14(4):617–27.

26. Miyoshi T, Aokage K, Katsumata S, et al. Ground-glass opacity is a strong prognosticator for pathologic stage IA lung adenocarcinoma. Ann Thorac Surg 2019;108(1):249–55.

27. Hur J, Lee H-J, Nam JE, et al. Diagnostic accuracy of CT fluoroscopy-guided needle aspiration biopsy of ground-glass opacity pulmonary lesions. AJR Am J Roentgenol 2009;192(3): 629–34.

28. Kim TJ, Lee J-H, Lee C-T, et al. Diagnostic accuracy of CT-guided core biopsy of ground-glass opacity pulmonary lesions. AJR Am J Roentgenol 2008; 190(1):234–9.

29. Inoue D, Gobara H, Hiraki T, et al. CT fluoroscopy-guided cutting needle biopsy of focal pure ground-glass opacity lung lesions: diagnostic yield in 83 lesions. Eur J Radiol 2012;81(2):354–9.

30. Kobayashi Y, Fukui T, Ito S, et al. How long should small lung lesions of ground-glass opacity be followed? J Thorac Oncol 2013;8(3):309–14.

31. Sawada S, Yamashita N, Sugimoto R, et al. Long-term outcomes of patients with ground-glass opacities detected using computed tomography. Chest 2017;151(2):308–15.

32. Hiramatsu M, Inagaki T, Inagaki T, et al. Pulmonary Ground-Glass Opacity (GGO) lesions-large size and a history of lung cancer are risk factors for growth. J Thorac Oncol 2008;3(11): 1245–50.

33. Takahashi S, Tanaka N, Okimoto T, et al. Long term follow-up for small pure ground-glass nodules: implications of determining an optimum follow-up period and high-resolution CT findings to predict the growth of nodules. Jpn J Radiol 2012;30(3):206–17.

34. Kobayashi Y, Mitsudomi T. Management of ground-glass opacities: should all pulmonary lesions with ground-glass opacity be surgically resected? Transl Lung Cancer Res 2013;2(5):354–63.

35. Kobayashi Y, Mitsudomi T, Sakao Y, et al. Genetic features of pulmonary adenocarcinoma presenting with ground-glass nodules: the differences between nodules with and without growth. Ann Oncol 2015; 26:156–61.

36. Aoki T, Hanamiya M, Uramoto H, et al. Adenocarcinomas with predominant ground-glass opacity: correlation of morphology and molecular biomarkers. Radiology 2012;264(2):590–6.

37. Collado M, Gil J, Efeyan A, et al. Tumour biology: senescence in premalignant tumours. Nature 2005; 436(7051):642.

38. Ji H, Li D, Chen L, et al. The impact of human EGFR kinase domain mutations on lung tumorigenesis and in vivo sensitivity to EGFR-targeted therapies. Cancer Cell 2006;9(6):485–95.

39. Politi K, Zakowski MF, Fan PD, et al. Lung adenocarcinomas induced in mice by mutant EGF receptors found in human lung cancers respond to a tyrosine kinase inhibitor or to down-regulation of the receptors. Genes Dev 2006;20(11):1496–510.

40. Kim CF, Jackson EL, Woolfenden AE, et al. Identification of bronchioalveolar stem cells in normal lung and lung cancer. Cell 2005;121(6):823–35.

41. Yatabe Y, Borczuk AC, Powell CA. Do all lung adenocarcinomas follow a stepwise progression? Lung Cancer 2011;74(1):7–11.

42. Hasegawa M, Sone S, Takashima S, et al. Growth rate of small lung cancers detected on mass CT screening. Br J Radiol 2000;73(876):1252–9.

43. Detterbeck F, Gibson C. Turning gray: the natural history of lung cancer over time. J Thorac Oncol 2008;3(7):781–92.

44. de Hoop B, Gietema H, van de Vorst S, et al. Pulmonary ground-glass nodules: increase in mass as an early indicator of growth. Radiology 2010;255(1): 199–206.

45. Lindell RM, Hartman TE, Swensen SJ, et al. Five-year lung cancer screening experience: CT appearance, growth rate, location, and histologic features of 61 lung cancers. Radiology 2007;242(2):555–62.

46. Cho J, Kim E, Kim S, et al. Long-term follow-up of small pulmonary ground-glass nodules stable for 3 years: implications of the proper follow-up period and risk factors for subsequent growth. J Thorac Oncol 2016;11(9):1453–9.

47. Yoshizawa A, Motoi N, Riely GJ, et al. Impact of proposed IASLC/ATS/ERS classification of lung adenocarcinoma: prognostic subgroups and implications for further revision of staging based on analysis of 514 stage I cases. Mod Pathol 2011; 24(5):653–64.

48. Murakawa T, Konoeda C, Ito T, et al. The ground glass opacity component can be eliminated from the T-factor assessment of lung adenocarcinoma. Eur J Cardiothorac Surg 2013;43(5):925–32.

49. Sawabata N, Kanzaki R, Sakamoto T, et al. Clinical predictor of pre- or minimally invasive pulmonary adenocarcinoma: possibility of sub-classification of clinical T1a. Eur J Cardiothoracic Surg 2014;45(2): 256–61.

50. Ito M, Miyata Y, Kushitani K, et al. Prediction for prognosis of resected pT1a-1bN0M0 adenocarcinoma based on tumor size and histological status: relationship of TNM and IASLC/ATS/ERS classifications. Lung Cancer 2014;85(2):270–5.

51. Hattori A, Matsunaga T, Takamochi K, et al. Oncological characteristics of radiological invasive adenocarcinoma with additional ground-glass nodules on initial thin-section computed tomography: comparison with solitary invasive adenocarcinoma. J Thorac Oncol 2016;11(5):729–36.

52. Hattori A, Matsunaga T, Takamochi K, et al. Prognostic impact of a ground glass opacity component in the clinical T classification of non-small cell lung cancer. J Thorac Cardiovasc Surg 2017;154(6): 2102–10.e1.

53. Hattori A, Hirayama S, Matsunaga T, et al. Distinct clinicopathologic characteristics and prognosis based on the presence of ground glass opacity component in clinical stage IA lung adenocarcinoma. J Thorac Oncol 2019;14(2):265–75.

54. Rami-Porta R, Bolejack V, Crowley J, et al. The IASLC lung cancer staging project: proposals for the revisions of the T descriptors in the forthcoming eighth edition of the TNM classification for lung cancer. J Thorac Oncol 2015;10(7):990–1003.

55. Hattori A, Matsunaga T, Takamochi K, et al. Neither maximum tumor size nor solid component size is prognostic in part-solid lung cancer: impact of tumor size should be applied exclusively to solid lung cancer. Ann Thorac Surg 2016;102(2):407–15.

56. Berry MF, Gao R, Kunder CA, et al. Presence of even a small ground-glass component in lung adenocarcinoma predicts better survival. Clin Lung Cancer 2018;19(1):e47–51.

57. Aokage K, Miyoshi T, Ishii G, et al. Influence of ground glass opacity and the corresponding pathological findings on survival in patients with clinical stage I non-small cell lung cancer. J Thorac Oncol 2018;13(4):533–42.

58. Nakata M, Sawada S, Saeki H, et al. Prospective study of thoracoscopic limited resection for ground-glass opacity selected by computed tomography. Ann Thorac Surg 2003;75:1601–6.

59. Yamada S, Kohno T. Video-assisted thoracic surgery for pure ground-glass opacities 2 cm or less in diameter. Ann Thorac Surg 2004;77(6):1911–5.

60. Yoshida J, Nagai K, Yokose T, et al. Limited resection trial for pulmonary ground-glass opacity nodules: Fifty-case experience. J Thorac Cardiovasc Surg 2005;129(5):991–6.

61. Mun M, Kohno T. Efficacy of thoracoscopic resection for multifocal bronchioloalveolar carcinoma showing pure ground-glass opacities of 20 mm or less in diameter. J Thorac Cardiovasc Surg 2007;134(4):877–82.

62. Nakamura H, Saji H, Ogata A, et al. Lung cancer patients showing pure ground-glass opacity on computed tomography are good candidates for wedge resection. Lung Cancer 2004;44(1):61–8.

63. Park JH, Lee KS, Kim JH, et al. Malignant pure pulmonary ground-glass opacity nodules: prognostic implications. Korean J Radiol 2009;10(1):12–20.

64. Asamura H, Hishida T, Suzuki K, et al. Radiographically determined noninvasive adenocarcinoma of the lung: survival outcomes of Japan Clinical Oncology Group 0201. J Thorac Cardiovasc Surg 2013;146(1):24–30.

65. Hattori A, Matsunaga T, Hayashi T, et al. Prognostic impact of the findings on thin-section computed tomography in patients with subcentimeter non-small cell lung cancer. J Thorac Oncol 2017;12(6):954–62.

66. Hattori A, Matsunaga T, Takamochi K, et al. Importance of ground glass opacity component in clinical Stage IA radiologic invasive lung cancer. Ann Thorac Surg 2017;104(1):313–20.

67. Matsunaga T, Suzuki K, Takamochi K, et al. What is the radiological definition of part-solid tumour in lung cancer?dagger. Eur J Cardiothorac Surg 2017;51(2):242–7.

68. Yanagawa M, Kusumoto M, Johkoh T, et al. Radiologic-pathologic correlation of solid portions on thin-section CT images in lung adenocarcinoma: a multicenter study. Clin Lung Cancer 2018;19(3):e303–12.

69. Libby DM, Wu N, Lee I-J, et al. CT screening for lung cancer. Chest 2006;129(4):1039–42.

70. Lee HW, Jin KN, Lee JK, et al. Long-term follow-up of ground-glass nodules after 5 years of stability. J Thorac Oncol 2019;14(8):1370–7.

71. Revel M-P, Bissery A, Bienvenu M, et al. Are two-dimensional CT measurements of small noncalcified pulmonary nodules reliable?1. Radiology 2004;231(2):453–8.

72. Nietert PJ, Ravenel JG, Leue WM, et al. Imprecision in automated volume measurements of pulmonary nodules and its effect on the level of uncertainty in volume doubling time estimation. Chest 2009;135(6):1580–7.

73. Kakinuma R, Ashizawa K, Kuriyama K, et al. Measurement of focal ground-glass opacity diameters on CT images: interobserver agreement in regard to identifying increases in the size of ground-glass opacities. Acad Radiol 2012;19(4):389–94.

74. Kim H, Park CM, Woo S, et al. Pure and part-solid pulmonary ground-glass nodules: measurement variability of volume and mass in nodules with a solid portion less than or equal to 5 mm. Radiology 2013;269(2):585–93.

75. MacMahon H, Naidich DP, Goo JM, et al. Guidelines for management of incidental pulmonary nodules detected on CT images: from the Fleischner Society 2017. Radiology 2017;284(1):228–43.

76. National Comprehensive CN. NCCN clinical practice guidelines in oncology (NCCN Guidelines) non-small cell lung cancer Version 7.2019 - August 30 2019. Available at: https://www.nccn.org/professionals/physician_gls/pdf/nscl.pdf. Accessed October 5, 2019.

77. National Comprehensive CN. NCCN Clinical Practice Guidelines in Oncology (NCCN Guidelines) Lung Cancer Screening. Version 1.2020-May 14, 2019. Available at: https://www.nccn.org/professionals/physician_gls/pdf/lung_screening.pdf. Accessed October 5, 2019.

78. Detterbeck FC. Achieving clarity about lung cancer and opacities. Chest 2017;151(2):252–4.

79. Maeyashiki T, Suzuki K, Hattori A, et al. The size of consolidation on thin-section computed tomography is a better predictor of survival than the maximum tumour dimension in resectable lung cancer. Eur J Cardiothorac Surg 2013;43(5):915–8.

80. Tsutani Y, Miyata Y, Nakayama H, et al. Prognostic significance of using solid versus whole tumor size on high-resolution computed tomography for predicting pathologic malignant grade of tumors in clinical stage IA lung adenocarcinoma: a multicenter study. J Thorac Cardiovasc Surg 2012;143(3):607–12.

81. Tsutani Y, Miyata Y, Nakayama H, et al. Appropriate sublobar resection choice for ground glass opacity-dominant clinical stage IA lung adenocarcinoma: wedge resection or segmentectomy. Chest 2013;145(1):66–71.

82. Yanagawa N, Shiono S, Abiko M, et al. New IASLC/ATS/ERS classification and invasive tumor size are predictive of disease recurrence in Stage I lung adenocarcinoma. J Thorac Oncol 2013;8(5):612–8.

83. Detterbeck F, Khandani AH. The role of PET imaging in solitary pulmonary nodules. Clin Pulm Med 2009;16(2):81–8.

84. Nomori H, Watanabe K, Ohtsuka T, et al. Evaluation of F-18 fluorodeoxyglucose (FDG) PET scanning for pulmonary nodules less than 3 cm in diameter, with special reference to the CT images. Lung Cancer 2004;45(1):19–27.

85. Suzuki K, Watanabe S, Wakabayashi M, et al. A nonradomized confirmatory phase III study of sublobar

surgical resection for peripheral ground glass opacity dominant lung cancer defined with thoracic thin-section computed tomography. Paper presented at: ASCO2017. Chicago, IL, June 2-6, 2017.

86. Yoshida J, Ishii G, Yokose T, et al. Possible delayed cut-end recurrence after limited resection for ground-glass opacity adenocarcinoma, intraoperatively diagnosed as Noguchi Type B, in three patients. J Thorac Oncol 2010;5(4):546–50.

87. Nakao M, Yoshida J, Goto K, et al. Long-term outcomes of 50 cases of limited-resection trial for pulmonary ground-glass opacity nodules. J Thorac Oncol 2012;7(10):1563–6.

88. Eguchi T, Kameda K, Lu S, et al. Lobectomy is associated with better outcomes than sublobar resection in spread through air spaces (STAS)-positive T1 lung adenocarcinoma: a propensity score-matched analysis. J Thorac Oncol 2019;14(1):87–98.

89. Toyokawa G, Yamada Y, Tagawa T, et al. Computed tomography features of resected lung adenocarcinomas with spread through air spaces. J Thorac Cardiovasc Surg 2018;156(4):1670–6.e4.

90. Suzuki K, Saji H, Aokage K, et al. Comparison of pulmonary segmentectomy and lobectomy: safety results of a randomized trial. J Thorac Cardiovasc Surg 2019;158(3):895–907.

91. Altorki NK, Wang X, Wigle D, et al. Perioperative mortality and morbidity after sublobar versus lobar resection for early-stage non-small-cell lung cancer: post-hoc analysis of an international, randomised, phase 3 trial (CALGB/Alliance 140503). Lancet Respir Med 2018;6(12):915–24.

92. Ginsberg RJ, Rubinstein LV, for the Lung Cancer Study Group. Randomized trial of lobectomy versus limited resection for T1 N0 non-small cell lung cancer. Ann Thorac Surg 1995;60(3):615–23.

93. Howington J, Blum M, Chang A, et al. Treatment of Stage I and II non-small cell lung cancer. Chest 2013;432(5 Suppl):e278S–313S.

94. Detterbeck F, Nicholson F, Franklin W, et al. The IASLC lung cancer staging project:summary of proposal revisions of the classification of lung cancers with multiple pulmonary sites of involvement in the forthcoming eighth ediiton of the TNM classification. J Thorac Oncol 2016;11(5):639–50.

95. Detterbeck F, Arenberg D, Asamura H, et al. The IASLC lung cancer staging project: background data and proposals for the application of TNM staging rules to lung cancer presenting as multiple nodules with ground glass or lepidic features or a pneumonic-type of involvement in the forthcoming eight edition of the TNM classification. J Thorac Oncol 2016;11(5):666–80.

96. Chen K, Chen W, Cai J, et al. Favorable prognosis and high discrepancy of genetic features in surgical patients with multiple primary lung cancers. J Thorac Cardiovasc Surg 2018;155(1):371–9.e1.

97. Naidich DP, Bankier AA, MacMahon H, et al. Recommendations for the management of subsolid pulmonary nodules detected at CT: a statement from the Fleischner Society. Radiology 2013;266(1):304–17.

Biomarkers in Lung Cancer

Catherine R. Sears, MD[a],*, Peter J. Mazzone, MD, MPH, FCCP[b]

KEYWORDS

- Lung cancer screening • Lung nodules • Next-generation sequencing • Radiomics • Clinical utility
- Trial design

KEY POINTS

- Biomarkers can be used for risk assessment, detection, diagnosis, and prognosis and to personalize treatment in lung cancer.
- Clinically useful biomarkers for selection of high-risk patients for lung cancer screening and to differentiate early lung cancer from benign pulmonary nodules are needed.
- Biomarkers for nodule management and determination of high-risk groups for lung cancer screening are at all phases of development, from discovery to clinical utility studies.
- Current trends in lung cancer biomarker development include the integration of clinical and radiologic features with molecular biomarkers, the application of artificial intelligence to molecular and imaging biomarker development, the use highly sensitive technologies such as next-generation sequencing for molecular exploration, and a commitment to high-quality clinical validation and utility studies.

INTRODUCTION

Lung cancer is diagnosed in more than 1.8 million people yearly and remains the leading cause of cancer deaths in both developing and developed countries, with survival at 5 years a disappointing 19%.[1,2] This poor survival rate is attributable to many factors, including lung cancer diagnosis at a late stage, when cure is uncommon with currently available therapies.[3] Biomarkers that accurately predict lung cancer risk may aid in targeting intensive preventative interventions to those at the highest risk of lung cancer development. Lung cancer screening (LCS) by low-dose computed tomography of the chest (LDCT) decreases mortality by diagnosing lung cancers at an early stage, when treatment is potentially curative.[4] The population for whom LCS would be most beneficial is not definitively identified.[5] A biomarker that better identifies patients likely to benefit from LCS, particularly healthy patients at high lung cancer risk not currently offered LCS,

would be beneficial.[5–7] In addition, LDCT identifies both cancerous and noncancerous lung nodules. A biomarker that distinguishes between benign and malignant nodules can help to avoid potentially dangerous procedures for those without cancer.[8,9] Particularly in non–small cell lung cancer (NSCLC), much progress has been made to classify lung cancers by molecular markers, some of which can be used to personalize therapy. Now many are actively developing and testing the utility of predictive, diagnostic, and prognostic lung cancer biomarkers (**Fig. 1**). This article focuses on the development, current utilization, and future trends of lung cancer biomarkers and provides specific examples of how these can impact management.

BIOMARKER DEVELOPMENT

Biomarkers to predict, diagnose, and prognosticate lung cancer are being developed at a rapid rate, fueled by an increasing knowledge of normal and malignant genetic, epigenetic, and

---

[a] Department of Medicine, Division of Pulmonary, Critical Care, Sleep and Occupational Medicine, Indiana University School of Medicine, 980 West Walnut Street, Room R3-C400, Indianapolis, IN, USA; [b] Lung Cancer Program, Respiratory Institute, Cleveland Clinic, 9500 Euclid Avenue, A90, Cleveland, OH 44195, USA
* Corresponding author.
E-mail address: crufatto@iu.edu

Clin Chest Med 41 (2020) 115–127
https://doi.org/10.1016/j.ccm.2019.10.004
0272-5231/20/© 2019 Elsevier Inc. All rights reserved.

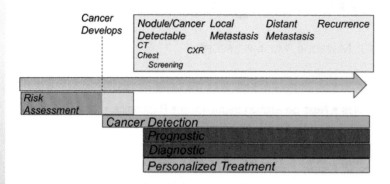

Fig. 1. Biomarker utility in lung cancer. CXR, chest radiograph.

immunologic signatures and increasingly available samples, big data, and methods with which to analyze them. The Institute of Medicine has developed a framework by which -omics-based tests can be developed and evaluated for scientific rigor.[10] The Centers for Disease Control and Prevention ACCE model of biomarker development includes 5 distinct phases: discovery, analytical validation, clinical validation, clinical utility, and associated implementation factors (including ethical, legal, and social implications, such as cost-effectiveness) (**Fig. 2**). These concepts have been applied to the development, implementation, and evaluation of biomarkers for lung cancer diagnosis and screening.[11]

Discovery

There is an accelerated pace to lung cancer biomarker discovery. In this phase, potential biomarkers are identified, confirmed, and prioritized for validation. The initial identification can use cell culture or human samples, available databases, or a combination of these resources. It is important at this very early stage of biomarker development to consider several factors. First, the biospecimen used for the assay must be easily accessible, simple to prepare and store, and available in sufficient amounts for biomarker measurement.[12] Lung cancer biomarkers have been developed from blood components, sputum, exhaled breath, urine, and oronasal and bronchial epithelium to measure molecular targets, such as tumor and immune antigens, autoantibodies, messenger RNA (mRNA) and microRNA (miRNA), DNA methylation, circulating free tumor DNA, and circulating tumor cells, among others.[13] The discovery phase has 3 components[10]: Component 1: quality control determines the accuracy and reproducibility of the measurement, including

Fig. 2. Stages of biomarker development.

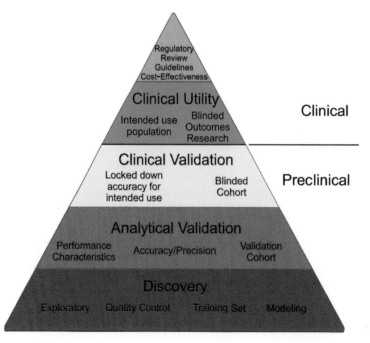

optimizing operating procedures (collection, storage, methods) and meeting minimally acceptable variations in results; Component 2: a training set is used to develop the modeling and fitting of the biomarker for its intended use; Component 3: confirmation of the computational modeling with a separate testing set. Although more fastidiously required during the later stages of biomarker development, use of specimens from the intended use population is favored during the biomarker discovery phase, because the use of appropriate samples for test development and validation may prevent failure of test validation. For instance, a serum biomarker that uses a cancer antigen to differentiate between patients with stage IV NSCLC and those without cancer in a test cohort may not be able to detect earlier stage NSCLC. Similarly, a lung nodule biomarker able to detect different serum miRNA signatures in a training set containing specimens from patients with lung cancer who are smokers compared with a control population comprising mostly non-smokers may select for a biomarker able to differentiate between smokers and non-smokers, but may be unable to differentiate between cancerous and noncancerous nodules.

Analytical Validation

After a biomarker has completed the discovery phase, the test must go through analytical validation, which establishes acceptable performance characteristics of a biomarker in the intended use population. At this point, the established methods and modeling are applied to a new validation cohort, separate from that used in the discovery phase, containing samples representing the intended use population. The analytical validation evaluates the reproducibility of a biomarker (low interlaboratory variability, repeatability over time, and from sample to sample). Accuracy and precision of the assay, analytical sensitivity/specificity, linearity, limits of detection, cutoff values, and intraassay and interassay coefficients of variation are assessed in this phase. For these measurements, recommendations for minimally acceptable standards are available.[14–17] Analytical validation requires collection of samples from patients for a specific purpose and requires institutional review board approval. Most biomarker developers will have consulted with the Food and Drug Administration (FDA) by this point.[10,11]

Clinical Validation

The clinical validation phase, sometimes referred to as the biological validation phase, is used to determine the diagnostic accuracy of a biomarker in the intended use population. Accuracy is compared with a relevant reference standard and must improve upon currently available assessment tools, making evaluation in the appropriate population essential. For instance, for a lung nodule management biomarker, the clinical validation phase would use specimens from patients with lung nodules determined to be lung cancer as well as specimens from patients with benign lung nodules. Analyzing clinical validity requires a blinded, intended-use specimen set, unique to the samples used in the discovery and analytical validation training sets. These specimens are usually obtained from different institutions as well to eliminate geographic and associated population differences as a potential bias. Using locked-down biomarker thresholds developed in the discovery and analytical validation phases, clinical validation determines performance characteristics of a biomarker in this population, including sensitivity, specificity, positive predictive value, negative predictive value, likelihood and hazard ratios, and area under the curve or receiver operating characteristic curve analysis.[16] Findings from a clinical validation study can be used to estimate the predicted clinical impact of using the test in the intended use population.[18] For instance, the clinically validated accuracy of a biomarker used to stratify intermediate risk pulmonary nodules into a high- and low-risk category could be used to estimate the potential impact of the results if it were used to impact clinical decisions. However, clinical utility assessment is needed to confirm these estimates.[11] Results from clinical validation studies have been used for FDA approval and coverage of a biomarker by public or private insurance sources.

Clinical Utility

Clinical utility is the ultimate determinant of a biomarker's performance, because it reflects how the results affect clinical decision making and patient outcomes. For this reason, a highly reliable and accurate biomarker may not always be clinically useful. There are many possible reasons for this. For one, clinical utility takes into consideration both the benefits and the harms of using a biomarker, and use in the appropriate context is necessary for a favorable benefit-to-harm ratio.[11,19] In **Fig. 3**, the authors provide an example of a highly accurate biomarker that is potentially harmful when applied to the wrong population.[20] Clinical utility takes into consideration how biomarker results affect clinical decisions beyond estimates extrapolated from clinical validation studies. Misinterpretation of the results or

LungRADS 2

	Cancer	Benign	Total
Biomarker +	36	996	1,032
Biomarker -	4	8,964	8,968
Total	40	9,960	10,000

LungRADS 4

	Cancer	Benign	Total
Biomarker +	639	929	1,568
Biomarker -	71	8,361	8,432
Total	710	9,290	10,000

Fig. 3. Potential harms of a biomarker in management of nodules detected by LDCT. A highly accurate biomarker (90% sensitivity and 90% specificity) is applied to solid pulmonary nodules classified as LungRADS 2 on LDCT (sized <6 mm).[20] The probability of this nodule being malignant is 0.4%; most positive biomarker results will be for those with benign disease, leading to a positive predictive value (PPV) of only 3%. If a positive test result leads to more aggressive evaluation of nodules, which would have otherwise been followed radiologically, the biomarker may lead to harm. Alternatively, if this same test is applied to solid pulmonary nodules 8 to 15 mm identified by LDCT (LungRADS 4A), the PPV increases to 41%.

mismanagement owing to inaccurate or incorrectly interpreted results can result in harm or increased costs to the patient. Finally, lung cancer biomarkers must improve upon currently available assessment tools to be clinically useful. There are several different ways to assess clinical utility.[21] More detailed examples of lung cancer biomarker clinical utility, including trial design, are available.[11]

Cost-Effectiveness, Implementation, and Policy Considerations

If a biomarker is determined to be clinically useful in a specific population for a defined purpose, the impact of widespread utilization is often evaluated before policy recommendations for implementation. One of the measurements to estimate societal impact is cost-effectiveness analysis (CEA). The measurement of biomarker cost-effectiveness is complex but important to determine the ultimate utility to society. Several groups have provided guidelines on the evaluation, reporting, and utilization of CEA.[22–25] CEA is commonly measured as quality-adjusted life-years (QALY), which takes into account not only the lives saved by a certain intervention but also the quality of life during that time, or as an incremental cost-effectiveness ratio, which compares the cost-effectiveness of a biomarker to the existing standard of care. CEA compares the net cost of implementing a biomarker to a specific outcome, most commonly on a societal scale. The cost of a test should account for all net expenditures, including fixed costs (eg, equipment and materials needed to perform the test), direct costs (eg, physician and technician time to perform and interpret the test), and indirect costs (eg, cost of additional studies based on test results, potential complications of the testing).

There are several potential confounders to CEA, including cost variability, type of outcome measured, demographics, geography, and resource availability. It is important to use large,

well-designed trials that include the appropriate intended use population for CEA. For instance, the cost-effectiveness of LCS by LDCT is estimated at $81,000/QALY gained, within the range typically considered cost-effective.[26] However, the confidence interval ranges from $52,000 to $186,000/QALY gained, depending on the lung cancer risk of the population by variation of sex, age, and smoking status at the time of screening.[26–28] These calculations highlight how defining a particular population may alter cost-effectiveness measures. Biomarkers may serve as adjunctive tools to further improve cost-effectiveness of LCS by LDCT by (1) defining a higher-risk population for screening or (2) improving the management of lung nodules, thereby limiting additional workup, including procedural, surgical, or radiologic follow-up. Examples of calculations to assess favorable CEA in lung cancer biomarkers have been previously outlined.[11,19]

In addition, other less quantifiable factors should be considered in biomarker implementation, including resources needed to perform and interpret the analysis and the impact on the individual (eg, pain, distress, time, and loss or gain in productivity). On a larger scale, policy decisions may consider allocation of resources (eg, in the distribution of research funds for biomarker development) and implementation considerations, which are not directly addressed in most CEA, but are important when determining the impact of the biomarker in an intended use population.

CLINICAL UTILITY EVALUATION
Lung Cancer Prevention

There have been extensive efforts to determine those at high risk for lung cancer development. Several risk calculators for lung cancer development are available that use clinical data.[11,29] All major lung cancer risk calculators include age and tobacco smoking history, and variably other risk factors, including asbestos exposure, family history, presence of chronic obstructive pulmonary disease, prior cancers, prior pneumonia, low level of education, and race/ethnicity, with some models including sex/gender. The impact of other exposures and diseases associated with increased lung cancer risk, including exposure to radon, polycyclic aromatic hydrocarbons, heavy metals, human immunodeficiency virus infection, and the presence of interstitial lung disease, are not routinely included in risk calculators.[30–33] Although no single biomarker has been found that accurately predicts the risk of developing lung cancer, specific genetic polymorphisms, including those in the nicotinic acetylcholine receptor gene, are strongly associated with nicotine addiction and increased risk of lung cancer.[34] Intervention on this finding is cessation of tobacco smoking. However, tobacco smoking is one of the 2 strongest risk factors for lung cancer development (age being the other). Because of this factor alone, in addition to the high morbidity associated with other tobacco-related diseases, aggressive tobacco cessation efforts should be offered to all smokers regardless of biomarker results, making this a poor target for development of a preventative biomarker development when used alone. However, a biomarker that could improve upon currently available clinical risk prediction tools may be beneficial in the selection of cohorts for chemoprevention studies or as a surrogate endpoint in prevention intervention studies.

Lung Cancer Screening

The National Lung Screening Trial (NLST) randomized more than 53,000 patients (30 pack-year current or former smokers who quit within the last 15 years, aged 55–74) to either LDCT or chest radiographs yearly for 3 years. Those who were randomized to LDCT had a 20% relative risk reduction of lung cancer death.[4] This finding has led to the recommendation for LCS in high-risk smokers by several specialty- and disease-specific societies and led to the decision by the Centers for Medicare and Medicaid Services (CMS) to cover LCS services.[35] Another large randomized controlled trial in Europe suggests an even greater survival benefit from LCS using LDCT extending beyond 3 years.[36] However, LCS is associated with both direct and indirect risks, many of which are associated with a large number of benign nodules (false positives) identified by LDCT.[9] Nodules were identified on 24% of LDCTs, most of which (96%) are ultimately discovered to be benign, but may lead to invasive surgical and nonsurgical diagnostic procedures, associated with morbidity and less

likely death.[4,9] Additional risks and concerns raised have included patient quality of life, overdiagnosis, risks and costs of unnecessary procedures, the quality, compliance, and cost of widespread implementation, and secondary malignancies from radiation exposure from imaging.[9,37] Furthermore, there is also concern about patient selection for LCS: (1) that the NLST criteria may exclude populations at high risk for lung cancer development, which may benefit but are excluded from LCS; and (2) that certain patient populations included in NLST criteria may be less likely to benefit and more likely to have complications of LCS.[20,38–40]

A biomarker may therefore benefit LCS in several ways. First, a biomarker of lung cancer risk may aid in discussions of individual risk-to-benefit ratio for LCS. In order to do this, the biomarker would need to be more accurate at identifying those at high or low risk of having/developing potentially curative lung cancer than currently available risk stratification criteria (eg, current LCS enrollment criteria or available clinical risk assessment tools), either alone or in combination with these tools.[29] Compared with the standard of care, that biomarker must either (a) lead to fewer lung cancer deaths in a screened population without increasing harms or expense or (b) lead to a similar number of lung cancer deaths in a screened population but decrease harms or expense.[11] For instance, a biomarker may be able to select for a population at high risk of lung cancer development not included in the currently screened population, who would benefit from LCS. Similarly, a biomarker that predicted those at highest risk for lung cancer could select a population within those currently offered LCS, which will most benefit while excluding, and thereby reducing potential risks, to those unlikely to benefit. Alternatively, a biomarker that would predict those at lowest risk of lung cancer may identify a patient, currently considered for LCS but with an unfavorable benefit-to-risk ratio, reducing potential harms and costs associated with LCS. Specific ways in which an LCS biomarker can be tested against a standard of care to determine clinical utility are available.[11]

Nodule Management

The increased use of chest computed tomography (CT) scans, for both LCS and diagnostic indications, has led to an increase in the identification of pulmonary nodules.[41] Although some of these nodules are immediately identified as high or low risk of lung cancer based on imaging characteristics, many are considered intermediate risk.[42]

Subsolid nodules have a higher risk of malignancy than solid nodules, but typically behave in a more indolent fashion. For this reason, they can be followed radiologically for growth or development of a solid component, at which time surgical resection is the preferred treatment.[42–45] For solid, noncalcified nodules measuring 8 to 30 mm in diameter without benign characteristics, a biomarker that could differentiate benign from malignant would be beneficial. Several lung nodule risk calculators have been developed for risk assessment of these intermediate-risk nodules, with utility variable by cohort.[46,47] Malignancy risk, determined by nodule risk calculators or physician estimation, is then used to determine initial management strategies based on malignant risk stratification into very low ($\leq$10%), intermediate ($\sim$11%–64%), and high risk (>65%), with cutoffs variable depending on patient preference and comorbidities.[42,48] Very low-risk nodules are typically managed by close radiologic follow-up. High-risk nodules are managed by definitive treatment (surgical resection or stereotactic radiotherapy). Intermediate-risk nodules require further evaluation, which can include additional imaging (eg, PET) or biopsy (percutaneous or bronchoscopic). PET combined with CT, although highly sensitive ($\sim$90%), has a lower specificity (61%–77%), which is even lower in areas with a high incidence of endemic mycoses.[49] Percutaneous nodule biopsies have a high diagnostic yield, but are associated with a risk of complications, including pneumothorax, particularly in this patient population that may have tobacco-associated emphysematous changes.[42,50] Bronchoscopic biopsy, although having a lower risk of pneumothorax, is performed in selected individuals based on nodule characteristics and has variable diagnostic yields even when performed by highly experienced proceduralists.[42,51] It is these intermediate-risk nodules that would most benefit from further risk stratification by a pulmonary nodule biomarker.

A few considerations are important in a nodule management biomarker. In order to be clinically useful, a lung nodule management biomarker must be more accurate than existing pulmonary nodule risk assessment tools (nodule risk calculators, PET) or improve accuracy when combined with these risk assessment tools. Although theoretically a biomarker could identify a nodule as either high or low likelihood of malignancy, most current nodule management biomarkers are classified as either rule-in (high likelihood of malignancy) or rule-out (low likelihood of malignancy). As such, a potentially useful rule-in lung nodule biomarker will increase the probability of malignancy in an intermediate-risk pulmonary nodule above the threshold for recommending definitive therapy (surgery or stereotactic body radiation therapy [SBRT]). The benefit of this biomarker would be to avoid possible delay or complications associated with diagnostic procedures. A potentially useful rule-out lung nodule biomarker decreases the probability of a malignancy in an intermediate-risk pulmonary nodule low enough to warrant radiologic surveillance. The potential benefit of such a biomarker would be to avoid complications and costs of invasive diagnostic procedures in those with benign nodules. In both of these scenarios, it is important to stress that clinical validity does not equate to clinical utility. Clinical utility in a nodule management biomarker requires either (a) that lung cancers are diagnosed earlier without significantly increasing procedures performed on benign nodules or (b) that fewer procedures are performed on benign nodules without a clinically significant delay in the diagnosis of lung cancer in those with malignant pulmonary nodules.[11] However, even if those criteria are fulfilled, a lung nodule biomarker may have limited clinical utility. For instance, a patient with a very early or slow-growing lung cancer, correctly identified as malignant by a lung nodule biomarker, may have a complication during a surgery or intervention for a cancer that would have remained indolent (ie, never cause the patient's death). Alternatively, a false negative biomarker result on a very small, early lung cancer that is followed by close radiologic surveillance may result in a delay in diagnosis that is not associated with any increase in mortality. For this reason, it is important that these biomarkers are applied to the intended use population and trials to address clinical utility are designed with these specific outcomes in mind. Another publication gives detailed examples of such clinical utility trial designs.[11]

Lung Cancer Prognosis and Prediction of Response to Therapy

In patients already diagnosed with lung cancer, there are several ways in which a biomarker may be of benefit. It can be used to predict tumor behavior, often measured by the surrogate of patient survival. The best prognostic marker in NSCLC is TMN stage, which takes into consideration tumor size and metastasis.[3] Other tumor characteristics are associated with poor survival, including gross and microscopic evidence of lymphatic vessel invasion.[52] Additional tumor characteristics, particularly expression levels of oncogenes and tumor suppressors, have been associated with favorable (*EGFR* mutant and *ERCC1*, *RRM1* overexpression) and unfavorable (*Kras*, *p53* mutations and *p53*, *Her2* overexpression) prognostic value in early NSCLC.[53] A rapidly growing list of biomarkers can be used to predict response to therapy, particularly because the available therapies are tailored to specific tumor mutations and characteristics expand. Among this list is expression of immune antigens and ligands (such as PD-1/PD-L1 and CTLA-4 expression), tumor characteristics such as mutational burden, and presence of tumor infiltrating lymphocyte.[53–55] Characterization and quantification of circulating tumor cells, which increase with advancing stages of lung cancer, have been used to evaluate for response to therapy and to diagnose early, preclinical recurrence.[56,57] Similarly, circulating tumor DNA (ctDNA) has been used to diagnose and predict response to targeted therapies.[58,59] Many of these biomarkers are covered in another article in this issue.

CURRENT UTILIZATION OF BIOMARKERS

Many lung cancer biomarkers are currently in development, most in the early stages (**Table 1**),

with few progressed beyond clinical validation studies (**Table 2**). Most biomarkers designed for use as risk prediction and diagnostic biomarkers have been developed using histologically agnostic cohorts. However, most available specimens represent NSCLCs, particularly adenocarcinomas and squamous cell carcinomas as the most common histologic classifications, with small cell and other less common lung cancers less commonly the focus of biomarker development or utilization. Many lung cancer biomarkers have been used to guide therapy, such as when genetic alterations driving tumor growth can be targeted by available drug therapies (EGFR, ALK, ROS1, HER2, BRAF/MEK, MET, and RET mutation and aberrancies), to prognosticate tumor aggressiveness or response to treatment, or to predict response to immune checkpoint inhibition (PD-L1, CTLA-4 expressions, genomic alterations).[53,60] Most other molecular biomarkers, which have reached the clinical validation phase of development, have been designed for patient selection in LCS or to guide lung nodule management (see **Table 2**). These biomarkers measure different molecules, often in panels that include proteins, autoantibodies, methylated DNA, mRNA, miRNA, and

---

Table 1
Lung cancer biomarkers: candidate markers post-discovery phase

Biologic Source	Measured Molecule(s)	Assay
Blood: Serum/plasma	Protein	6 protein panel (CA125, CEA, CYFRA21-1, NSE, ProGRP, SCC)[81]
		3 protein + AAb panel (CEA, CYRFA21-1, CA125, HGF, NY-ESO-1)[82]
		Complement C4d[83]
	miRNA	2 miRNA signature[84]
	"Liquid Biopsy" ctDNA and cfDNA	ctDNA NGS
		mPCR[68,74]
		CAPP-Seq[58]
		Ion proton cfDNA and targeted Seq[69]
		TEC-Seq[71]
		ctDNA mutations + 8 proteins (CancerSEEK)[72]
		ctDNA methylation[59]
	PBMC RNA	29 gene signature[85]
Airway/oral epithelium	Buccal cell structure	Partial wave spectroscopic Nanocytology[86]
Sputum	Sputum cytology: flow cytometry	TCPP affinity[87]
	miRNA	13 miRNA[88]
BAL fluid	DNA methylation	SHOX2 and RASF1A[89]
Exhaled breath	Volatile organic Compounds	VOC-NBT[90]
		VOC-FAIMS[91]
Urine	Metabolites	3 protein panel (IGFBP-1, sIL-1Ra, CEACAM-1)[92]

Abbreviations: CAPP-Seq, cancer personalized profiling by deep sequencing; cfDNA, cell-free DNA; ctDNA, circulating tumor DNA; FAIMS, field asymmetric ion mobility spectrometry; NBT, nanoparticle biometric tagging; TCCP, tetra (4-carboxyphenyl) porphine; TEC-Seq, tagged error correction sequencing; VOC, volatile organic compounds.

Table 2
Lung cancer biomarkers by intended use: post-discovery phase

Name	Company	Biomarker	Source	Approval	Complete	Ongoing	Planned
Lung cancer screening							
Early CDT-Lung	Oncimmune[c]	7 AAb panel: ELISA	Blood	CLIA	Clinical validation	ECLS NCT01700257	Clinical utility
Lung EpiCheck	Nucleix	6 DNA methylation	Blood	N/A	Discovery	N/A	Clinical validation
miR-Test	—	13 miRNA	Blood	N/A	Clinical validation	COSMOS II Trial	Clinical utility
MicroRNA Signature Classifier (MSC)	—	24 miRNA	Blood	N/A	Clinical validation	BIOMILD NCT02247453	Clinical utility
PAULA's test	Genesys	3 antigen, 1 AAb panel: ELISA	Blood	CLIA	Clinical validation	N/A	N/A
RespiraGene	Synergenx	20 SNPs + clinical	Blood	N/A	Clinical validation	N/A	N/A
Nodule management							
Xpresys Lung 2	Biodesix	2 proteins MRM mass spectrometry + clinical	Blood	CMS	Clinical validation	Registry	Clinical utility
Percepta	Veracyte	23 mRNA/gene expression profile	Bronchial epithelial cells (brush)	CMS	Clinical validation: 2nd and 3rd generation	Registry	Clinical utility[b]
Epi proLung	Epigenomics AG	DNA methylation	Bronchial aspirate	No[a]	Clinical validity	N/A	N/A
REVEAL	MagArray	Tumor Ag and AAb	Blood	CLIA	Discovery	Clinical Validation	Clinical utility
DetermaVu Lung	OncoCyte	15 mRNA + size	Blood	CLIA	Discovery	Clinical Validation	Clinical utility

Abbreviations: AAb, autoantibodies; ELISA, enzyme-linked immunosorbent assay; MRM, multiple reaction monitoring; N/A, not applicable; SNP, single nucleotide polymorphism.
[a] Previously available in Europe.
[b] Ongoing second- to third-generation discovery studies.
[c] in partnership with Biodesix (United States).

single nucleotide polymorphisms alone or in combination with clinical factors. Most of the early biomarkers were developed using blood components, collected at the time of routine blood sampling and preserved, relying on systemic changes caused by lung cancer.[18,61–64] Two assays were developed for use in bronchial epithelial specimens obtained during diagnostic bronchoscopy performed to evaluate pulmonary nodules, which rely on altered genetic and epigenetic characteristics of noncancerous bronchial epithelial cells in patients with lung cancer (field cancerization effect).[65–67] Some of these tests are commercially available, and a few are approaching clinical utility testing.[13,18,61–66]

CURRENT TRENDS AND FUTURE DIRECTIONS

Paralleling the rapid advances in the understanding of lung cancer biology is the development of novel biomarkers. The number of biomarkers in early development for risk prediction and diagnostic evaluation of lung cancers is too expansive to cover individually, but there are exciting trends and novel directions for biomarkers currently under development.

Initial efforts at biomarker development focused on single genes, proteins, or pathways or combining a handful of promising biomarkers to improve accuracy. However, as the clinical needs for lung cancer biomarkers have become further defined, banked specimens to use in training sets and for further biomarker validation are increasingly available. Because of this, analytical and clinical validation studies have become larger, more comprehensive, and multi-institutional. These newer biomarkers are increasingly combining quantitative biomarker measurements with clinical features, such as tumor size, smoking status, and age, often incorporating previously validated clinical risk assessment calculators to improve accuracy.

The availability of advanced biologic assays, such as next-generation sequencing (NGS), has led to rapid advances in the understanding of tumor biology and comprehensive assessment of the tumor genome. NGS is increasingly applied to the molecular characterization of cancers, allowing for personalization of treatment decisions. It is now being developed for use in lung cancer diagnosis and management (see **Table 1**). The ability of NGS to detect even rare mutations and clonal changes has expanded its utility to assess ctDNA in the serum of even early lung cancers.[68] This technology is already in use for identifying specific driver mutations with available targeted treatments, and there are promising data that ctDNA could serve as a useful tool in monitoring for treatment response, for drug resistance, and in diagnosing early recurrence.[58,60,68,69] ctDNA signatures are being developed for application in the LCS and lung nodule management setting.[58,59,70–74] Attempts to improve the limits of detection of circulating tumor cells as an early lung cancer detection biomarker are ongoing.

Several biomarker advances require a high level of technological expertise for assay operation and interpretation, requiring performance in CLIA-certified laboratories. Some are working to simplify this process, either by streamlining the collection, by processing and interpretation of these assays, or by developing assays that can be determined by point-of-care kits. Novel assays use biological specimens that can be collected noninvasively, require little processing, opening opportunities to adapt them for collection at home (eg, sputum, exhaled breath volatile organic compounds [by digital noses], buccal mucosal swabs, and urine) (see **Table 1**).[75]

Radiomics refers to using databases containing large numbers of medical images combined with computer deep learning to find quantitative and qualitative image features, which correlate with disease states.[76] For lung cancer, radiomic biomarkers can be developed from imaging, such as chest CT and PET. Combinations of these radiomic markers with clinical characteristics, and molecular signatures may improve the accuracy of prognostic, diagnostic, and therapeutic biomarkers. Perhaps one of the most promising uses for radiomics is diagnostic evaluation of pulmonary nodules.[77] Modeling by artificial intelligence (AI) holds great promise in distinguishing benign from malignant pulmonary nodules. Recently, 3-dimensional modeling, developed from almost 30,000 LDCTs for LCS, was able to predict the probability of malignancy as accurately, and in some cases better than, trained chest radiologists.[78] Because these computer-aided detection models rely on deep learning, and program algorithms are designed to improve with additional samples, one might expect even greater accuracy in the future. In addition to nodule detection and characterization, AI-based radiologic tools may aid in monitoring for response to treatment, detecting early recurrence, and may be combined with other biospecimens to further improve diagnostic, prognostic, and therapeutic accuracy.[79,80]

Clinical utility studies of clinically validated biomarkers for further selection of a high-risk population for LCS or for pulmonary nodule management are being planned or currently enrolling (see **Table 1**). Prospective trials may compare a biomarker-stratified strategy against a management standard of care, in which the standard of care is either the biomarker-negative population (enrichment) or the agnostic to biomarker results as a separate control population (biomarker strategy).[11] Acceleration of biomarker development may be possible by ongoing efforts to bank specimens from these clinical utility studies so that additional biomarkers can be evaluated retrospectively on prospectively collected samples in the intended use population.[11,12] Larger, multi-institutional clinical utility trials in combination with registry-collected outcomes data may also aid in the understanding of biomarker utility in less well-studied ethnic populations and in rarer lung cancer subtypes.

SUMMARY

The development of biomarkers in lung cancer is rapidly evolving. Of particular need are accurate and clinically useful biomarkers to differentiate malignant from benign pulmonary nodules and to identify those at highest risk for lung cancer development. Advances in the scientific understanding of lung cancer have led to the development of biomarkers that show potentially useful accuracies in clinical validation studies. Further investigation in large registries and well-designed clinical utility studies are anticipated. Promising trends in lung cancer biomarker development include using easily collected biospecimens, along with highly sensitive and increasingly available technologies, such as radiomics and NGS, in combination with clinical and tumor characteristics to advance biomarker development for the diagnosis and risk assessment of lung cancer.

DISCLOSURE

Scientific and Medical Advisory Board, Biodesix. Scientific and Medical Advisory Board, bioAffinity Technologies Inc (C.R. Sears). Research support to institution: Veracyte, OncoCyte, Exact Sciences, SEER, PCORI (P.J. Mazzone).

REFERENCES

1. Torre LA, Bray F, Siegel RL, et al. Global cancer statistics, 2012. CA Cancer J Clin 2015;65(2):87–108.
2. Siegel R, Miller K, Jemal A. Cancer statistics, 2019. CA Cancer J Clin 2019;69(1):7–34.
3. Goldstraw P, Chansky K, Crowley J, et al. The IASLC lung cancer staging project: proposals for revision of the TNM stage groupings in the forthcoming (eighth) edition of the TNM classification for lung cancer. J Thorac Oncol 2016;11(1):39–51.
4. Aberle DR, Adams AM, Berg CD, et al. The National Lung Screening Trial Research Team. Reduced lung-cancer mortality with low-dose computed tomographic screening. N Engl J Med 2011; 265(5):395–409.
5. Mazzone PJ, Silvestri GA, Patel S, et al. Screening for lung cancer: CHEST guideline and expert panel report. Chest 2018;153(4):954–85.
6. Tammemagi MC, Ten Haaf K, Toumazis I, et al. Development and validation of a multivariable lung cancer risk prediction model that includes low-dose computed tomography screening results: a secondary analysis of data from the national lung screening trial. JAMA Netw Open 2019;2(3): e190204.
7. Mazzone P. Lung cancer screening: examining the issues. Cleve Clin J Med 2012;79(Electronic Suppl 1):eS1–6.
8. Tanner NT, Aggarwal J, Gould MK, et al. Management of pulmonary nodules by community pulmonologists: a multicenter observational study. Chest 2015;148(6):1405–14.
9. Bach PB, Mirkin JN, Oliver TK, et al. Benefits and harms of CT screening for lung cancer: a systematic review. JAMA 2012;307(22):2418–29.
10. Institute of Medicine. Evolution of translational Omics: lessons learned and the path forward. In: Micheel CM, Nass S &, Omenn GS, editors. Washington (DC): National Academies Press; 2012.
11. Mazzone PJ, Sears CR, Arenberg DA, et al. Evaluating molecular biomarkers for the early detection of lung cancer: when is a biomarker ready for clinical use? An official American Thoracic Society Policy Statement. Am J Respir Crit Care Med 2017; 196(7):e15–29.
12. Moore HM, Kelly A, Jewell SD, et al. Biospecimen reporting for improved study quality. Biopreserv Biobank 2011;9(1):57–70.
13. Seijo LM, Peled N, Ajona D, et al. Biomarkers in lung cancer screening: achievements, promises, and challenges. J Thorac Oncol 2019;14(3):343–57.
14. Sandberg S, Fraser CG, Horvath AR, et al. Defining analytical performance specifications: consensus statement from the 1st strategic conference of the European Federation of Clinical Chemistry and Laboratory Medicine. Clin Chem Lab Med 2015;53(6):833–5.
15. Sturgeon CM, Hoffman BR, Chan DW, et al. National Academy of Clinical Biochemistry Laboratory medicine practice guidelines for use of tumor markers in clinical practice: quality requirements. Clin Chem 2008;54(8):e1–10.
16. Duffy MJ, Sturgeon CM, Soletormos G, et al. Validation of new cancer biomarkers: a position statement from the European group on tumor markers. Clin Chem 2015;61(6):809–20.

17. Cohen JF, Korevaar DA, Altman DG, et al. STARD 2015 guidelines for reporting diagnostic accuracy studies: explanation and elaboration. BMJ Open 2016;6(11):e012799.

18. Silvestri GA, Tanner NT, Kearney P, et al. Assessment of plasma proteomics biomarker's ability to distinguish benign from malignant lung nodules: results of the PANOPTIC (Pulmonary Nodule Plasma Proteomic Classifier) trial. Chest 2018;154(3): 491–500.

19. Pepe MS, Janes H, Li CI, et al. Early-phase studies of biomarkers: what target sensitivity and specificity values might confer clinical utility? Clin Chem 2016; 62(5):737–42.

20. Pinsky PF, Gierada DS, Black W, et al. Performance of lung-RADS in the national lung screening trial: a retrospective assessment. Ann Intern Med 2015; 162(7):485–91.

21. Pepe MS, Etzioni R, Feng Z, et al. Phases of biomarker development for early detection of cancer. J Natl Cancer Inst 2001;93:1054–61.

22. Russell LB, Gold MR, Siegel JE, et al, Medicine ftPoC-EiHa. The role of cost-effectiveness analysis in health and medicine. JAMA 1996;276:1172–7.

23. Siegel JE, Weinstein MC, Russell LB, et al, Medicine ftPoC-EiHa. Recommendations for reporting cost-effectiveness analyses. JAMA 1996;276: 1339–41.

24. Weinstein MC, Siegel JE, Gold MR, et al, Medicine ftPoC-EiHa. Recommendations of the panel on cost-effectiveness in health and medicine. JAMA 1996;276:1253–8.

25. World Health Organization, Baltussen RMPM, Adam T, et al. Making choices in health: WHO guide to cost-effectiveness analysis. In: Tan-Torres Edejer T, editor. Geneva (Switzerland): WHO; 2003.

26. Black WC, Gareen IF, Soneji SS, et al. Cost-effectiveness of CT screening in the national lung screening trial. N Engl J Med 2014;371(19):1793–802.

27. McMahon PM, Kong CY, Bouzan C, et al. Cost-effectiveness of computed tomography screening for lung cancer in the United States. J Thorac Oncol 2011;6(11):1841–8.

28. Villanti AC, Jiang Y, Abrams DB, et al. A cost-utility analysis of lung cancer screening and the additional benefits of incorporating smoking cessation interventions. PLoS One 2013;8(8):e71379.

29. Ten Haaf K, Jeon J, Tammemagi MC, et al. Risk prediction models for selection of lung cancer screening candidates: a retrospective validation study. PLoS Med 2017;14(4):e1002277.

30. Simard EP, Engels EA. Cancer as a cause of death among people with AIDS in the United States. Clin Infect Dis 2010;51(8):957–62.

31. Celik I, Gallicchio L, Boyd K, et al. Arsenic in drinking water and lung cancer: a systematic review. Environ Res 2008;108(1):48–55.

32. Lubin JH, Boice JD. Lung cancer risk from residential radon: meta-analysis of eight epidemiologic studies. J Natl Cancer Inst 1997;89:49–57.

33. Daniels CD, Jett JR. Does interstitial lung disease predispose to lung cancer? Curr Opin Pulm Med 2005;11:431–7.

34. Thorgeirsson TE, Geller F, Sulem P, et al. A variant associated with nicotine dependence, lung cancer and peripheral arterial disease. Nature 2008; 452(7187):638–42.

35. Moyer VA, Force USPT. Screening for lung cancer: U.S. Preventative services task force recommendation statement. Ann Intern Med 2014; 160(5):330–8.

36. De Koning H, Van Der Aalst C, Ten Haaf K, et al. PL02.05 Effects of volume CT lung cancer screening: mortality results of the NELSON randomized-controlled population based trial. J Thorac Oncol 2018;13(10):S185.

37. Wiener RS, Gould MK, Arenberg DA, et al. An official American Thoracic Society/American College of Chest Physicians policy statement: implementation of low-dose computed tomography lung cancer screening programs in clinical practice. Am J Respir Crit Care Med 2015;192(7):881–91.

38. Kovalchik SA, Tammemagi M, Berg CD, et al. Targeting of low-dose CT screening according to the risk of lung-cancer death. N Engl J Med 2013;369(3): 245–54.

39. Caverly TJ, Cao P, Hayward RA, et al. Identifying patients for whom lung cancer screening is preference-sensitive: a microsimulation study. Ann Intern Med 2018;169(1):1–9.

40. Katki HA, Kovalchik SA, Berg CD, et al. Development and validation of risk models to select ever-smokers for CT lung cancer screening. JAMA 2016;315(21):2300–11.

41. Gould MK, Tang T, Liu I-LA, et al. Recent trends in the identification of incidental pulmonary nodules. Am J Respir Crit Care Med 2015;192(10):1208–14.

42. Gould MK, Donington J, Lynch WR, et al. Evaluation of individuals with pulmonary nodules: when is it lung cancer? Diagnosis and management of lung cancer, 3rd ed: American College of Chest Physicians evidence-based clinical practice guidelines. Chest 2013;143(5 Suppl):e93S–120S.

43. Sawada S, Yamashita N, Sugimoto R, et al. Long-term outcomes of patients with ground-glass opacities detected using computed tomography. Chest 2017;151(2):308–15.

44. Henschke CI, Yankelevitz DF, Mirtcheva R, et al. CT screening for lung cancer: frequency and significance of part-solid and nonsolid nodules. Am J Roentgenol 2002;178:1053–7.

45. Nomori H, Watanabe K, Ohtsuka T, et al. Evaluation of F-18 fluorodeoxyglucose (FDG) PET scanning for pulmonary nodules less than 3 cm in diameter, with

special reference to the CT images. Lung Cancer 2004;45(1):19–27.

46. Tanner NT, Porter A, Gould MK, et al. Physician assessment of pretest probability of malignancy and adherence with guidelines for pulmonary nodule evaluation. Chest 2017;152(2):263–70.

47. Choi HK, Ghobrial M, Mazzone PJ. Models to estimate the probability of malignancy in patients with pulmonary nodules. Ann Am Thorac Soc 2018; 15(10):1117–26.

48. Ost DE, Gould MK. Decision making in patients with pulmonary nodules. Am J Respir Crit Care Med 2012;185(4):363–72.

49. Deppen S, Putnam JB Jr, Andrade G, et al. Accuracy of FDG-PET to diagnose lung cancer in a region of endemic granulomatous disease. Ann Thorac Surg 2011;92(2):428–32 [discussion: 433].

50. Cox JE, Chiles C, McManus CM, et al. Transthoracic needle aspiration biopsy: variables that affect risk of pneumothorax. Radiology 1999;212:165–8.

51. Mehta AC, Hood KL, Schwarz Y, et al. The evolutional history of electromagnetic navigation bronchoscopy: state of the art. Chest 2018;154(4): 935–47.

52. Shimada Y, Saji H, Kato Y, et al. The frequency and prognostic impact of pathological microscopic vascular invasion according to tumor size in non-small cell lung cancer. Chest 2016;149(3):775–85.

53. Burotto M, Thomas A, Subramaniam D, et al. Biomarkers in early-stage non-small-cell lung cancer: current concepts and future directions. J Thorac Oncol 2014;9(11):1609–17.

54. Hellmann MD, Ciuleanu T-E, Pluzanski A, et al. Nivolumab plus Ipilimumab in lung cancer with a high tumor mutational burden. N Engl J Med 2018;378(22): 2093–104.

55. Biton J, Ouakrim H, Dechartres A, et al. Impaired tumor-infiltrating T cells in patients with chronic obstructive pulmonary disease impact lung cancer response to PD-1 blockade. Am J Respir Crit Care Med 2018;198(7):928–40.

56. Pantel K, Speicher MR. The biology of circulating tumor cells. Oncogene 2016;35(10):1216–24.

57. Gorges TM, Penkalla N, Schalk T, et al. Enumeration and molecular characterization of tumor cells in lung cancer patients using a novel in vivo device for capturing circulating tumor cells. Clin Cancer Res 2016;22(9):2197–206.

58. Newman AM, Bratman SV, To J, et al. An ultrasensitive method for quantitating circulating tumor DNA with broad patient coverage. Nat Med 2014;20(5): 548–54.

59. Weiss G, Schlegel A, Kottwitz D, et al. Validation of the SHOX2/PTGER4 DNA methylation marker panel for plasma-based discrimination between patients with malignant and nonmalignant lung disease. J Thorac Oncol 2017;12(1):77–84.

60. Saarenheimo J, Eigeliene N, Andersen H, et al. The value of liquid biopsies for guiding therapy decisions in non-small cell lung cancer. Front Oncol 2019;9:129.

61. Sozzi G, Boeri M. Potential biomarkers for lung cancer screening. Transl Lung Cancer Res 2014;3(3): 139–48.

62. Jett JR, Peek LJ, Fredericks L, et al. Audit of the autoantibody test, EarlyCDT(R)-lung, in 1600 patients: an evaluation of its performance in routine clinical practice. Lung Cancer 2014;83(1):51–5.

63. Doseeva V, Colpitts T, Gao G, et al. Performance of a multiplexed dual analyte immunoassay for the early detection of non-small cell lung cancer. J Transl Med 2015;13:55.

64. Montani F, Marzi MJ, Dezi F, et al. miR-Test: a blood test for lung cancer early detection. J Natl Cancer Inst 2015;107(6):djv063.

65. Schmidt B, Liebenberg V, Dietrich D, et al. SHOX2 DNA methylation is a biomarker for the diagnosis of lung cancer based on bronchial aspirates. BMC Cancer 2010;10:600.

66. Silvestri GA, Vachani A, Whitney D, et al. A bronchial genomic classifier for the diagnostic evaluation of lung cancer. N Engl J Med 2015;373(3):243–51.

67. Kadara H, Wistuba II. Field cancerization in non-small cell lung cancer: implications in disease pathogenesis. Proc Am Thorac Soc 2012;9(2):38–42.

68. Aravanis AM, Lee M, Klausner RD. Next-generation sequencing of circulating tumor DNA for early cancer detection. Cell 2017;168(4):571–4.

69. Guo N, Lou F, Ma Y, et al. Circulating tumor DNA detection in lung cancer patients before and after surgery. Sci Rep 2016;6:33519.

70. Chorostowska-Wynimko J, Horváth I, Shitrit D, et al. P2.11-20 lung EpiCheck TM–results of the training and test sets of a methylation-based blood test for early detection of lung cancer. J Thorac Oncol 2018;13(10):S786.

71. Phallen J, Sausen M, Adleff V, et al. Direct detection of early-stage cancers using circulating tumor DNA. Sci Transl Med 2017;9:eaan2415.

72. Cohen JE, Li L, Wang Y, et al. Detection and localization of surgically resectable cancers with a multi-analyte blood test. Science 2018;359:926–30.

73. Calabrese F, Lunardi F, Pezzuto F, et al. Are there new biomarkers in tissue and liquid biopsies for the early detection of non-small cell lung cancer? J Clin Med 2019;8(3) [pii:E414].

74. Abbosh C, Birkbak NJ, Swanton C. Early stage NSCLC–challenges to implementing ctDNA-based screening and MRD detection. Nat Rev Clin Oncol 2018;15(9):577–86.

75. Mazzone PJ, Wang XF, Lim S, et al. Progress in the development of volatile exhaled breath signatures of lung cancer. Ann Am Thorac Soc 2015;12(5): 752–7.

76. Gillies RJ, Kinahan PE, Hricak H. Radiomics: images are more than pictures, they are data. Radiology 2016;278(2):563–77.

77. Liu Z, Wang S, Dong D, et al. The applications of radiomics in precision diagnosis and treatment of oncology: opportunities and challenges. Theranostics 2019;9(5):1303–22.

78. Ardila D, Kiraly AP, Bharadwaj S, et al. End-to-end lung cancer screening with three-dimensional deep learning on low-dose chest computed tomography. Nat Med 2019;25(6):954–61.

79. Fave X, Zhang L, Yang J, et al. Delta-radiomics features for the prediction of patient outcomes in non-small cell lung cancer. Sci Rep 2017;7(1):588.

80. Lee G, Lee HY, Park H, et al. Radiomics and its emerging role in lung cancer research, imaging biomarkers and clinical management: state of the art. Eur J Radiol 2017;86:297–307.

81. Liu L, Teng J, Zhang L, et al. The combination of the tumor markers suggests the histological diagnosis of lung cancer. Biomed Res Int 2017;2017:2013989.

82. Mazzone PJ, Wang XF, Han X, et al. Evaluation of a serum lung cancer biomarker panel. Biomark Insights 2018;13. 1177271917751608.

83. Ajona D, Okroj M, Pajares MJ, et al. Complement C4d-specific antibodies for the diagnosis of lung cancer. Oncotarget 2018;9(5):6346–55.

84. Yanaihara N, Caplen N, Bowman E, et al. Unique microRNA molecular profiles in lung cancer diagnosis and prognosis. Cancer Cell 2006;9(3):189–98.

85. Showe MK, Vachani A, Kossenkov AV, et al. Gene expression profiles in peripheral blood mononuclear cells can distinguish patients with non-small cell lung cancer from patients with nonmalignant lung disease. Cancer Res 2009; 69(24):9202–10.

86. Subramanian H, Viswanathan P, Cherkezyan L, et al. Procedures for risk-stratification of lung cancer using buccal nanocytology. Biomed Opt Express 2016;7(9):3795–810.

87. Patriquin L, Merrick DT, Hill D, et al. Early detection of lung cancer with meso Tetra (4-carboxyphenyl) porphyrin-labeled sputum. J Thorac Oncol 2015; 10(9):1311–8.

88. Xing L, Su J, Guarnera MA, et al. Sputum microRNA biomarkers for identifying lung cancer in indeterminate solitary pulmonary nodules. Clin Cancer Res 2015;21(2):484–9.

89. Zhang C, Yu W, Wang L, et al. DNA methylation analysis of the SHOX2 and RASSF1A panel in bronchoalveolar lavage fluid for lung cancer diagnosis. J Cancer 2017;8(17):3585–91.

90. Song G, Qin T, Liu H, et al. Quantitative breath analysis of volatile organic compounds of lung cancer patients. Lung Cancer 2010;67(2):227–31.

91. Westhoff M, Litterst P, Freitag L, et al. Ion mobility spectrometry for the detection of volatile organic compounds in exhaled breath of patients with lung cancer: results of a pilot study. Thorax 2009;64(9): 744–8.

92. Nolen BM, Lomakin A, Marrangoni A, et al. Urinary protein biomarkers in the early detection of lung cancer. Cancer Prev Res (Phila) 2015;8(2):111–9.

Bronchoscopic Diagnostic Procedures Available to the Pulmonologist

A. Cole Burks, MD*, Jason Akulian, MD, MPH

KEYWORDS

- Lung cancer • Bronchoscopy • Convex probe EBUS • Radial probe EBUS • EMN bronchoscopy
- Robotic bronchoscopy • Cone-beam CT • Augmented fluoroscopy

KEY POINTS

- Linear, convex probe endobronchial ultrasonography is highly sensitive and specific for diagnosis and staging of lymph node metastasis in lung cancer.
- Radial probe ultrasonography can provide proof of nodule localization but requires extensive knowledge of distal airway anatomy and computed tomography (CT)–anatomic correlation.
- Virtual bronchoscopic navigation, electromagnetic navigation bronchoscopy, and transthoracic needle aspiration improve correct airway selection and ability to find nodules, respectively, but do not provide real-time tools-to-target colocalization.
- Robotic bronchoscopy seeks to increase tool control and precision in the lung periphery but requires additional study of its effect on lung cancer diagnosis.
- Cone-beam CT and augmented fluoroscopy may provide improved imaging-based confirmation of location of bronchoscopy tools in relationship to the target nodule.

INTRODUCTION

Lung cancer (LC) remains the most lethal form of cancer in the United States, leading to a projected 155,870 deaths in 2017/2018, more than the next 3 most common causes of cancer death combined.[1] In addition to high mortality, the incidence of new LC cases remains high and is increasingly borne by women and nonsmokers. Despite improvements in thoracic imaging, the rate of false-positive and false-negative findings precludes their use as sole diagnostic modalities and instead aids in the risk stratification of those abnormal findings potentially in need of tissue confirmation.[2–7] Coupled with an aging population, this increase in significant comorbidities among patients at risk for LC and screen eligible patients and the need for advanced molecular/biomarker testing have led to advances in bronchoscopic technology geared toward the care of patients with known or suspected LC.[8,9]

As the tools evolve to include intrathoracic/extrathoracic perioperative imaging and virtual and/or visual endoluminal navigation, it is apparent that the data available to support the use of these technologies range from robust to absent. This article presents a brief overview of historical diagnostic bronchoscopy tools and focuses discussion on maturing and emerging technologies as well as the available data for their use.

FLEXIBLE BRONCHOSCOPY

The conventional flexible bronchoscope (FB) and its uses in LC diagnosis have been well described since its introduction in 1965 by Dr Shigeto Ikeda.

Section of Interventional Pulmonology, Division of Pulmonary and Critical Care Medicine, University of North Carolina at Chapel Hill, Burnett Womack Building, Room 8008, CB 7219, 160 Dental Circle, Chapel Hill, NC 27599, USA
* Corresponding author.
E-mail address: acole_burks@med.unc.edu

Clin Chest Med 41 (2020) 129–144
https://doi.org/10.1016/j.ccm.2019.11.002
0272-5231/20/© 2020 Elsevier Inc. All rights reserved.

Although the introduction of the FB constituted a major advancement in the care of patients with known or suspected LC, new challenges were quickly uncovered. These challenges included newly found biopsy targets outside the reach of FBs and inadequate evaluation of regional sites of metastasis. Attempts to overcome these challenges have included the introduction of transbronchial tools for biopsy and the use of monoplane fluoroscopy. Despite early reports of success, FBs have found limited use outside the central airways and in biopsy of large or diffuse peripheral lung lesions, with poor results when attempting diagnosis of lesions with the following characteristics: subsolid, less than 20 mm, lack of an air-bronchus sign on CT, and a lack of transbronchial needle aspiration (TBNA) use.[10–14]

CONVEX (LINEAR) PROBE ENDOBRONCHIAL ULTRASOUND–GUIDED TRANSBRONCHIAL NEEDLE ASPIRATION

Introduced in 2004, the endobronchial ultrasound (EBUS) transbronchial needle aspiration (TBNA) bronchoscope (**Fig. 1**) allows real-time, ultrasound-guided needle aspiration of mediastinal, hilar, and central lung lesions under either moderate conscious sedation or general anesthesia. Among the tools available to pulmonologists, the data associated with EBUS-TBNA are the most robust in terms of safety and efficacy when applied to the diagnosis and staging of LC.[7] These data show EBUS having equivalent sensitivity, specificity, and access to a wider array of lymph node stations to mediastinoscopy for LC diagnosis, and subsequently led to its recommendation as the first-line approach in the diagnosis and staging of suspected LC.[7,15–17]

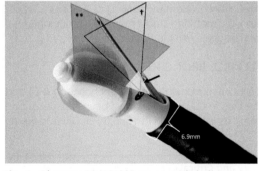

Fig. 1. Olympus BF-UC180F scope with balloon. Forward oblique viewing angle is 35° with 80° field of view (*dagger*). Ultrasound angular view is 50° (*double asterisks*). Needle exit angle is 20° (*yellow triangle with arrow*). (*Courtesy of* Olympus Medical, Tokyo, Japan.)

Advances in Endobronchial Ultrasound Bronchoscope Technology

Until recently there had been little change in EBUS bronchoscope technology aside from an increase in the working channel size from 2.0 to 2.2 mm. This situation seems to be changing with the introduction of a hybrid EBUS scope that offers a higher degree of flexion, narrower external diameter, larger ultrasound scanning angle (50°), and a 120° field of view at a 10° forward oblique viewing field compared with conventional EBUS (C-EBUS) bronchoscopes. These advances were shown in a randomized controlled trial comparing the H-EBUS scope with a C-EBUS scope, which found use of H-EBUS to be associated with improved visualization of airway segments and a significantly decreased need to convert to an FB during airway inspection.[18] Further advances seem on the horizon with the recent reports of a thin EBUS scope featuring a narrower outer diameter and improved flexion angle (170°) compared with C-EBUS. Publications in porcine and ex vivo human lung models reported an improved ability to insert the thin EBUS scope into deeper bronchi and upper lobe segments compared with C-EBUS.[19,20] Although these advances have not resulted in an improvement in TBNA diagnostic yield or specimen adequacy, studies evaluating how their reach may affect the sampling of targets unreachable by C-EBUS are needed.

Advances in Endobronchial Ultrasonography Sampling Tools

As EBUS-TBNA use has grown, a variety of needle sizes have been introduced (19–25 gauge). Multiple publications evaluating the effect of needle gauge on diagnostic yield and specimen adequacy have reported conflicting results, with most data suggesting little or no clinical difference.[21–25] In addition to diagnostic success, EBUS-TBNA has reproducibly shown a high degree of adequacy for LC subtyping and molecular/biomarker testing.[17,26,27] Despite this, a recommendation for a minimum number of passes needed for advanced molecular testing has not been established, nor have best methods/practices been determined for ensuring adequacy of EBUS-TBNA samples for performance of the entire compendium of testing now required from a single procedure (diagnosis, subtyping, staging, programmed death-ligand 1 (PDL-1) biomarker status, molecular markers, and/or next-generation sequencing [NGS]).

The perceived need for increasing quantities of tissue for advanced testing has led to exploration into new device concepts and designs. Biopsy needles adapted from the gastrointestinal (GI) endoscopy space with additional cutting edges are being introduced to the EBUS-TBNA market in hopes that they will allow improved specimen acquisition (**Fig. 2**). Current GI literature suggests that these fine-needle biopsy needles may provide higher diagnostic yields; better-quality samples for histology; and qualitative data not obtainable by fine-needle aspiration, such as tissue architecture, degree of differentiation, metastatic origin, and rate of proliferation.[28–30] In addition to new needle design, GI miniaturized forceps have been adapted for use in the lung (**Fig. 3**). Intranodal forceps biopsies (IFBs) are performed via passage of miniforceps into a target lymph node through a previously performed TBNA puncture site. Herth and colleagues[31] reported significant improvement in diagnostic yield in 75 patients compared with 19-gauge and 22-gauge TBNA needles (88% vs 49% vs 36%, respectively) in patients without high suspicion of LC; yield was highest in sarcoidosis (88% vs 35% for TBNA) and lymphoma (81% vs 35%). Chrissian and colleagues[32] prospectively evaluated IFB in 50 patients and reported a significant improvement in diagnostic yield when combining techniques (IFB and TBNA). Further study is needed to fully evaluate the benefit of these new needle designs and IFB with regard to the diagnosis and treatment of patients with known or suspected LCA.

APPROACHES TO SAMPLING PERIPHERAL PULMONARY LESIONS

The management of peripheral pulmonary nodules (PPNs) remains a challenging clinical situation. Publication of the National Lung Screening Trial reporting an associated reduction in LC mortality with application of chest low-dose CT (LDCT) screening in a high-risk population, the increasing rates of nodules (>4 mm and <30 mm) detected on chest CT scanning (up to 30.6% in 2012), and the subsequent US Preventive Services Task Force recommendation endorsing LDCT in at-risk populations has driven increased interest in this issue.[5,9,33]

Radial Probe Endobronchial Ultrasonography

Historically, fluoroscopy (monoplanar and/or biplanar) alone as a method of bronchoscope/tool guidance in the evaluation of PPNs has been largely abandoned because of poor

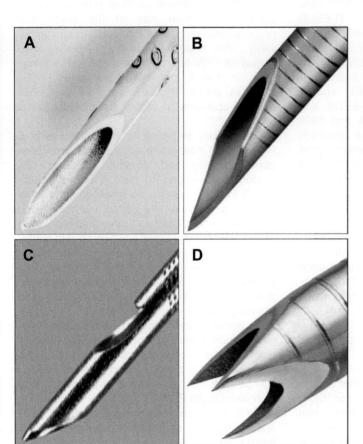

Fig. 2. Comparison of EBUS-TBNA needles. (*A, B*) Single-cutting-edge needles (*A*) Vizishot II, *Courtesy of* Olympus Medical, Tokyo, Japan; (*B*) Expect, *Courtesy of* Boston Scientific, Boston MA). (*C*) Reverse-bevel needle (Procore, Permission for use granted by Cook Medical, Bloomington, Indiana). (*D*) Multiple-cutting-edge needle (Acquire needle with Franseen tip geometry, *Courtesy of* Boston Scientific, Boston MA).

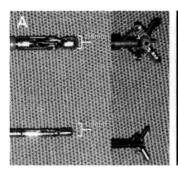
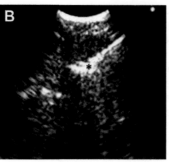

Fig. 3. Intranodal forceps biopsy tools. (*A*) Transbronchial biopsy forceps (*Top,* Radial Jaw 4, *Courtesy of* Boston Scientific, Boston MA), Intranodal biopsy forceps (*Bottom,* CoreDx, *Courtesy of* Boston Scientific, Boston MA). (*B*) EBUS image of intranodal biopsy forceps open within lymph node (*asterisk*). *Courtesy of* Boston Scientific, Boston MA.

localization and diagnostic rates, particularly with decreasing target size and/or location in the outer one-third of the lung. Introduced in the 1990s, radial probe EBUS (R-EBUS) was first used to assess tracheobronchial wall integrity and mediastinal adenopathy.[34] Since then, R-EBUS has been adapted for the evaluation of PPN because its radial side-scanning properties are able to produce a high-resolution 360° ultrasonography image of the surrounding lung parenchyma. Since 2002, use of R-EBUS (plus or minus guide sheath [GS] and/or ultrathin bronchoscope [UTB]) to evaluate and diagnose PPN has reported diagnostic yield ranging from 58% to 85%.[35–40] Comparative trials of R-EBUS (plus or minus GS) and electromagnetic navigation bronchoscopy (ENB) reported comparable diagnostic yields of 69% and 63% respectively.[41,42] A later study by Eberhardt and colleagues[43] evaluated R-EBUS, ENB, and a combination of the two. Alone, R-EBUS and ENB had diagnostic yields of 69% and 59% respectively; however, the combined approach significantly improved the diagnostic yield (88%). Subsequent meta-analyses of R-EBUS have reported diagnostic yields ranging from 56.3% to 60.9% for lesions smaller than 20 mm versus 77.7% to 82.5% for lesions larger than 20 mm.[44,45] The American College of Chest Physicians' (ACCP) AQuIRE (ACCP Quality Improvement Registry, Evaluation, and Education) registry, a retrospective multi-center evaluation of peripheral bronchoscopy, confirmed incremental improvement of diagnostic yield when combining R-EBUS with ENB (38.5% for ENB alone vs 47.1% with ENB plus R-EBUS). However, these results revealed diagnostic yields significantly lower than previously reported, which may be explained by the elimination of biases previously associated with earlier single-center retrospective studies.[13] Most recently, a multicenter, prospective, randomized trial comparing PPN biopsy using FB plus fluoroscopy or R-EBUS plus UTB found R-EBUS to be

associated with a significantly higher diagnostic yield of 49% compared with 37% with FB. Of note, this study did not include the use of peripheral TBNA, which may have contributed to the lower than previously reported yields.[46]

When considering use of R-EBUS for PPN sampling, factors that have been shown to significantly affect PPN visualization and diagnostic yield include lesion size, presence of bronchus sign, distance from the hilum, lobar distribution, the presence of malignancy, and positioning of the probe in relation to the lesion (eccentric vs within /concentric) (**Fig. 4**).[47–50] Of these, the characteristics most reproducibly reported have been size of the lesion and probe positioning within the lesion (a concentric view). With regard to safety, R-EBUS–guided biopsy of PPN has been reported to be favorable. In the 2 previously mentioned meta-analyses, pneumothorax rates of 1% and 1.5% and no episodes of significant bleeding were reported.[44,45]

The primary limitation to the applicability of R-EBUS has been its reliance on the bronchoscopist's ability and comfort in using CT-anatomic correlation to pilot a bronchoscope and R-EBUS probe to the intended PPN while navigating increasingly small airways and numerous branch points, often without direct visualization.[51] The other most prominent limitation of R-EBUS involves the ultrasound image and the reflective properties of the lung. Although solid PPNs create a well-demarcated interface between themselves and normally aerated lung parenchyma, ground-glass nodules return poor or no ultrasound signals, which leads to poor representations of these lesions during localization. Despite these limitations, the reported pooled diagnostic yields comparable with other forms of peripheral lung navigation make R-EBUS–guided bronchoscopy, alone or in combination with an additional guidance modality, an attractive option to PPN biopsy.

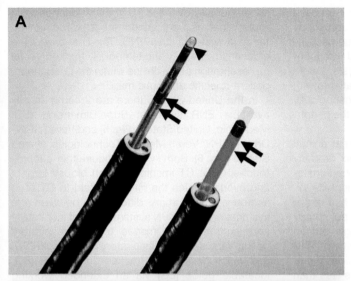

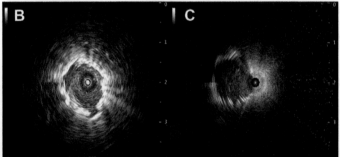

Fig. 4. (*A*) Radial probe EBUS (*arrowhead*) within guide sheath (*double arrows*). (*B*) Radial EBUS image within nodule, concentric view. (*C*) Radial EBUS image adjacent to nodule, eccentric view. (*Courtesy of* Olympus Medical, Tokyo, Japan.)

Virtual Navigation Bronchoscopy

Virtual airway reconstruction software/platforms for navigation bronchoscopy provide pre- and peri-procedural guidance for the bronchoscopist by assisting in plotting an appropriate course through the bronchial tree to the target lesion. Pre-procedural CT scanning is required, with specific requirements for scan resolution and image thickness per manufacturer guidelines. After uploading CT data to the virtual navigation bronchoscopy (VNB) platform, a three-dimensional (3D) bronchial tree and roadmap is created. During procedural planning, the target, or region of interest (ROI), is identified and software provides a virtual roadmap of the bronchial tree, providing a potential bronchus-by-bronchus route access to the ROI. Multiple different views are often available, including views of the vascular tree, virtual fluoroscopy, and the ability to rotate an ROI in almost any plane or direction. These software platforms are available as stand-alone platforms or in conjunction with tracked navigation systems. The term VNB is used here to refer to those stand-alone systems. Intraprocedural VNB requires an additional operator to advance through the planned virtual route (akin to a navigator providing map-based directions to a driver), but has shown improvement in appropriate pathway selection in a simulated patient setting.[52]

The Bf-NAVI system (not available in the United States; Olympus, Tokyo, Japan) and the Lung-Point system (Broncus, Mountain View, CA) are the two VNB systems available that have been studied in humans, with varied data regarding their efficacy. Of the 2 systems, the Bf-NAVI has a more extensive dataset in human patients, including 2 randomized trials in patients undergoing bronchoscopy for PPNs. The initial feasibility study of the Bf-NAVI VNB system suggested good success. Subsequent trials, including a prospective Bf-NAVI trial, identified no improvement in diagnostic yield when comparing R-EBUS alone with R-EBUS with VNB in PPNs.[53] This trial was followed by a large randomized trial using the same comparison, which reported a significant increase in diagnostic yield for both malignant and nonmalignant diseases in the combined technique arm.[54]

In contrast, another large, randomized controlled trial (n = 334) compared VNB with fluoroscopy versus standard bronchoscopy with fluoroscopy. No overall difference in diagnostic yield was identified; however, in subgroup analysis, there seemed to be some improvement in patients with lesions in the right upper lobe, fluoroscopically invisible lesions, and lesions located in the peripheral one-third of the lung field.[55]

LungPoint VNB has several preclinical animal studies suggesting improved ability to properly select bronchial pathways and locate phantom lesions.[52,56] Limitations of these studies include the use of a 24-mm ROI lesions and that half of the participating bronchoscopists were pulmonary fellow trainees.[52,56] The system's single human study (n = 25) was a pilot feasibility study of VNB use in a patient cohort with 18F-fluorodeoxyglucose–avid peripheral pulmonary lesions less than 42 mm (mean size, 28 mm) assessing sensitivity, specificity, and overall accuracy of the system. Using VNB and an ultrathin bronchoscope, more than 50% of the lesions were directly visualized and the reported overall diagnostic yield was 80% (all patients with a directly visualized lesion obtained a diagnosis).[57] In addition, a recent meta-analysis of peripheral lung biopsy has suggested an overall diagnostic yield of 72% when using VNB.[45]

In addition, the use of VNB seems to offer no advantage compared with standard fluoroscopy for bronchoscopists with advanced training.[55] However, VNB may offer improvements with regard to bronchoscopy training or bronchoscopists with less experience. Anecdotally, the primary drawback to using VNB technology is its lack of instrument tracking in space and time. This lack of real-time guidance was shown in a porcine model of VNB. The wedging of the bronchoscope near an ROI was associated with significant anatomic displacement, and "the wedging maneuver could pose a substantive problem as one could risk that no part of the tumor is within the preoperative CT image location."[58]

These limitations have resulted in the limited adoption of VNB for peripheral bronchoscopy, whereas ENB has grown in use. Further study of VNB is required alone or in combination of other advanced diagnostic procedures, although it seems that bronchoscopy has moved on in other directions.

Electromagnetic Navigation Bronchoscopy

ENB uses the creation of a magnetic field around the patient to detect spatially tracked devices to display device position within the magnetic field superimposed over the 3D virtual bronchoscopic route; that is, an integrated electromagnetic tracking system within VNB. The final product is a dynamic, spatially and temporally tracked virtual representation of the device within the preplanned, patient-specific anatomic map.

In the United States, there are 2 commercially available ENB systems: SuperDimension (SD; Medtronic, United States) (**Fig. 5**) and Veran SPiN-Drive (VSPN; Veran Medical Technologies, United States) (**Fig. 6**). Both systems require thin-cut protocol-specific CT imaging to plan biopsy targets and overlay/match the magnetic field to CT scan anatomy. The primary differences between the systems are the VSPN system's use of inspiratory and expiratory CT images to add respiratory gating versus a static inspiratory breath hold (SD) and which devices are tracked during ENB (SD, locatable guide [LG] via an extended working channel [EWC]; VSPN, tip-tracked biopsy instruments). The SD LG is similar to a probe that passes through the EWC, which requires a minimum FB working channel size of 2.6 mm. The EWC comes in various angles (45°, 90°, 180°), offers steerability during navigation, and remains in place after the LG is removed. Standard PPN biopsy instruments are then used to sample the lesion in question and/or R-EBUS is used for real-time confirmation of the target lesion. Although the VSPN system has recently introduced its own version of an LG/EWC combination, the platform is primarily predicated on the use of always-on tipped track biopsy instruments (forceps, brush, and needle) allowing continuous direct navigation of the biopsy instrument. Both platforms use similar planning systems and computer software to generate four-dimensional (4D) reconstructions of the patient's chest CT and allowing PPN targeting and pathway building.

A plethora of studies have sought to define the clinical effectiveness of ENB in PPN sampling, and reported diagnostic yields have ranged from 39% to 94%.[13,59] Two meta-analyses have been done on ENB for PPN, both of which included many studies of poor methodologic quality. Gex and colleagues[60] found the pooled diagnostic yield of ENB to be 64.9% (95% confidence interval [CI], 59.2–70.3) and a negative predictive value of 52.1% (95% CI, 43.5–60.6), whereas Zhang and colleagues[59] reported the pooled sensitivity, specificity, and positive and negative likelihood ratios to be 82%, 100%, 19.36, and 0.23 respectively, indicating a prohibitively high false-negative rate when attempting to rule out malignant disease. The largest prospective randomized controlled trial with 3 arms comparing ENB, R-EBUS, and combined ENB with R-EBUS found similar results for

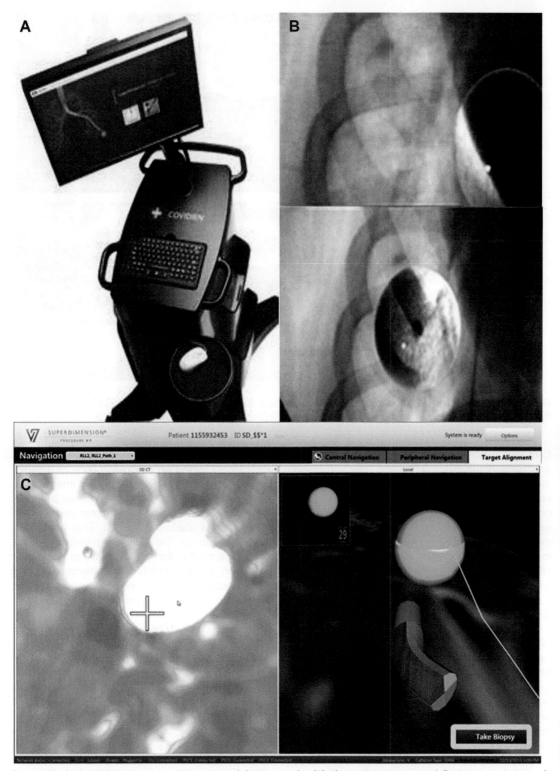

Fig. 5. SD electromagnetic navigation system. (*A*) SD console. (*B*) FluoroNav augmented fluoroscopic image of nodule. (*C*) Screenshot of navigation via the SD software. (*Courtesy of* Medtronic, Dublin, Ireland.)

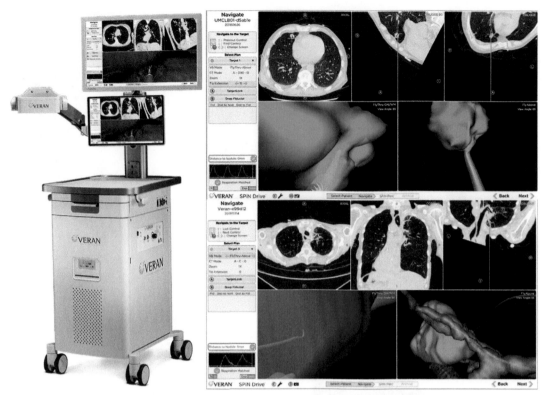

Fig. 6. Veran SpinDrive electromagnetic navigation system console with screenshot of navigation software. (*Courtesy of* Veran Medical, St. Louis, MO.)

ENB and R-EBUS with diagnostic yields of 59% and 69% respectively. However, the combined technology arm had a significant increase in diagnostic yield (88%) compared with either R-EBUS or ENB alone.[43] To date, there have been no multicenter prospective trials of ENB published; however, one such study using the VSPN platform is in active enrollment (ClinicalTrials.gov ID NCT03338049). ENB has a comparable risk profile with that of PPN biopsy using a standard FB and is superior to CT needle biopsy with regard to incidence of pneumothorax.[59–62]

Several factors have been identified that may positively influence ENB yield: (1) PPN location in the upper or middle lobe, (2) presence of a bronchus sign on CT imaging, (3) combined use of radial EBUS, (4) catheter suctioning as a sampling technique, (5) lower registration error, (6) deep sedation, and (7) large PPN size.[60,63] Of note, nodule size has been a consistent determinant of biopsy success, with a significant decrement in diagnostic yield reproducibility seen in PPNs less than 20 mm.[45,64,65]

Each ENB system also offers a unique differentiating approach to PPN biopsy. The SD system has recently introduced the Fluoroscopic Navigation software, which enables periprocedural

reregistration of the tracked LG in relation to the PPN target based on reconstructions of a series of two-dimensional (2D) fluoroscopy images processed into a pseudo-3D image (similar to tomosynthesis) that is then back-integrated on the original preprocedure CT scan. This extra step seeks to reduce the CT image-to-body divergence, account for scope-induced anatomic distortion, and improve final tool alignment during PPN biopsy. Each image obtained as part of the fluoroscopic C-arm scan requires approximately 30 seconds of scan time and the associated radiation exposure. There are currently no data regarding the efficacy of the addition of fluoroscopy navigation in clinical use. The VSPN platform offers electromagnetic-guided transthoracic needle aspiration (EM-TTNA; SPiNPerc, Veran Medical, St Louis, MO) using a tracked needle stylet similar to CT-guided needle biopsy (**Fig. 7**). Unlike CT needle biopsy, the images are not in real time; the system uses the preprocedural CT scan to offer the user navigation assistance for skin insertion and needle alignment before and while advancing toward the target lesion. This technique allows bronchoscopists to perform EBUS-TBNA, ENB, and EM-TTNA in the same procedure, as appropriate. Two published studies of EM-TTNA

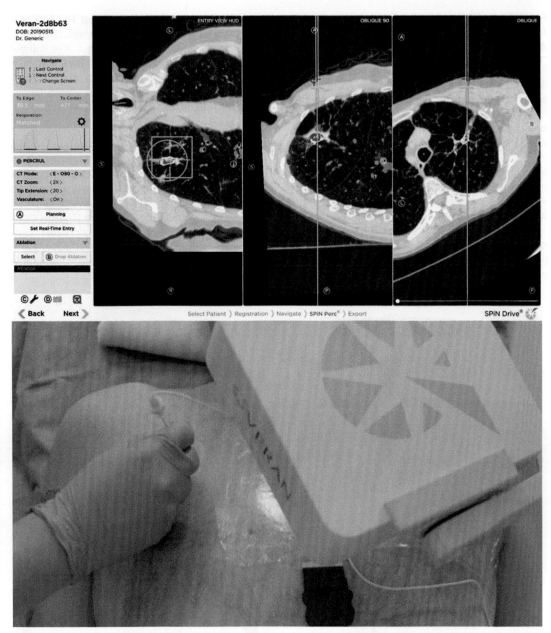

Fig. 7. Veran SpinPerc electromagnetic-guided transthoracic needle biopsy. (*Courtesy of* Veran Medical, St. Louis, MO.)

have reported diagnostic yields ranging between 73% and 83% and pneumothorax rates similar to those reported in the CT-guided biopsy literature.[66,67] However, EM-TTNA is currently limited to anteriorly located lesions, because repositioning the patient introduces the possibility for increased CT-body divergence.

Although both technologies are impressive in their engineering and concept, there remain limited high-quality data on their performance and both seem to be limited by a lack of real-time confirmation during the biopsy maneuver. This situation is concerning, because of the difficulty with assessing strengths and limitations of different systems as well as when and/or how to best apply ENB. Further investigations of these technologies are needed, specifically multicenter prospective singular and comparative trials. In addition, there are no studies directly comparing nonbronchoscopic biopsy modalities such as CT-guided needle biopsy with ENB.

EMERGING TECHNOLOGIES
Bronchoscopic Transparenchymal Nodule Access

Bronchoscopic transparenchymal nodule access (BTPNA; Archimedes, Broncus, San Jose, CA) is a technology that is meant to allow biopsy of peripheral nodules not accessible through traditional bronchoscopy. The principle behind BTPNA is navigation software generation of a 4D map including both airways and pulmonary vasculature. Following this, a path is generated that includes an airway exit point and a computer-enhanced fluoroscopic interface to allow transparenchymal guidance to the target (**Fig. 8**).

In a pilot study of BTPNA on canine models, 10 canines underwent the procedure (44 tunnels) with no reports of pneumothorax.[68] A study by Herth and colleagues[69] of BTPNA in 12 patients followed immediately by resection found that 10 of 12 procedures were successful in achieving a diagnosis, the resected specimens were intact and without laceration or significant signs of bleeding, and there were no adverse events reported. A multicenter prospective trial of BTPNA (ClinicalTrials.gov ID NCT02867371) is currently ongoing.

Augmented Fluoroscopy

Augmented fluoroscopy (LungVision, Body Vision Medical Ltd, Israel) uses a software platform that overlays a computer-derived airway pathway to target lesions planned from preprocedural CT scan images onto an intraoperative C-arm–based fluoroscopy image. This technology creates a virtual, visible nodule on fluoroscopy to allow intraprocedural tracking of a proprietary, steerable biopsy tool in relation to the target lesion. The

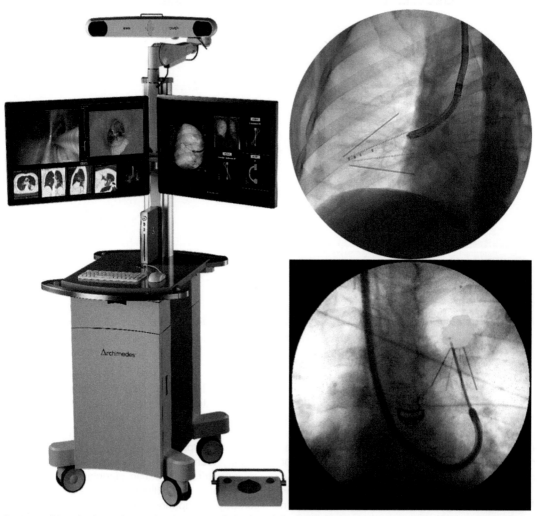

Fig. 8. Archimedes bronchoscopic transparenchymal nodule access system. (*Courtesy of* Broncus Medical, San Jose, CA.)

data on this technology currently exist only in abstract form, with reported localization success (defined as R-EBUS confirmation or definitive diagnosis) of 86%, and a diagnostic yield of 78%. Although this technology may be an improvement on conventional fluoroscopy, its reliance on a virtual projection of the target nodule onto real-time fluoroscopic imaging is concerning for the potential to introduce image-body divergence. Continued study is needed to more fully understand the potential of this technology.

Robotic Bronchoscopy

Two robotic bronchoscopy platforms Monarch (MA; Auris Health, Redwood City, CA) and Ion Endoluminal Platform (IEP; Intuitive, Sunnyvale, CA) have recently become commercially available for use in the diagnosis of PPN. Given their novelty, this article describes in as much detail as possible the technology similarities and differences as well as the limited data currently available regarding their clinical performance.

The MA platform (**Fig. 9**) is composed of 2 distinct pieces: the robotic bronchoscope and the navigation software platform. The robotic bronchoscope is made up of 2 independently articulating robotic scopes nested within one another. The outer scope has a 5.9-mm outer diameter and is responsible for directing the inner scope into a lobar or segmental bronchus. The second or inner scope has an outer diameter of 4.2 mm, 2.0-mm working channel, light source, and camera. The arms can be controlled simultaneously or independently with a remote control modeled after popular console video-gaming systems. Endobronchial navigation is provided by a combination of ENB, scope lengthening, and carina/orifice registration. Under ENB guidance, based on thin-cut CT images, the outer sheath (with the inner scope withdrawn to its distal tip) is steered to and locked into position at the smallest accessible bronchus on the computer-generated route. At this point, the inner scope is advanced and driven distally along the route and subsequently locked into position as proximal to the lesion as the anatomy-scope relationship allows. Fine adjustments to the trajectory of the tools advanced through the working channel can then be made. Bronchoalveolar lavage, brushings, forceps biopsies, and needle aspirations can all be performed through the working channel of the

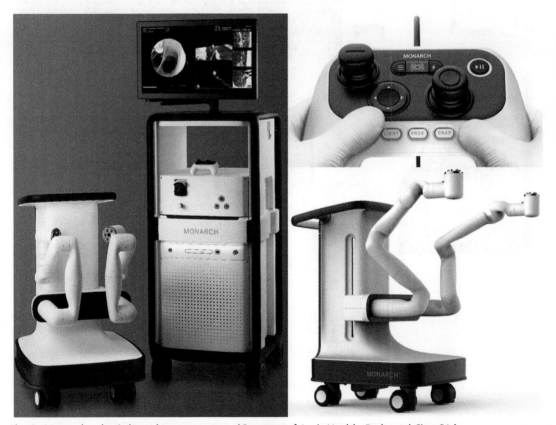

Fig. 9. Monarch robotic bronchoscopy system. (*Courtesy of* Auris Health, Redwood City, CA.)

scope. The proof-of-concept study of the ability to drive the scope more distally than conventional bronchoscopy, hypothetically because of the mechanical advantage of a nested scope-in-scope design, showed an ability to pass the inner scope a mean difference of 3.5 to 4.5 bronchi generations more distal than conventional bronchoscopy with a 4.2-mm bronchoscope (P-190, Olympus, Tokyo, Japan).[70] A feasibility study of using the MA platform for lung biopsy in 15 patients at a single institution reported successful biopsy attempts in 93%, and an overall diagnostic yield reported to be 93.3% (9 out of 15 malignant, 5 out of 15 benign features).[71]

The IEP (Fig. 10) is a single 3.5-mm outer diameter fully articulating scope controlled by a single robotic arm. The tip is capable of 180° movement in all planes and directions and visualization is achieved via a video camera passed through the catheter during the navigation phase of the procedure. Navigation of the IEP is not ENB based; the scope is guided by the novel application of a fiber-optic–based position-sensing technology that continuously monitors the entire length and shape of the catheter. This information is overlaid on proprietary virtual bronchoscopic software, creating a pathway based on thin-cut CT scan images. The IEP-user interface is a track ball for directional aiming and a wheel to advance or retract the scope. The scope is designed to automatically lock into place when the user is not in contract with the controls via a touch capacitance interaction. On arrival at the biopsy target, the camera is removed and replaced with biopsy tools deployed down the same working channel. A proprietary flexible needle has been developed by the

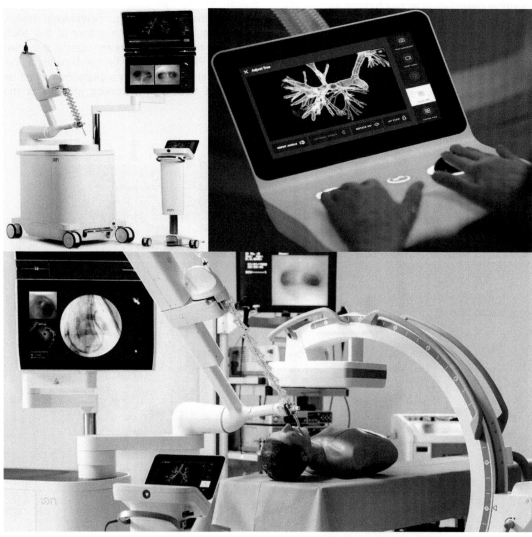

Fig. 10. Ion endoluminal robotic platform. (*Courtesy of* Intuitive Medical, Sunnyvale, CA.)

manufacturer with an emphasis on easy passage and the ability to negotiate tight-radius bends. Both platforms are cross-compatible with existing fluoroscopy and R-EBUS technologies, with the ability to incorporate those external images into 1 integrated user heads-up display. At the time of this publication, there are no published data on the use of the Ion platform in humans or otherwise.

Cone-beam Computed Tomography

As with global positioning systems (GPSs), one limitation to guided bronchoscopy is that navigation is based on a virtual (not real-time) map, resulting in an inability to account for changes to the target or map that may have occurred since the CT data were obtained. In addition, none of the systems currently used (or proposed) for peripheral lung navigation have the ability to provide real-time confirmation of target-to-tool colocalization. As such, intraprocedural imaging and bronchoscopists have begun to develop/apply a new technology in cone-beam CT to provide real-time target to tool colocalization.

Cone-beam CT (CBCT) is an advanced imaging modality using a round or rectangular cone-shaped beam of electrons to create a single 200° (180° plus fan/cone angle) scan in which the area detector and x-ray source rotate simultaneously around the patient to generate volumetric imaging.[72] The cone-shaped x-ray beam eliminates the need for the patient to be physically moved through the beam to obtain the images. It provides nearly 10 times less radiation exposure (~ 1 mSv) compared with conventional CT scans and has been adapted for use with a C-arm, providing standard 2D fluoroscopy-like images as well as CT-like multidimensional imaging.[73,74] The data regarding the use of CBCT during bronchoscopy are limited. In a prospective study (n = 33), Hohenforst-Schmidt and colleagues[75] described a diagnostic yield during peripheral nodule biopsy while using CBCT of 70% (mean diameter of 15 ± 3 mm). This finding was subsequently supported by Park and colleagues[76] in a retrospective study of 59 patients with an average lesion diameter of 3.1 ± 1.0 cm, which reported a diagnostic yield of 71.2%. Another, much smaller study (n = 14) evaluated the use of CBCT with ENB for lesions without a bronchus sign and reported an overall diagnostic yield of 71%.[77] Larger, higher-quality studies are needed to fully evaluate the potential impact of CBCT in the acquisition of diagnostic material during peripheral bronchoscopy.

Although early work with CBCT is encouraging, particularly given its potential to provide confirmation of biopsy target-to-tool colocalization, there are potential limitations that may prevent its widespread adoption. Currently available CBCT systems require dedicated rooms in which to operate, which may result in both increased cost and space prohibition at many institutions. Although many institutions currently use CBCT for the treatment and diagnosis of a spectrum of malignancies, this too creates an economy of time, which many pulmonologists may find themselves lacking. In addition, the workflow, increase in procedural time, and radiation exposure (to both patient and proceduralist) required for incorporation of CBCT into the bronchoscopy space must be taken into account.

SUMMARY

Just as humans have advanced in their ability to navigate into the unknown with various skills and technological advances, so have significant technological skills and tools been developed to aid pulmonologists in the diagnosis of LC. With advances in the care of patients with known or suspected cancer, the targets of interest are increasingly becoming smaller and are in remote locations requiring advanced techniques not only to reach but to biopsy meaningfully. The ability to reach these small PPNs in a minimally invasive fashion via bronchoscopy continues to improve; however, the goal of greater than 90% diagnostic yield remains unrealized. With this in mind, technology continues to progress at an ever-increasing pace, making the future of advanced diagnostic bronchoscopy an exciting destination.

DISCLOSURE

Dr Burks has no financial relationships with any commercial companies related to the subject matter or materials discussed within this article. Dr Akulian has received consulting fees, honoraria, and/or grant funding from Veran Medical, Medtronic, Becton Dickinson, Boston Scientific, Intuitive Surgical, FujiFilm and Cook Medical.

REFERENCES

1. Siegel RL, Miller KD, Jemal A. Cancer statistics, 2017. CA Cancer J Clin 2017;67(1):7–30.
2. Ambrose J. CT scanning: a backward look. Semin Roentgenol 1977;12(1):7–11.
3. Schellinger D, Di Chiro G, Axelbaum SP, et al. Early clinical experience with the ACTA scanner. Radiology 1975;114(2):257–61.
4. Henschke CI, McCauley DI, Yankelevitz DF, et al. Early Lung Cancer Action Project: overall design and findings from baseline screening. Lancet 1999;354(9173):99–105.

5. National Lung Screening Trial Research Team, Aberle DR, Adams AM, et al. Reduced lung-cancer mortality with low-dose computed tomographic screening. N Engl J Med 2011;365(5): 395–409.

6. van Tinteren H, Hoekstra OS, Smit EF, et al. Effectiveness of positron emission tomography in the preoperative assessment of patients with suspected non-small-cell lung cancer: the PLUS multicentre randomised trial. Lancet 2002;359(9315):1388–93.

7. Silvestri GA, Gonzalez AV, Jantz MA, et al. Methods for staging non-small cell lung cancer: diagnosis and management of lung cancer, 3rd ed: American College of Chest Physicians evidence-based clinical practice guidelines. Chest 2013;143(5 Suppl): e211S–50S.

8. Rivera MP, Tanner NT, Silvestri GA, et al. Incorporating coexisting chronic illness into decisions about patient selection for lung cancer screening. An Official American Thoracic Society Research Statement. Am J Respir Crit Care Med 2018;198(2):e3–13.

9. Gould MK, Tang T, Liu IL, et al. Recent trends in the identification of incidental pulmonary nodules. Am J Respir Crit Care Med 2015;192(10):1208–14.

10. Rivera MP, Mehta AC, Wahidi MM. Establishing the diagnosis of lung cancer: diagnosis and management of lung cancer, 3rd ed: American College of Chest Physicians evidence-based clinical practice guidelines. Chest 2013;143(5 Suppl):e142S–65S.

11. Baaklini WA, Reinoso MA, Gorin AB, et al. Diagnostic yield of fiberoptic bronchoscopy in evaluating solitary pulmonary nodules. Chest 2000;117(4): 1049–54.

12. Shure D, Fedullo PF. Transbronchial needle aspiration of peripheral masses. Am Rev Respir Dis 1983;128(6):1090–2.

13. Ost DE, Ernst A, Lei X, et al. Diagnostic yield and complications of bronchoscopy for peripheral lung lesions. results of the AQuIRE registry. Am J Respir Crit Care Med 2016;193(1):68–77.

14. Okachi S, Imai N, Imaizumi K, et al. Factors affecting the diagnostic yield of transbronchial biopsy using endobronchial ultrasonography with a guide sheath in peripheral lung cancer. Intern Med 2016;55(13): 1705–12.

15. Herth FJ, Eberhardt R, Krasnik M, et al. Endobronchial ultrasound-guided transbronchial needle aspiration of lymph nodes in the radiologically and positron emission tomography-normal mediastinum in patients with lung cancer. Chest 2008;133(4): 887–91.

16. Yasufuku K, Pierre A, Darling G, et al. A prospective controlled trial of endobronchial ultrasound-guided transbronchial needle aspiration compared with mediastinoscopy for mediastinal lymph node staging of lung cancer. J Thorac Cardiovasc Surg 2011;142(6): 1393–400.e1.

17. Rooper LM, Nikolskaia O, Carter J, et al. A single EBUS-TBNA procedure can support a large panel of immunohistochemical stains, specific diagnostic subtyping, and multiple gene analyses in the majority of non-small cell lung cancer cases. Hum Pathol 2016;51:139–45.

18. Yarmus L, Akulian J, Ortiz R, et al. A randomized controlled trial evaluating airway inspection effectiveness during endobronchial ultrasound bronchoscopy. J Thorac Dis 2015;7(10):1825–32.

19. Patel P, Wada H, Hu HP, et al. First evaluation of the new thin convex probe endobronchial ultrasound scope: a human ex vivo lung study. Ann Thorac Surg 2017;103(4):1158–64.

20. Wada H, Hirohashi K, Nakajima T, et al. Assessment of the new thin convex probe endobronchial ultrasound bronchoscope and the dedicated aspiration needle: a preliminary study in the porcine lung. J Bronchology Interv Pulmonol 2015;22(1):20–7.

21. Chaddha U, Ronaghi R, Elatre W, et al. Comparison of sample adequacy and diagnostic yield of 19- and 22-G EBUS-TBNA needles. J Bronchology Interv Pulmonol 2018;25(4):264–8.

22. Pickering EM, Holden VK, Heath JE, et al. Tissue acquisition during EBUS-TBNA: comparison of cell blocks obtained from a 19G versus 21G needle. J Bronchology Interv Pulmonol 2019;26(4):237–44.

23. Yarmus LB, Akulian J, Lechtzin N, et al. Comparison of 21-gauge and 22-gauge aspiration needle in endobronchial ultrasound-guided transbronchial needle aspiration: results of the American College of Chest Physicians Quality Improvement Registry, Education, and Evaluation Registry. Chest 2013;143(4): 1036–43.

24. Oki M, Saka H, Kitagawa C, et al. Randomized study of 21-gauge versus 22-gauge endobronchial ultrasound-guided transbronchial needle aspiration needles for sampling histology specimens. J Bronchology Interv Pulmonol 2011;18(4):306–10.

25. Nakajima T, Yasufuku K, Takahashi R, et al. Comparison of 21-gauge and 22-gauge aspiration needle during endobronchial ultrasound-guided transbronchial needle aspiration. Respirology 2011;16(1): 90–4.

26. Yarmus L, Akulian J, Gilbert C, et al. Optimizing endobronchial ultrasound for molecular analysis. How many passes are needed? Ann Am Thorac Soc 2013;10(6):636–43.

27. Labarca G, Folch E, Jantz M, et al. Adequacy of samples obtained by endobronchial ultrasound with transbronchial needle aspiration for molecular analysis in patients with non-small cell lung cancer. Systematic review and meta-analysis. Ann Am Thorac Soc 2018;15(10):1205–16.

28. Rodrigues-Pinto E, Jalaj S, Grimm IS, et al. Impact of EUS-guided fine-needle biopsy sampling with a new core needle on the need for onsite cytopathologic

assessment: a preliminary study. Gastrointest Endosc 2016;84(6):1040–6.

29. Kandel P, Tranesh G, Nassar A, et al. EUS-guided fine needle biopsy sampling using a novel fork-tip needle: a case-control study. Gastrointest Endosc 2016;84(6):1034–9.

30. Khoury T, Sbeit W, Ludvik N, et al. Concise review on the comparative efficacy of endoscopic ultrasound-guided fine-needle aspiration vs core biopsy in pancreatic masses, upper and lower gastrointestinal submucosal tumors. World J Gastrointest Endosc 2018;10(10):267–73.

31. Herth FJ, Morgan RK, Eberhardt R, et al. Endobronchial ultrasound-guided miniforceps biopsy in the biopsy of subcarinal masses in patients with low likelihood of non-small cell lung cancer. Ann Thorac Surg 2008;85(6):1874–8.

32. Chrissian A, Misselhorn D, Chen A. Endobronchial-ultrasound guided miniforceps biopsy of mediastinal and hilar lesions. Ann Thorac Surg 2011;92(1):284–8.

33. Final recommendation statement: lung cancer: screening. 2013. Available at: https://www.uspreventiveservicestaskforce.org/Page/Document/RecommendationStatementFinal/lung-cancer-screening. Accessed July 1, 2019.

34. Hurter T, Hanrath P. Endobronchial sonography in the diagnosis of pulmonary and mediastinal tumors. Dtsch Med Wochenschr 1990;115(50):1899–905 [in German].

35. Herth FJ, Ernst A, Becker HD. Endobronchial ultrasound-guided transbronchial lung biopsy in solitary pulmonary nodules and peripheral lesions. Eur Respir J 2002;20(4):972–4.

36. Shirakawa T, Imamura F, Hamamoto J, et al. Usefulness of endobronchial ultrasonography for transbronchial lung biopsies of peripheral lung lesions. Respiration 2004;71(3):260–8.

37. Yang MC, Liu WT, Wang CH, et al. Diagnostic value of endobronchial ultrasound-guided transbronchial lung biopsy in peripheral lung cancers. J Formos Med Assoc 2004;103(2):124–9.

38. Kikuchi E, Yamazaki K, Sukoh N, et al. Endobronchial ultrasonography with guide-sheath for peripheral pulmonary lesions. Eur Respir J 2004;24(4):533–7.

39. Kurimoto N, Miyazawa T, Okimasa S, et al. Endobronchial ultrasonography using a guide sheath increases the ability to diagnose peripheral pulmonary lesions endoscopically. Chest 2004;126(3):959–65.

40. Asano F, Matsuno Y, Tsuzuku A, et al. Diagnosis of peripheral pulmonary lesions using a bronchoscope insertion guidance system combined with endobronchial ultrasonography with a guide sheath. Lung Cancer 2008;60(3):366–73.

41. Becker HC, Herth F, Ernst A. Bronchoscopic biopsy of peripheral lung lesions under electromagnetic guidance: a pilot study. J Bronchology Interv Pulmonol 2005;12:9–13.

42. Asahina H, Yamazaki K, Onodera Y, et al. Transbronchial biopsy using endobronchial ultrasonography with a guide sheath and virtual bronchoscopic navigation. Chest 2005;128(3):1761–5.

43. Eberhardt R, Anantham D, Ernst A, et al. Multimodality bronchoscopic diagnosis of peripheral lung lesions: a randomized controlled trial. Am J Respir Crit Care Med 2007;176(1):36–41.

44. Steinfort DP, Khor YH, Manser RL, et al. Radial probe endobronchial ultrasound for the diagnosis of peripheral lung cancer: systematic review and meta-analysis. Eur Respir J 2011;37(4):902–10.

45. Wang Memoli JS, Nietert PJ, Silvestri GA. Meta-analysis of guided bronchoscopy for the evaluation of the pulmonary nodule. Chest 2012;142(2):385–93.

46. Tanner NT, Yarmus L, Chen A, et al. Standard bronchoscopy with fluoroscopy vs thin bronchoscopy and radial endobronchial ultrasound for biopsy of pulmonary lesions: a multicenter, prospective, randomized trial. Chest 2018;154(5):1035–43.

47. Tay JH, Irving L, Antippa P, et al. Radial probe endobronchial ultrasound: factors influencing visualization yield of peripheral pulmonary lesions. Respirology 2013;18(1):185–90.

48. Huang CT, Ho CC, Tsai YJ, et al. Factors influencing visibility and diagnostic yield of transbronchial biopsy using endobronchial ultrasound in peripheral pulmonary lesions. Respirology 2009;14(6):859–64.

49. Yoshikawa M, Sukoh N, Yamazaki K, et al. Diagnostic value of endobronchial ultrasonography with a guide sheath for peripheral pulmonary lesions without X-ray fluoroscopy. Chest 2007;131(6):1788–93.

50. Yamada N, Yamazaki K, Kurimoto N, et al. Factors related to diagnostic yield of transbronchial biopsy using endobronchial ultrasonography with a guide sheath in small peripheral pulmonary lesions. Chest 2007;132(2):603–8.

51. Chen AC, Loiselle A, Zhou L, et al. Localization of peripheral pulmonary lesions using a method of computed tomography-anatomic correlation and radial probe endobronchial ultrasound confirmation. Ann Am Thorac Soc 2016;13(9):1586–92.

52. Dolina MY, Cornish DC, Merritt SA, et al. Interbronchoscopist variability in endobronchial path selection: a simulation study. Chest 2008;133(4):897–905.

53. Oshige M, Shirakawa T, Nakamura M, et al. Clinical application of virtual bronchoscopic navigation system for peripheral lung lesions. J Bronchology Interv Pulmonol 2011;18(2):196–202.

54. Ishida T, Asano F, Yamazaki K, et al. Virtual bronchoscopic navigation combined with endobronchial ultrasound to diagnose small peripheral pulmonary lesions: a randomised trial. Thorax 2011;66(12):1072–7.

55. Asano F, Shinagawa N, Ishida T, et al. Virtual bronchoscopic navigation combined with ultrathin bronchoscopy. A randomized clinical trial. Am J Respir Crit Care Med 2013;188(3):327–33.

56. Merritt SA, Gibbs JD, Yu KC, et al. Image-guided bronchoscopy for peripheral lung lesions: a phantom study. Chest 2008;134(5):1017–26.

57. Eberhardt R, Kahn N, Gompelmann D, et al. Lung-Point-a new approach to peripheral lesions. J Thorac Oncol 2010;5(10):1559–63.

58. Leira HO, Lango T, Sorger H, et al. Bronchoscope-induced displacement of lung targets: first in vivo demonstration of effect from wedging maneuver in navigated bronchoscopy. J Bronchology Interv Pulmonol 2013;20(3):206–12.

59. Zhang W, Chen S, Dong X, et al. Meta-analysis of the diagnostic yield and safety of electromagnetic navigation bronchoscopy for lung nodules. J Thorac Dis 2015;7(5):799–809.

60. Gex G, Pralong JA, Combescure C, et al. Diagnostic yield and safety of electromagnetic navigation bronchoscopy for lung nodules: a systematic review and meta-analysis. Respiration 2014;87(2):165–76.

61. Leong S, Ju H, Marshall H, et al. Electromagnetic navigation bronchoscopy: a descriptive analysis. J Thorac Dis 2012;4(2):173–85.

62. Wilson DS, Bartlett RJ. Improved diagnostic yield of bronchoscopy in a community practice: combination of electromagnetic navigation system and rapid on-site evaluation. J Bronchology Interv Pulmonol 2007;14(4):227–32.

63. Seijo LM, de Torres JP, Lozano MD, et al. Diagnostic yield of electromagnetic navigation bronchoscopy is highly dependent on the presence of a Bronchus sign on CT imaging: results from a prospective study. Chest 2010;138(6):1316–21.

64. Savage C, Morrison RJ, Zwischenberger JB. Bronchoscopic diagnosis and staging of lung cancer. Chest Surg Clin N Am 2001;11(4):701–21. vii-viii.

65. Schreiber G, McCrory DC. Performance characteristics of different modalities for diagnosis of suspected lung cancer: summary of published evidence. Chest 2003;123(1 Suppl):115S–28S.

66. Mallow C, Lee H, Oberg C, et al. Safety and diagnostic performance of pulmonologists performing electromagnetic guided percutaneous lung biopsy (SPiNperc). Respirology 2019;24(5):453–8.

67. Yarmus LB, Arias S, Feller-Kopman D, et al. Electromagnetic navigation transthoracic needle aspiration for the diagnosis of pulmonary nodules: a safety and feasibility pilot study. J Thorac Dis 2016;8(1):186–94.

68. Silvestri GA, Herth FJ, Keast T, et al. Feasibility and safety of bronchoscopic transparenchymal nodule access in canines: a new real-time image-guided approach to lung lesions. Chest 2014;145(4):833–8.

69. Herth FJ, Eberhardt R, Sterman D, et al. Bronchoscopic transparenchymal nodule access (BTPNA): first in human trial of a novel procedure for sampling solitary pulmonary nodules. Thorax 2015;70(4):326–32.

70. Chen AC, Gillespie CT. Robotic endoscopic airway challenge: REACH assessment. Ann Thorac Surg 2018;106(1):293–7.

71. Rojas-Solano JR, Ugalde-Gamboa L, Machuzak M. Robotic bronchoscopy for diagnosis of suspected lung cancer: a feasibility study. J Bronchology Interv Pulmonol 2018;25(3):168–75.

72. Orth RC, Wallace MJ, Kuo MD, Technology Assessment Committee of the Society of Interventional Radiology. C-arm cone-beam CT: general principles and technical considerations for use in interventional radiology. J Vasc Interv Radiol 2009;20(7 Suppl):S538–44.

73. Hohenforst-Schmidt W, Banckwitz R, Zarogoulidis P, et al. Radiation exposure of patients by cone beam CT during endobronchial navigation - a phantom study. J Cancer 2014;5(3):192–202.

74. Pritchett MA, Schampaert S, de Groot JAH, et al. Cone-beam CT with augmented fluoroscopy combined with electromagnetic navigation bronchoscopy for biopsy of pulmonary nodules. J Bronchology Interv Pulmonol 2018;25(4):274–82.

75. Hohenforst-Schmidt W, Zarogoulidis P, Vogl T, et al. Cone beam computertomography (CBCT) in interventional chest medicine - high feasibility for endobronchial realtime navigation. J Cancer 2014;5(3):231–41.

76. Park SC, Kim CJ, Han CH, et al. Factors associated with the diagnostic yield of computed tomography-guided transbronchial lung biopsy. Thorac Cancer 2017;8(3):153–8.

77. Bowling MR, Brown C, Anciano CJ. Feasibility and safety of the transbronchial access tool for peripheral pulmonary nodule and mass. Ann Thorac Surg 2017;104(2):443–9.

Therapeutic Bronchoscopic Techniques Available to the Pulmonologist

Emerging Therapies in the Treatment of Peripheral Lung Lesions and Endobronchial Tumors

Matt Aboudara, MD, FCCP[a], Otis Rickman, DO, FCCP[b], Fabien Maldonado, MD, FCCP[b],*

KEYWORDS

- Bronchoscopy • Peripheral lung cancers • Central airway obstruction • Treatment • Ablation

KEY POINTS

- Patients with central airway obstruction should be evaluated by individuals trained in interventional pulmonology to achieve the best outcome based on patient selection and the intended objectives of the procedure.
- Relief of central airway obstruction improves clinically important outcomes such as health-related quality of life, lung function, functional status, and, in some cases, survival. Spray cryotherapy, endobronchial injection of chemotherapy drugs, photodynamic therapy, and monopolar radiofrequency ablation catheter are emerging techniques that may achieve durable treatment responses in the correct patient population.
- Bronchoscopic treatment of peripheral lung cancers is a rapidly evolving area with microwave ablation, radiofrequency ablation, laser, and thermal vapor ablation currently being studied.
- The patient population suitable for endobronchial ablative technologies, both for central and peripheral airway lesions, has yet to be defined.

INTRODUCTION

With the advent of lung cancer screening and the increase of incidentally discovered pulmonary nodules, it is expected that the number of early stage lung cancers identified will continue to increase. Current guideline recommendations for the management of early stage lung cancer include surgical resection and stereotactic body radiation therapy (SBRT) for high-risk surgical patients. Percutaneous radiofrequency ablation is also recommended as an alternative to SBRT in selected patients with lesions in a suitable anatomic location and who have met maximal radiation doses in the course of their treatment.[1] Recent developments in percutaneous ablation techniques include cryotherapy and microwave ablation. However, all percutaneous techniques carry a substantial complication rate (pneumothorax, hemorrhage, and hemoptysis), which has hindered widespread adoption. As a result, and

[a] Division of Pulmonary and Critical Care, St. Luke's Health System, 4321 Washington Street, Suite 6000, Kansas City, MO 64111, USA; [b] Division of Allergy, Pulmonary, and Critical Care, Vanderbilt University Medical Center, 1161 21st Avenue South, T-1218 Medical Center North, Nashville, TN 37232, USA
* Corresponding author.
E-mail address: Fabien.maldonado@vumc.org

Clin Chest Med 41 (2020) 145–160
https://doi.org/10.1016/j.ccm.2019.11.003
0272-5231/20/© 2019 Elsevier Inc. All rights reserved.

in conjunction with the recent explosion of more accurate diagnostic bronchoscopy platforms, some with near real-time imaging and localization, the delivery of bronchoscopy-guided ablation procedures is generating considerable interest, aiming for similar efficacy at a lower complication rate.

In addition, it is estimated that up to 30% of patients diagnosed with lung cancer will initially present with central airway obstruction (CAO).[2] Although surgical resection of the airway tumor is considered the definitive management option, this is often not possible because most patients presenting with an endobronchial mass have advanced stage of disease, poor performance status, complete or partial atelectasis of the affected lung, and are not suitable to undergo an operation. Although most of the endobronchial ablation techniques are used primarily to relieve symptoms of obstruction and improve quality of life (QOL), there is emerging evidence that therapeutic bronchoscopy can also improve survival when used alone or in combination with systemic therapy and is effective at controlling and palliating locally advanced disease.

In this review, the authors attempt to address 5 practical clinical questions that arise when considering therapeutic bronchoscopy for patients with endobronchial tumor or peripheral lung cancer (**Box 1**). Although many therapies have been around for decades, this review focuses on recent evidence on patient selection, outcomes, and developing technologies in the areas of endobronchial and peripheral lung ablation that would be of interest to the pulmonologist.

WHAT PATIENTS BENEFIT FROM THERAPEUTIC INTERVENTIONS TO THE CENTRAL AIRWAYS?

When considering an endoscopic intervention for CAO, it is of first importance to clearly define the

---

Box 1
Practical clinical questions in approaching central airway obstruction and treatment of peripheral lung cancers
What patients benefit from therapeutic interventions to the central airways?
Does relieving CAO improve clinically meaningful outcomes?
What are the new and emerging therapies available for treatment of endobronchial tumors?
What options are available for treatment of peripheral lung cancers by bronchoscopy?

---

goals of the procedure, as appropriate patient selection will be directly related to these objectives. Is the goal to liberate a patient with CAO from the ventilator? Alternatively, is the objective to relieve dyspnea, clear postobstructive pneumonia, or treat hemoptysis, thus improving performance status and permitting a patient to undergo systemic therapy? Or is the goal to relieve the obstruction and simultaneously provide definitive local treatment of the disease? It is worth pointing out that in the absence of such indications, attempts at endobronchial ablation have inherently little utility.

In clinical practice, it is common for patients with malignant CAO, respiratory failure, and mechanical ventilation to be transitioned to hospice and comfort care without consideration of therapeutic bronchoscopy, and this is particularly true in the absence of dedicated interventional pulmonology (IP) services. With the recent development and accreditation of more than 30 specialized IP training programs in the United States, it is expected that advanced therapeutic bronchoscopy will become increasingly available.[3] It is also incorrectly assumed that patients with advanced lung cancer and CAO have a uniformly poor clinical course and that further intervention would have no impact on QOL or clinical outcome. Published literature contradicts such nihilism. Recent data suggest that CAO adequately managed bronchoscopically may not portend a worse survival prognosis than similarly staged patients without CAO.[4] It is also imperative that patients presenting with acute respiratory failure requiring mechanical ventilation be evaluated for the possibility of rigid bronchoscopy to restore luminal patency. This intervention allows rapid relief of the obstruction, improvement in symptoms, and reduction in the level of care in 71% to 94% of patients.[5,6] Although this can be performed with flexible bronchoscopy techniques, rigid bronchoscopy allows a broader range of therapeutic options, better airway control, and safety, as these procedures are often complicated by significant endobronchial bleeding. Therapeutic bronchoscopy should be also considered as a purely palliative intervention, as it was demonstrated to significantly improve QOL even in the terminally ill.[7–9]

Although external beam radiation therapy (XRT) is often a reasonable option for these patients, bronchoscopic intervention should be attempted when possible before radiation treatment. Although comparative data are sparse, one study of patients who only received radiation therapy and who were mechanically ventilated due to CAO showed that only 27% (7/26) of patients were successfully extubated with time to extubation ranging from 4 to 22 days.[10] In an older study from Desai and colleagues,[11] the survival benefit of laser ablation compared with XRT alone was evaluated using a historical control of patients with CAO who only underwent XRT. Patients who underwent emergency laser ablation had a better survival than those who underwent XRT alone (267 days vs 150 days, $P = .04$); however, there was no difference in overall survival when patients with nonurgent malignant CAO were analyzed (312 days vs 258 days, $P = .44$). These patients frequently have coexisting atelectasis or postobstructive pneumonia, which complicates simulation plans by making it difficult to distinguish atelectatic lung from tumor, potentially exposing healthy lung tissue to the toxic effects of radiation. In addition, because these tumors are in central airways, radiation injury to adjacent vascular structures and noninvolved airways are more likely. Because radiation therapy is not immediately effective, rigid bronchoscopy facilitates relief of the obstruction and liberation from mechanical ventilation more quickly than radiation therapy, thus, in theory, reducing the daily incremental risk of ventilator-associated pneumonia. Once the obstruction has been treated bronchoscopically, the lung reinflated, and any postobstructive purulent secretions removed, the patient can then undergo more effective radiation therapy, chemotherapy, or even possibly surgery.

Patient selection is straightforward in most circumstances. There is little doubt that the symptomatic patients with CAO, and either dyspnea, hemoptysis, or, obviously, impending suffocation are prime candidates for therapeutic bronchoscopy, and this approach is supported by current guidelines.[12] Some data suggest that early intervention may improve survival, although this may admittedly represent lead-time bias resulting from the selection of patients with less severe disease and higher performance status.[13] However, patients with minimal symptoms, who are asymptomatic, or who have significantly reduced performance status can be a more challenging situation. Limited data exist to guide the pulmonologist in these types of situations. In general, it is unlikely that a moribund patient with poor performance status will benefit from general anesthesia and therapeutic bronchoscopy. It is also often claimed that once a lobe has been atelectatic for 4 to 6 weeks, the probability of recovery of this lobe is low. In actuality, lung that has been atelectatic for more than 6 weeks is occasionally reexpandable (**Fig. 1**), although this is difficult to predict until after the time of bronchoscopy. As such, it is important that these patients be evaluated by

interventional pulmonologists to ascertain the probable success of an intervention.

Endoluminal obstruction does not necessarily entail that a tumor is unresectable. Based on updated tumor classification (T) for lung cancer staging, a tumor with invasion of the bronchus is classified as T2a tumor regardless of distance from the main carina or if partial or complete atelectasis is observed.[14] As such, if neither lymph node involvement (N0) nor hilar disease is identified (N1), the patient could be classified from stage IB through IIB, assuming no metastatic disease and no features consistent with T3 or T4 status. Thus, proper assessment of staging should be done around the time of the procedure, defining as accurately as possible the location of the tumor in relation to the secondary carinas, main carina, and any mucosal involvement. This intervention and localization will allow the patient the best benefit not only from a symptomatic palliative standpoint but in providing optimal staging to guide therapy.

Recent data have provided more insight into who may benefit from a therapeutic intervention. The multicenter registry AQuIRE investigators reported on the technical success and predictive factors of success and health-related QOL (HRQOL) in more than a thousand therapeutic procedures.[8] They defined technical success of the procedure as greater than 50% recanalization of the airway, which was achieved in 93% of patients with a combination of different techniques (rigid bronchoscopy, flexible bronchoscopy, thermal therapies, and airway stenting). Predictors of success were an endobronchial obstruction and stent placement. Factors associated with failure included an American Society of Anesthesiology (ASA) score of greater than 3, renal failure, tracheal esophageal fistula, left main disease, and primary lung cancer. The greatest improvement in HRQOL occurred in individuals with the highest baseline Borg scores (dyspnea scale), a higher ASA, and higher Zubrod scores (performance status metric). Those least likely to notice an improvement in symptoms were those with lobar obstruction. Interestingly, although greater than 90% of patients had a successful procedure, only 48% noticed an improvement in their dyspnea, implying that technical success does not necessarily translate into clinically meaningful patient-centered outcomes. Complications were low (3.9%), and procedure-specific mortality was less than 1%. Although patients with an ASA score greater than 3 and Zubrod score greater than 1 had a noticeable improvement in their HRQOL following bronchoscopy; they were also the most likely to experience complications.

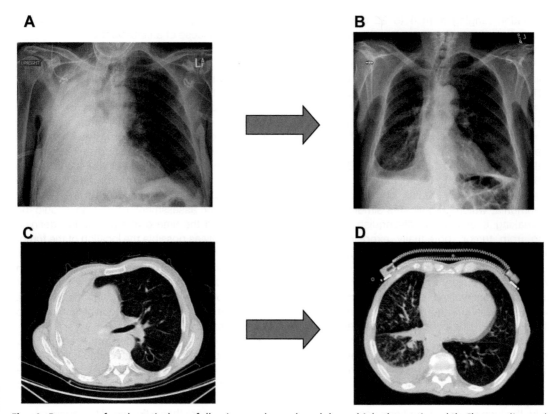

Fig. 1. Recovery of atelectatic lung following prolonged endobronchial obstruction. (*A*) Chest radiograph 3 months before intervention. (*B*) Chest radiograph 3 weeks after removal of right mainstem obstruction. (*C*) CT of chest 3 months before intervention. (*D*) SBRT simulation CT 3 weeks after intervention. CT, computed tomography; SBRT, stereotactic body radiation therapy.

DOES RELIEVING CENTRAL AIRWAY OBSTRUCTION IMPROVE CLINICALLY MEANINGFUL OUTCOMES?

Although the relief of impending suffocation and liberation from mechanical ventilation are obvious clinical benefits derived from therapeutic bronchoscopy, the benefit is less certain in the minimally symptomatic patient. However, recent data have confirmed that therapeutic bronchoscopy in patients with functional and symptomatic limitations can experience an improvement in lung function, QOL, and survival (**Table 1**).

In a prospective study by Mahmood and colleagues,[9] 67 patients were observed who had both benign and malignant CAO (defined as a central airway through which a therapeutic bronchoscope [outer diameter 6.3 mm] could not be passed—trachea, right and left mainstem, bronchus intermedius, and lobar bronchi) and who underwent therapeutic rigid bronchoscopy with ablative therapy with or without stent placement. The technical success of the procedure was defined as luminal patency of greater than 50%, which was achieved in 90.5% (43/53). Study subjects performed spirometry, dyspnea, and QOL evaluations (Shortness of Breath Questionnaire [SOBQ] and the Short Form Health Survey questionnaire [SF36]) both pre- and postbronchoscopy. The forced expiratory volume in the first second of expiration and forced vital capacity improved by 0.4 L and 0.5 L, respectively ($P = .002$ and $P = .009$). Patients had improvements in most domains of the SF36 (physical functioning, role limitations—physical health and energy/fatigue). Dyspnea score (SOBQ) also showed a significant improvement (55.8–37.9, $P = .002$). In addition, overall survival was better in those patients with malignant CAO who underwent successful therapeutic bronchoscopy versus those who had a nonsuccessful intervention with a difference in survival of 114 days (229 vs 115).

Similarly, a study performed by Oviatt and colleagues[15] demonstrated an improvement in 6-minute walk distance of more than 100 m following a therapeutic bronchoscopy that persisted up to 6 months postprocedure. They also observed sustained and clinically significant improvements in dyspnea scores, QOL, and spirometry.

Table 1
Studies reporting quality of life, physiologic improvement, and/or survival following intervention for symptomatic central airway obstruction

Study	Type of Study	HRQOL	Dyspnea	Variables		
				FEV1	6-Minute Walk	Survival
Chhajed et al,[4,49] 2006	Retrospective	NR	NR	Increased by 0.5 L	NR	8.4 mo[a]
Ost et al,[8] 2015	Retrospective, multicenter registry	Δutility,0.023 ± 0.107[b]	ΔBorg−0.9 ± 2.2[c]	NR	NR	NR
Oviatt et al,[15] 2011	Prospective observational	Improved at days 90, 180[d]	Improved at 30, 90, and 180 d[e]	Increased by 0.4 L at 30 d	Improved by 99.7 m at 30 d	NR
Ong et al,[16] 2019	Prospective observational	Δutility,0.047 (0.23–0.71)[b]	ΔBorg −1.8 (−2.2 to −1.3)[c]	NR	NR	109 quality-adjusted life days
Amjadi et al,[50] 2008	Prospective observational	No improvement in global QOL[d]	ΔBorg −2.5[c]	NR	NR	NR
Mahmood et al,[9] 2015	Prospective observational	Improved at 8 wk[f]	Improved at 8 wk[g]	Increased by 0.4 L	NR	242 d[a]
Stratakos et al,[51] 2016	Prospective observational	Improvement up to 6 mo[c]	Improved up to 6 mo[c]	NR	NR	10 mo[h]
Venuta et al,[52] 2002	Retrospective	Improvement noted, $P<.001$[d]	NR	Increased by 0.8 L	NR	12 mo[i]
Jeon et al,[5] 2006	Retrospective	NR	Improved in 94% (34/36)[j]	NR	NR	38 mo[k]

Abbreviations: FEV1, forced expiratory volume in the first second of expiration; NR: not reported.

a Reported as median.
b SF-6D measure used, statistically significant.
c Negative changes in Borg score indicate improved dyspnea, statistically significant.
d European Organization for Research and Treatment of Cancer Quality of Life Questionnaire (EORTC QLQ-C30) and lung cancer-specific module (LC13) were used.
e Resting and 6-minute walk test, Borg scale, lung cancer module questionnaire (LC13), and C30 dyspnea scale were used.
f SF-36 measure used.
g University of California San Diego Shortness of Breath Questionnaire (SOBQ) used.
h Reported as mean.
i Palliation only and no chemotherapy or radiation.
j Dyspnea scale used not reported.
k Reported as median, when combined with chemotherapy ± radiation

In a detailed study analyzing the magnitude of therapeutic bronchoscopy on quality-adjusted survival, investigators reviewed data on 102 patients with malignant CAO.[16] Median survival was 179 days, and the number of quality-adjusted life days was 109. This effect was maintained from the baseline prebronchoscopy up to and beyond 180 days. Factors that were associated with quality-adjusted survival included better baseline performance status, treatment naive tumor, less baseline dyspnea, follow-up chemotherapy, and endobronchial disease. The investigators highlighted that this improvement in HRQOL was one and half times that observed following placement of indwelling pleural catheters for malignant pleural effusions, an intervention that is widely considered an excellent choice at improving QOL in metastatic malignancy.

High-quality, comparative studies demonstrating improved outcomes with therapeutic bronchoscopy alone or in combination with additional therapies (chemotherapy, radiation, surgery, or other ablative techniques) are lacking. However, the available data do suggest that there may be a potential survival benefit when endobronchial intervention is combined with conventional therapies. For example, in the study mentioned earlier by Ong and colleagues,[16] sustained HRQOL was achieved by a multimodality approach to treatment and resulted in a prolonged control in dyspnea that was originally achieved with bronchoscopy. In a retrospective study by Han and colleagues,[17] 110 patients underwent 153 laser treatments; patients were allocated to 2 groups: laser therapy alone (30 patients) and neodymium:yttrium aluminum garnet (Nd:YAG) laser combined with multimodality therapy (66 patients; stent, chemotherapy, radiation therapy). Median length of survival was longer with multimodality therapy versus single modality therapy (6.99 months vs 3.77 months, $P = .002$) for all types of malignancies. This was also observed for non-small cell lung cancer, with survival favoring a multimodality approach (7.17 vs 2.27 months, $P<.001$).

It is clear that therapeutic bronchoscopy improves clinically important outcomes. Dyspnea, hemoptysis, functional status, lung function, HRQOL, and survival can all be positively affected in properly selected patients and, in most instances, via a combination of modalities.

WHAT NEW AND EMERGING THERAPIES ARE AVAILABLE FOR THE TREATMENT OF ENDOBRONCHIAL TUMORS?

Several therapies, many of which have been around for decades, are available to the pulmonologist when managing an endobronchial tumor (**Table 2**). These ablative technologies have well-established safety and efficacy profiles for the palliation of malignant CAO. The choice of modality will depend on the size and location of the tumor, provider experience, training, institutional availability, and goals of the procedure.

Although SBRT, systemic chemotherapy, and immunotherapy are effective therapies, recurrent or progression of disease does occur, and not infrequently with concurrent endobronchial tumor involvement. Recurrence may be at the previous surgical stump site, or within a previously irradiated field, limiting treatment options. If the goal is to provide definitive, local control of tumor rather than simple airway palliation, it is important that the pulmonologist recognizes that there are limited data to guide treatment decisions. Current guidelines recommend photodynamic therapy (PDT), brachytherapy, electrocautery, or cryotherapy as an option to treat superficial limited mucosal cancer that is not suitable for resection.[18] This is based on only 13 studies of PDT, 3 studies evaluating brachytherapy, and one study each assessing electrocautery and cryotherapy, highlighting the paucity of data informing current practice. Endobronchial ablation as curative intent is rare and controversial but is sometimes considered in cases of unresectable carcinoid tumors. In these situations, assessing the degree of cartilaginous invasion and lymph node involvement is paramount as extension beyond the mucosal and submucosal layers will most likely predict a poor response to endobronchial therapy. The use of radial or convex ultrasound is a valuable tool in these circumstances.

The following section briefly reviews new therapies aimed at achieving sustained treatment response, new data on established therapies, and information on new ablative technologies.

Photodynamic Therapy

PDT is a nonthermal ablative technique that applies light energy of a specific wavelength to photosensitized tissue. It is primarily used in patients with superficial mucosal malignancies, carcinoma in situ, bronchial stump R1 resection (residual microscopic tumor following resection), or bronchial stump recurrence. Although one study from Japan demonstrated 5-year and 10-year survival rates of 81% and 71%, respectively, in operable patients with radiographically occult squamous cell carcinoma of the central airway,[19] PDT is primarily used in the United States when SBRT and surgery are considered nonviable options. In the studies mentioned earlier, it seems to be most

Table 2
Immediate and delayed ablative modalities for malignant endobronchial tumor

Immediate Effect	Indications	Contraindications	Complications	Training Requirements[53,54] (n = Number of Procedures)
Laser[a]	Exophytic tumor; hemostasis; granulation tissue	Fio_2 >40%; extrinsic tumor compression with normal mucosa; proximity to silicone stent, metal stents, and hybrid, fully covered metal stents	Bleeding, airway perforation, airway fire, gas embolism, myocardial infarction, stroke, death	15–20
APC[b]	Exophytic tumor; hemostasis; granulation tissue	Fio_2 >40%; extrinsic tumor compression with normal mucosa; covered ultraflex stent	Bleeding, airway perforation, airway fire, pneumothorax, pneumomedia-stinum, gas embolism, stroke, cardiac arrest, death	10–15
Electrocautery	Exophytic tumor; hemostasis; granulation tissue; treatment of early stage carcinoma in situ	Fio_2 >40%; extrinsic tumor compression with normal mucosa; caution in patients with pacemakers or internal defibrillators; proximity to silicone stent, metal stents, and hybrid, fully covered metal stents	Bleeding, airway perforation, airway fire, bronchospasm, pneumothorax, death	10–15

Delayed Effect	Indications	Contraindications	Complications	Training Requirements[53,54]
Cryotherapy[c]	Exophytic tumor; granulation tissue; treatment of early stage carcinoma in situ	Symptomatic critical airway obstruction; massive hemorrhage	Bleeding, bronchospasm, pneumothorax, arrhythmias, cardiac arrest, death	10
PDT[d]	Exophytic tumor ≤2 cm; superficial early stage lung cancer, R1 disease[e]	Lesion >2 cm, critical airway obstruction; porphyria, allergy to photosensitizer	Bleeding, airway obstruction, respiratory failure, photosensitivity, death	10
Brachytherapy	Palliation of malignant endobronchial, submucosal, and peribronchial obstruction; early stage lung cancer; granulation tissue	Tumor involvement of major arteries and mediastinum; upper lobe tumors; squamous histology; risk of bronchovascular fistula	Radiation bronchitis and bronchial stenosis, bronchovascular fistula, tracheoesophageal fistula, death	5

[a] Types of laser include Nd:YAG, neodymium:yttrium-aluminum-perovskite (ND:YAP), potassium titanyl phosphate (KTP), carbon dioxide (CO_2), and holmium.
[b] Argon plasma eoagulation—noncontact modality.
[c] Contact cryoprobe; complications from SCT are unique—see section on SCT for more details.
[d] Photodynamic therapy.
[e] Microscopic disease at bronchial margin following resection.

effective in early stage, centrally located tumors that are less than 2 cm in size. A complete response has been seen in 80% of lesions 10 mm to 20 mm but drops to 38% to 44% for lesions greater than 2 cm. The 5-year overall survival for PDT is 58%.[18]

Recent data published by Mehta and colleagues[20] assessed the response and survival rates of patients undergoing PDT for residual microscopic tumor at the resected bronchial margin (R1 disease). They identified 15 patients through a multidisciplinary tumor board that underwent PDT (3 with carcinoma in situ, 8 with mucosal residual disease, and 4 with peribronchial residual disease). The local control rate was 91% and the median time to recurrence after PDT was 26 months. The median overall survival was 45 months. There were no severe complications related to the procedure, such as airway obstruction, massive hemoptysis, or fistula formation. One patient had a photosensitivity reaction and another developed pneumonia postprocedure and required admission. Because R1 disease occurs on average in 4% to 5% of operations, and the data on SBRT and repeat resection in these patients are limited, the use of PDT seems reasonable in a highly selected patient population who have undergone a multidisciplinary tumor board discussion.

PDT has also recently been investigated as a potential ablative modality in peripheral lesions (see later discussion).[21]

Spray Cryotherapy

The concept of cryo-cytodestruction has been known for decades with the first reported use of a contact cryoprobe for tumor debulking within the airway in 1968 in an animal model.[22] Until recently, cryotherapy was only delivered by a contact mechanism via semirigid probe to facilitate tumor debulking and achieve a delayed tumor destructive effect. Nitrous oxide or carbon dioxide is delivered through the probe and is rapidly released, causing a drop in temperature at the tip of the probe to $-89°C$ (for nitrous oxide). The cytodestructive effects of cryosurgery are achieved by rapid cooling of the tissue, repeated freeze-thaw cycles, and resultant cell membrane degeneration and destruction that results from direct organelle damage and intracellular dehydration from extracellular ice crystal formation. For tissue destruction effect, the tissue is cooled for 30 to 60 seconds, the probe tip and tissue then dethaw, and the cycle is immediately repeated. Because it is a contact method, only the tissue touching and up to 5 to 8 mm circumferential to the probe

undergoes cytodestruction. The effect, although, is delayed, and a repeat bronchoscopy is needed to remove the sloughed necrotic tissue. Advantages of cryoablation include (1) no risk of airway fire; (2) safe use in close proximity to all types of stents; and (3) reduced risk of damage to underlying cartilage, fat, and connective tissue (hence reducing the risks of airway perforation, malacia, and stenosis). However, for larger tissue areas, multiple overlapping freeze-thaw cycles are needed to achieve adequate tissue destruction. This can become cumbersome in regions of the airways where it is difficult to achieve good overlapping "freeze-kill" zones (eg, right upper lobe secondary carina) or large tumor burden.

Spray cryotherapy (SCT) is a noncontact mode of cryosurgery that uses liquid nitrogen as its cryogen. The low boiling point of liquid nitrogen causes a rapid cooling to temperatures of $-196°C$ when it is exposed to room temperature, resulting in flash freeze of tissues, intracellular formation of ice crystals, and cell death. The noncontact method allows for a larger area to be treated more effectively and quickly. The uniform delivery of cryogen to the targeted tissues and the preservation of underlying tissue architecture have made it a potentially appealing option for management of benign and malignant airway stenosis. The main safety concern with SCT is the rapid expansion of nitrogen gas formation (by a factor of 700) with the risk of pneumothorax and air embolism when the egress of gas (ie, passive venting) is compromised. With proper training of both the proceduralist and the procedural staff (anesthesia, bronchoscopy technician), this complication can generally be prevented.

SCT was first used in the gastrointestinal tract to treat high-grade dysplasia in Barrett esophagus with good results. Reported rates of resolution of esophageal dysplasia of 97% and successful treatment of T1 esophageal tumors of 72% led to investigations into its use in the airway.[23]

Early reports using the first-generation system described its effectiveness in benign airway strictures such as tracheal, subglottic, and glottic stenosis and malignant CAO with a reasonable safety profile.[24–26] In these series, a total of 42 patients were treated with SCT, 93% of whom (39/42) had benign strictures. Of the 7% (3/42) of patients with malignant disease, good endoscopic results were noted but repeat bronchoscopies every 4 to 6 weeks with repeated treatments were required (the investigators did not report the number of procedures and treatments).[26] When taken in aggregate, complications were minimal, with a pneumothorax rate of 2.4% (1/42). However, a multicenter registry study in 2012 tempered enthusiasm, as a higher-than-expected complication rate was reported. In this registry, a total of 80 patients were treated with SCT for high-grade malignant airway obstruction.[27] Airway patency was achieved in all but one patient who had 100% obstruction before treatment. Most patients required an additional technique at the time of the initial bronchoscopy to restore airway patency. Intraprocedural complication rates occurred in 19% of patients (n = 22: hypotension, bradycardia, tachycardia, ST elevation, hypoxemia, and airway tear). One patient developed a pneumothorax requiring an emergent chest tube and one patient had an intraprocedural cardiac arrest but was successfully resuscitated and discharged home the next day. Alarmingly, five deaths occurred (4.4%), with 2 occurring intraoperatively within 5 to 30 minutes of treatment and were preceded by significant bradycardia and hypoxemia. The investigators appropriately concluded that although SCT held promise, the high risk of serious complications required further refinement of the technology.

In 2012, the Food and Drug Administration (FDA) granted approval to the current, third-generation version of SCT (TrueFreeze, CSA Medical Inc, USA) for destruction of abnormal tissue within the airway (**Fig. 2**). This upgrade incorporated 2 adjustable flow rates: 25 W (normal flow) and 12.5 W (reduced flow). By reducing the flow rate,

the amount of gaseous expansion is expected to decrease, thus hopefully mitigating the risk of complications. The company now requires face-to-face didactic training and observation of cases performed by experienced users to ensure patient safety. A key component of the procedure is to allow adequate passive ventilation of the nitrogen gas. In order to achieve this, all procedures should occur under general anesthesia with either an endotracheal tube or rigid bronchoscopy. Suspension laryngoscopy has also been used safely with subglottic stenosis.[28] At the time of treatment, ventilation is ceased, the airway circuit is disconnected (if an endotracheal tube is used, cap is removed from the rigid bronchoscope), and visualization of gas egressing from the circuit is mandatory. If the patient cannot tolerate this maneuver or egress of gas is not visualized, the procedure is immediately terminated. In order to prevent trapping of the nitrogen gas, treatment of lobar and distal bronchi should be avoided.

Since the approval of the upgraded device and specific training requirements and standardization was implemented, 2 studies have been published that demonstrated an acceptable safety profile.[28,29] In one study including 27 patients who underwent 80 treatments for malignant airway obstruction, 3.7% (3/80) had complications (transient, intraprocedural hypoxia). Thirty-nine percent (31/80) required multimodality approach and 56%

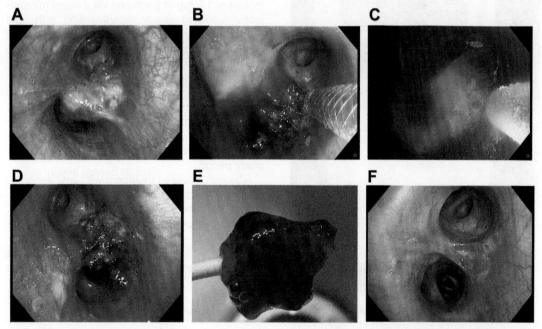

Fig. 2. SCT in the treatment of endobronchial carcinoid. (*A*) Carcinoid tumor at left secondary carina (LC2). (*B*) Alignment of SCT catheter to tumor via rigid bronchoscopy. (*C*) Application of SCT to tumor. (*D*) Appearance of tumor after SCT. (*E*) Patient expectorated tumor 1 week later. (*F*) Residual ulcer at LC2 on repeat bronchoscopy.

(45/80) were used in close proximity to silicone, hybrid, or metal stents without complication.

Although this technology is intriguing and holds promise (**Fig. 3**), particularly because it allows preservation of underlying cartilaginous architecture, its delayed effects on tissue destruction and restoration of airway patency preclude its use as an immediate ablative technology and should not be used in isolation for high-grade, symptomatic airway obstruction. The need for a second procedure to remove sloughed, necrotic tissue may be seen as a limitation, particularly in malignant airway obstruction, as many of these procedures are performed with palliative intention, and limiting the number and frequency of procedures should be prioritized. Further studies are needed to clarify the role of this technology in the management of malignant CAO.

Endobronchial Injection of Chemotherapy

Bronchoscopic injection of antineoplastic agents was first described in 1997 as a potential therapeutic option to relieve airway obstruction with prolonged effects.[30] In that study, 93 patients with primary lung cancer and metastatic disease with greater than 50% CAO were each treated with a combination of 5-fluorouracil, mitomycin, methotrexate, bleomycin, and mitoxantrone. They reported an immediate improvement in airway caliber in 87% (81/93), but the impact on long-term outcomes was unknown.

More recently, Mehta and colleagues[31] have described their experience with the intratumoral injection of cisplatin in 22 patients with metastatic endobronchial disease and primary lung cancer. They reported a response rate in 71% (15/21) with a median overall survival of 3 months, which was similar to other conventional ablative modalities.

In the only multicenter safety and feasibility study of intratumoral injection, 23 patients with non-small cell lung cancer and CAO underwent injection of 1.5 mg of paclitaxel via a novel microinjector following airway recanalization with rigid bronchoscopy.[32] The delivery device allowed near complete circumferential delivery of the drug into the tumor. Overall, 74% (17/23) of patients were either stage 3 or 4. Followed-up bronchoscopy at 6 weeks postintervention showed a sustained improvement in airway caliber. No serious events directly related to the therapy were identified. Interestingly, there was also a significant improvement in HRQOL over the 12-week study period.

Although localized treatment with antineoplastic agents is an intriguing option for patients, particularly if sustained results can be demonstrated, several questions (dose of drug needed to achieve and maintain efficacy, superiority to current approaches, etc.) need to be addressed before this being considered a routine option for patients with CAO.

Monopolar Radiofrequency Catheter

A monopolar radiofrequency catheter (CoreCath 2.7, Medtronic Advanced Energy, LLC, Portsmouth, USA) was recently approved in an attempt

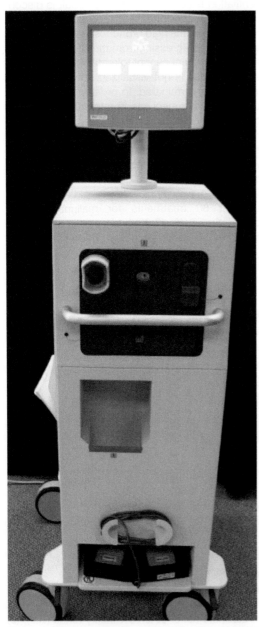

Fig. 3. Spray cryotherapy tower. (*Courtesy of* CSA Medical, Lexington, MA.)

to combine electrocautery cutting features, coagulation mode, and smoke evacuator into one instrument that can be used through the 2.8-mm working channel of a 6.2-mm flexible bronchoscope without the need for grounding pad (**Fig. 4**). At the time of this writing, only one animal study and one clinical study have been published in abstract form. In a preclinical study, the thermal ablation zone extent was assessed in 2 sheep. The penetration depth for both cut and coagulation modes at 5, 20, and 40 W were less than or equal to 1 mm. The extent of injury extended to the mucosal epithelium and submucosal tissue.[33] In comparison, the depth of penetration for Nd:YAG laser, electrocautery, and argon plasma coagulation (APC) is 6 to 10 mm, 2 mm, and less than or equal to 3 mm, respectively.[34,35] The smaller depth of penetration would in theory limit the possibility of airway perforation, damage to surrounding vascular structures, and the degree of airway cartilage injury and scar formation.

In data available in abstract form, this device was used in 41 patients for a total of 45 procedures.[36] Airway recanalization defined by greater than 50% patent airway caliber was achieved in all cases. In 96% of procedures, however, additional therapies were used: cryoprobe, balloon dilatation, APC, stent placement, rigid bronchoscopy and SCT.

Although this device may play a role in some cases of malignant CAO, its superiority to APC, electrocautery, and laser is yet to be demonstrated (**Fig. 5**). Also, it is a relatively stiff device that is not easily directed into more acutely angled airways, such as the upper lobes. The suction evacuator also becomes frequently clogged requiring removal from the airway for cleaning. Finally, it is a single-use device and the cost-effectiveness has yet to be established when compared with reusable instruments.

WHAT OPTIONS ARE AVAILABLE FOR THE TREATMENT OF PERIPHERAL LUNG CANCERS BY BRONCHOSCOPY?

The preferred treatment of early-stage lung cancer in nonoperable candidates is SBRT. Current guidelines recommend computed tomography (CT)-guided percutaneous radiofrequency ablation (RFA) for stage 1 non-small cell lung cancer in patients who are not candidates for either surgery or SBRT.[1] Although percutaneous PDT, microwave, and cryotherapy have also been used in these circumstances, RFA has the most robust data (although low quality) supporting its use. RFA achieves cell death by heat-induced coagulative necrosis delivered through an electrode placed within the tumor. Of the eight clinical studies to date, a primary tumor control rate of 58% to 87.5% and cancer-specific survival of 30% to 100% (over 1–3 years) with a median follow-up ranging from 14 to 30 months have been reported.[1] Complications are substantial, with pneumothorax rates ranging from 9% to

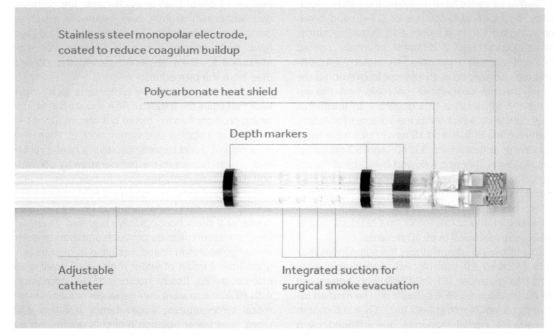

Stainless steel monopolar electrode, coated to reduce coagulum buildup

Polycarbonate heat shield

Depth markers

Adjustable catheter

Integrated suction for surgical smoke evacuation

Fig. 4. Monopolar radiofrequency catheter. (*Courtesy of* Medtronic, Plymouth, MN.)

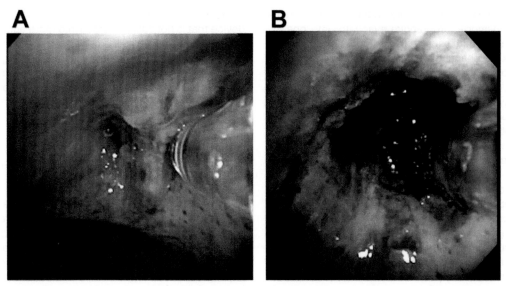

Fig. 5. Monopolar radiofrequency ablation of endobronchial tumor. (*A*) Catheter in direct contact with obstructing tumor in right upper lobe. (*B*) Recannulization of airway and coagulation of residual tumor following treatment. (*Courtesy of* B. Mahajan, MD, Falls Church, VA.)

63% and pleural effusions at a rate of 7% to 21%. In addition, massive hemoptysis, hemothorax, neuropathy, bronchopleural fistula, and pneumonia have also been reported.[37] Although the procedure-specific mortality rate is less than 1%, the rate of complications is often prohibitive in a patient population with compromised functional and cardiopulmonary status and hence bronchoscopic approaches have been considered.

Two case series have analyzed the safety, feasibility, and clinical outcomes of CT-guided bronchoscopic RFA. In a safety and feasibility study, investigators used 3 different internally cooled RFA catheters in 10 patients.[38] A cooled RFA catheter was developed in an attempt to overcome the rapid thermal coagulative necrosis and the increase in impedance that occurs with traditional RFA catheters, which limits the volume of ablation. Catheter tips of 5, 8, and 10 mm in size were used and were activated for 30, 40, and 50 seconds, respectively. This was followed by surgical resection. The catheters with a large tip and activated for 50 seconds had the largest RFA ablation zone; however, all the zones of ablation were smaller than the actual tumor and residual cancer cells were identified in all 10 patients.

In a follow-up clinical study, the same investigators followed 20 patients with inoperable non-small lung cancer (T1-2aN0M0) who underwent RFA with a cooled RFA catheter.[39] The median tumor size was 24 mm (12–45 mm). Over a 6-month period, the partial response rate (defined by a reduction in tumor size as classified by the

Response Evaluation Criteria in Solid Tumors) was 47.8% (11/23). Over the same time period, no change in tumor size occurred in 8 patients, indicating a local control rate of 82% (19/23). SBRT was added in 3 patients who progressed after treatment and chemotherapy was added in one other. The 5-year survival was 61.5% (95% confidence interval: 36–87 months). Importantly, no pneumothorax occurred. Two patients complained of chest pain in each case, the catheter was withdrawn slightly, and treatment resumed without complication. Three patients developed fever and consolidation on CT scan; this was attributed to acute ablation reaction. No patient died from the procedure.

Aerated lung around the tumor acts as an insulator that limits the extent of RFA-induced ablation, which protects healthy tissue but also reduces the margins of ablation and tumor control. Also, the proximity of blood vessels results in a heat-sink effect, which decreases the temperature by convection, limiting the ablation zone further.

Because of these limitations of RFA, microwave ablation has been investigated as both a percutaneous and bronchoscopically delivered modality. Electromagnetic waves produce agitation of polar water molecules in tissue, resulting in heat generation from friction of water molecules, leading to cell death via tissue necrosis.[40] As compared with RFA, microwave can generate higher intratumoral temperatures, larger tumor ablation volumes, and faster ablation times; is unaffected by impedance; and results in less procedural pain.

Microwave ablation has been applied to tumors in the kidney, liver, adrenal glands, pancreas, bone, and recently the lung by a CT-guided percutaneous approach.[41,42] In one study, 130 lesions were treated in 80 patients with pulmonary metastases.[42] The ablation success rate was 73.1%, with a lesion size of less than 3 cm and peripheral location (as compared with central) being predictive of more successful ablation. The 12- and 24-month survival rates were 91% and 75%, respectively.

The current status of bronchoscopic delivery of microwave ablation is evolving. In recently presented data from the United Kingdom in abstract form, 3 patients were treated with microwave ablation using the SuperDimension Navigational Bronchoscopy platform (Medtronic, Minneapolis, MN, USA) and a flexible microwave ablation catheter (Embrint, Medtronic) under cone beam CT (CBCT) guidance.[43] A total of 4 lesions were treated. An adequate ablation zone was confirmed by CBCT (Fig. 6). The only complication reported was mild chest pain in one patient that resolved

within 24 hours. No data are yet available on local control rates and progression-free and overall survival. A recent prospective multicenter trial evaluating safety, feasibility, and multiple other secondary outcomes with the NEUWAVE Flex microwave ablation system was temporarily suspended due to unexpected complications (ClinicalTrials.gov Identifier: NCT03603652).

PDT has also been studied in the treatment of peripheral lung tumors in small studies. An initial study involving CT-guided percutaneous treatment 48 hours after injection of a photosensitizer demonstrated the feasibility and safety of PDT.[44] Nine patients were included. No complete response was observed; however, all had a partial response. Two patients developed a pneumothorax, one requiring a chest tube. Musani and colleagues[21] recently described a preclinical study of electromagnetic navigation bronchoscopy–guided PDT in 3 dogs with peripheral adenocarcinoma. The photoradiation was delivered by the Veran ENB system (Veran Medical, St. Louis, MO, USA) 48 hours after injection of the photosensitizer

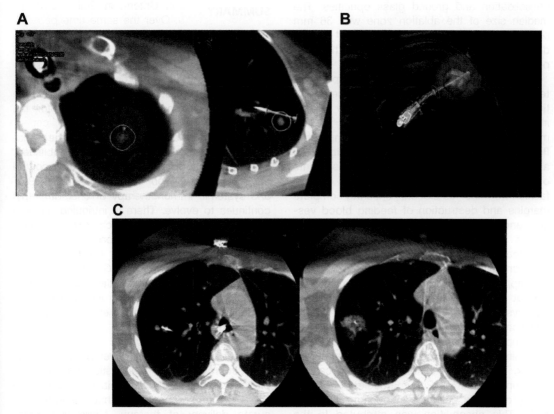

Fig. 6. Bronchoscopic microwave ablation of peripheral lung cancer. (*A*) Intraprocedural CBCT: Views along and perpendicular to the ablation catheter shows ablation zone completely encompasses the tumor and a 1 cm margin at every level. (*B*) Intraprocedural CBCT: 3-dimensional rendering of ablation zone encompassing tumor and a surrounding margin. (*C*) Before and 10 minutes after ablation. (*Courtesy of* K. Lau, Barts Thorax Center, London, UK.)

followed by resection of the affected lung tissue. Pathology demonstrated coagulative necrosis of the central tumor. Adenocarcinoma was located on the periphery of the treatment zone in all 3 specimens. PDT delivered by ENB under intraoperative CT localization was used in 3 patients who were deemed medically suitable to undergo the procedure.[45] The SuperDimension Navigational Bronchoscopy platform was used to deliver the treatment. The mean tumor size was 21.3 mm (8–36 mm). No immediate complications were noted, although one patient developed a photosensitivity reaction. At a mean of 14-month follow-up, 2 had partial response and 1 had complete response.

A preclinical study of a wide aperture diode laser fiber in a porcine model was performed to assess the safety and feasibility of this device.[46] Five pigs underwent ablation of normal lung tissue followed by a CT scan and then euthanasia and necropsy 72 hours after the procedure. They found that the round-tip laser fiber produced the most spherical ablation shape. CT findings showed central cavitation with surrounding consolidation and ground glass opacities. The median size of the ablation zone was 36 mm (24–38 mm) at day 1 and 34 mm (30–44 mm) at day 3. One pneumothorax occurred in the postprocedure period.

Finally, thermal vapor ablation, developed as a technique for bronchoscopic lung volume reduction in severe emphysema, was recently studied in a porcine model for tumor ablation.[47,48] Thermal energy is delivered via a catheter through a flexible bronchoscope positioned within an airway projecting to the lesion. Entire segments of the lung can thus be treated in a uniform fashion from the "outside in," ensuring complete margins and destruction of feeding blood vessels and lymphatics, resulting in a "bronchoscopic segmentectomy" (**Fig. 7**). In a safety and feasibility porcine model study, 11 pigs with normal lung were treated with escalating energy applications. Necrosis was uniformly identified at all energy levels. In animals alive at 30 days, necrosis was replaced by fibroblasts and scarred lung. Three animals had evidence of complications, with one dying. On necropsy, this animal was found to have bilateral pneumothorax. The 2 other animals had complications from pneumothorax. Pneumatoceles were uniformly observed on gross inspection in all animals. This observation was attributed to the pig's absence of collateral ventilation, which allowed for pressure build-up within the treated segment. As such, the application of this technology in humans is unknown, because the

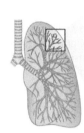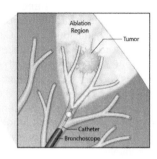

Fig. 7. Thermal vapor ablation. Bronchoscope is wedged into subsegmental airway that is directed toward target nodule. Catheter is directed to nodule and energy is applied to the nodule and surrounding lung tissue within that subsegment. (*From* Henne E, Ferguson JS, Mest R, Herth FJ. Thermal Vapor Ablation for Lung Lesions in a Porcine Model. Respiration 2015;90:146–54; with permission.)

distribution of thermal energy and the tumor ablative effect in lung segments with collateral ventilation is uncertain.

SUMMARY

Therapeutic bronchoscopy improves respiratory symptoms due to CAO, prolongs survival when used in conjunction with systemic therapy or surgical resection, and can improve HRQOL. Interventional pulmonologists should carefully evaluate patients to ensure the best outcome for the patient.

Endobronchial ablative therapies for the palliation of airway obstruction are well established. Their specific application to achieving local control of endobronchial tumor (as compared with SBRT and systemic immunotherapy or chemotherapy) continues to evolve. There is intriguing ongoing research into the delivery of chemotherapeutics into residual tumor and the proper role of PDT in the management of small, residual disease following surgical resection. SCT offers a unique therapeutic option for some patients too; however, further comparative research into these treatments is highly encouraged to elucidate their role in the care of these patients.

The treatment of peripheral lung cancers has entered a dynamic period, driven primarily by the rapid improvement in diagnostic bronchoscopy platforms (robotic, fluoroscopic navigation, and CBCT-guided bronchoscopy) that guarantees accurate delivery of therapy. Microwave, cryotherapy, RFA, PDT, vapor thermal ablation, and laser all have the potential to affect patient care. Although there are limitations and advantages to each of these modalities, it should be emphasized that well-designed, multicentered, comparative studies will be needed to determine the safest and most efficacious treatment.

DISCLOSURE

The authors have nothing to disclose.

REFERENCES

1. Donington J, Ferguson M, Mazzone P, et al. American College of Chest Physicians and Society of Thoracic Surgeons consensus statement for evaluation and management for high-risk patients with stage I non-small cell lung cancer. Chest 2012; 142:1620–35.

2. Cavaliere S, Venuta F, Foccoli P, et al. Endoscopic treatment of malignant airway obstructions in 2,008 patients. Chest 1996;110:1536–42.

3. Mullon JJ, Burkart KM, Silvestri G, et al. Interventional pulmonology fellowship accreditation standards: executive summary of the multisociety interventional pulmonology fellowship accreditation committee. Chest 2017;151:1114–21.

4. Chhajed PN, Baty F, Pless M, et al. Outcome of treated advanced non-small cell lung cancer with and without central airway obstruction. Chest 2006;130:1803–7.

5. Jeon K, Kim H, Yu CM, et al. Rigid bronchoscopic intervention in patients with respiratory failure caused by malignant central airway obstruction. J Thorac Oncol 2006;1:319–23.

6. Colt HG, Harrell JH. Therapeutic rigid bronchoscopy allows level of care changes in patients with acute respiratory failure from central airways obstruction. Chest 1997;112:202–6.

7. Vonk-Noordegraaf A, Postmus PE, Sutedja TG. Tracheobronchial stenting in the terminal care of cancer patients with central airways obstruction. Chest 2001;120:1811–4.

8. Ost DE, Ernst A, Grosu HB, et al. Therapeutic bronchoscopy for malignant central airway obstruction: success rates and impact on dyspnea and quality of life. Chest 2015;147:1282–98.

9. Mahmood K, Wahidi MM, Thomas S, et al. Therapeutic bronchoscopy improves spirometry, quality of life, and survival in central airway obstruction. Respiration 2015;89:404–13.

10. Louie AV, Lane S, Palma DA, et al. Radiotherapy for intubated patients with malignant airway obstruction: futile or facilitating extubation? J Thorac Oncol 2013;8:1365–70.

11. Desai SJ, Mehta AC, VanderBrug Medendorp S, et al. Survival experience following Nd:YAG laser photoresection for primary bronchogenic carcinoma. Chest 1988;94:939–44.

12. Simoff MJ, Lally B, Slade MG, et al. Symptom management in patients with lung cancer: diagnosis and management of lung cancer, 3rd ed: American College of Chest Physicians evidence-based clinical practice guidelines. Chest 2013;143:e455S–97S.

13. Razi SS, Lebovics RS, Schwartz G, et al. Timely airway stenting improves survival in patients with malignant central airway obstruction. Ann Thorac Surg 2010;90:1088–93.

14. Detterbeck FC, Boffa DJ, Kim AW, et al. The eighth edition lung cancer stage classification. Chest 2017;151:193–203.

15. Oviatt PL, Stather DR, Michaud G, et al. Exercise capacity, lung function, and quality of life after interventional bronchoscopy. J Thorac Oncol 2011;6:38–42.

16. Ong P, Grosu HB, Debiane L, et al. Long-term quality-adjusted survival following therapeutic bronchoscopy for malignant central airway obstruction. Thorax 2019;74:141–56.

17. Han CC, Prasetyo D, Wright GM. Endobronchial palliation using Nd:YAG laser is associated with improved survival when combined with multimodal adjuvant treatments. J Thorac Oncol 2007; 2:59–64.

18. Wisnivesky JP, Yung RC-W, Mathur PN, et al. Diagnosis and treatment of bronchial intraepithelial neoplasia and early lung cancer of the central airways: diagnosis and management of lung cancer, 3rd ed: American College of Chest Physicians evidence-based clinical practice guidelines. Chest 2013;143:e263S–77S.

19. Endo C, Miyamoto A, Sakurada A, et al. Results of long-term follow-up of photodynamic therapy for roentgenographically occult bronchogenic squamous cell carcinoma. Chest 2009;136:369–75.

20. Mehta HJ, Biswas A, Fernandez-Bussy S, et al. Photodynamic therapy for bronchial microscopic residual disease after resection in lung cancer. J Bronchology Interv Pulmonol 2019;26:49–54.

21. Musani AI, Veir JK, Huang Z, et al. Photodynamic therapy via navigational bronchoscopy for peripheral lung cancer in dogs. Lasers Surg Med 2018; 50:483–90.

22. Sheski FD, Mathur PN. Cryotherapy, electrocautery, and brachytherapy. Clin Chest Med 1999;20: 123–38.

23. Moore RF, Lile DJ, Abbas AE. Current status of spray cryotherapy for airway disease. J Thorac Dis 2017;9: S122–9.

24. Krimsky WS, Rodrigues MP, Malayaman N, et al. Spray cryotherapy for the treatment of glottic and subglottic stenosis. Laryngoscope 2010;120:473–7.

25. Fernando HC, Dekeratry D, Downie G, et al. Feasibility of spray cryotherapy and balloon dilation for non-malignant strictures of the airway. Eur J Cardiothoracic Surg 2011;40:1177–80.

26. Browning R, Parrish S, Sarkar S, et al. First report of a novel liquid nitrogen adjustable flow spray cryotherapy (SCT) device in the bronchoscopic

treatment of disease of the central tracheo-bronchial airways. J Thorac Dis 2013;5:E103–6.

27. Finley DJ, Dycoco J, Sarkar S, et al. Airway spray cryotherapy: initial outcomes from a multiinstitutional registry. Ann Thorac Surg 2012;94:199–203 [discussion: 4].

28. Bhora FY, Ayub A, Forleiter CM, et al. Treatment of benign tracheal stenosis using endoluminal spray cryotherapy. JAMA Otolaryngol Head Neck Surg 2016;142:1082–7.

29. Browning R, Turner JF Jr, Parrish S. Spray cryotherapy (SCT): institutional evolution of techniques and clinical practice from early experience in the treatment of malignant airway disease. J Thorac Dis 2015;7:S405–14.

30. Celikoglu SI, Karayel T, Demirci S, et al. Direct injection of anti-cancer drugs into endobronchial tumours for palliation of major airway obstruction. Postgrad Med J 1997;73:159–62.

31. Mehta HJ, Begnaud A, Penley AM, et al. Restoration of patency to central airways occluded by malignant endobronchial tumors using intratumoral injection of cisplatin. Ann Am Thorac Soc 2015;12:1345–50.

32. Yarmus L, Mallow C, Akulian J, et al. Prospective multicentered safety and feasibility pilot for endobronchial intratumoral chemotherapy. Chest 2019; 156(3):562–70.

33. Herdina KA, Howk KA, Andres D, et al. Performance of a novel electrosurgical device for cutting and coagulation of central airway obstructions. D61 imaging, interventions, and interventional pulmonology: the three "I's" of thoracic oncology:A7329-A.

34. van Boxem TJ, Westerga J, Venmans BJ, et al. Tissue effects of bronchoscopic electrocautery: bronchoscopic appearance and histologic changes of bronchial wall after electrocautery. Chest 2000;117: 887–91.

35. Mahmood K, Wahidi MM. Ablative therapies for central airway obstruction. Semin Respir Crit Care Med 2014;35:681–92.

36. Lum M, Krishna G. First in human evaluation of a novel monopolar radiofrequency electrosurgical device for cutting and coagulation of central airway obstruction. A30 what's new in interventional pulmonary and pleural disease:A1261-A.

37. Harris K, Puchalski J, Sterman D. Recent advances in bronchoscopic treatment of peripheral lung cancers. Chest 2017;151:674–85.

38. Tanabe T, Koizumi T, Tsushima K, et al. Comparative study of three different catheters for CT imaging-bronchoscopy-guided radiofrequency ablation as a potential and novel interventional therapy for lung cancer. Chest 2010;137:890–7.

39. Koizumi T, Tsushima K, Tanabe T, et al. Bronchoscopy-guided cooled radiofrequency ablation as a novel intervention therapy for peripheral lung cancer. Respiration 2015;90:47–55.

40. Carrafiello G, Lagana D, Mangini M, et al. Microwave tumors ablation: principles, clinical applications and review of preliminary experiences. Int J Surg 2008; 6(Suppl 1):S65–9.

41. Wolf FJ, Grand DJ, Machan JT, et al. Microwave ablation of lung malignancies: effectiveness, CT findings, and safety in 50 patients. Radiology 2008;247:871–9.

42. Vogl TJ, Naguib NN, Gruber-Rouh T, et al. Microwave ablation therapy: clinical utility in treatment of pulmonary metastases. Radiology 2011;261:643–51.

43. Lau K, Spiers A, Pritchett M, et al. P1.05-06 bronchoscopic image-guided microwave ablation of peripheral lung tumours-early results. J Thorac Oncol 2018;13:S542.

44. Okunaka T, Kato H, Tsutsui H, et al. Photodynamic therapy for peripheral lung cancer. Lung Cancer 2004;43:77–82.

45. Chen KC, Lee JM. Photodynamic therapeutic ablation for peripheral pulmonary malignancy via electromagnetic navigation bronchoscopy localization in a hybrid operating room (OR): a pioneering study. J Thorac Dis 2018;10:S725–30.

46. Casal RF, Walsh G, McArthur M, et al. Bronchoscopic laser interstitial thermal therapy: an experimental study in normal porcine lung parenchyma. J Bronchology Interv Pulmonol 2018;25:322–9.

47. Gompelmann D, Shah PL, Valipour A, et al. Bronchoscopic thermal vapor ablation: best practice recommendations from an expert panel on endoscopic lung volume reduction. Respiration 2018;95: 392–400.

48. Henne E, Ferguson JS, Mest R, et al. Thermal vapor ablation for lung lesions in a porcine model. Respiration 2015;90:146–54.

49. Chhajed PN, Eberhardt R, Dienemann H, et al. Therapeutic bronchoscopy interventions before surgical resection of lung cancer. Ann Thorac Surg 2006; 81:1839–43.

50. Amjadi K, Voduc N, Cruysberghs Y, et al. Impact of interventional bronchoscopy on quality of life in malignant airway obstruction. Respiration 2008;76:421–8.

51. Stratakos G, Gerovasili V, Dimitropoulos C, et al. Survival and quality of life benefit after endoscopic management of malignant central airway obstruction. J Cancer 2016;7:794–802.

52. Venuta F, Rendina EA, De Giacomo T, et al. Nd:YAG laser resection of lung cancer invading the airway as a bridge to surgery and palliative treatment. Ann Thorac Surg 2002;74:995–8.

53. Ernst A, Silvestri GA, Johnstone D. Interventional pulmonary procedures: guidelines from the American College of chest Physicians. Chest 2003;123: 1693–717.

54. Bolliger CT, Mathur PN, Beamis JF, et al. ERS/ATS statement on interventional pulmonology. European respiratory Society/American Thoracic Society. Eur Respir J 2002;19:356–73.

Moving?

Make sure your subscription moves with you!

To notify us of your new address, find your **Clinics Account Number** (located on your mailing label above your name), and contact customer service at:

Email: journalscustomerservice-usa@elsevier.com

800-654-2452 (subscribers in the U.S. & Canada)
314-447-8871 (subscribers outside of the U.S. & Canada)

Fax number: 314-447-8029

Elsevier Health Sciences Division
Subscription Customer Service
3251 Riverport Lane
Maryland Heights, MO 63043

Printed and bound by CPI Group (UK) Ltd, Croydon, CR0 4YY

08/05/2025

01864694-0016